CASES IN

Pre-Hospital and Retrieval Medicine

2nd Edition

For
Our families, our mentors and teachers, and for those patients who have benefited
and will continue to benefit from the ongoing development of Pre-Hospital and
Retrieval Medicine

CASES IN
Pre-Hospital and Retrieval Medicine
2nd Edition

Daniel Ellis
Matthew Hooper
Neel Bhanderi
Fran Lockie

ELSEVIER

Sydney Edinburgh London New York Philadelphia St Louis Toronto

Elsevier

Elsevier Australia. ACN 001 002 357
(a division of Reed International Books Australia Pty Ltd)
Tower 1, 475 Victoria Avenue, Chatswood, NSW 2067

Notice

Knowledge and best practice in this field are constantly changing. As new research and experience broaden our understanding, changes in research methods, professional practices or medical treatment may become necessary.

Practitioners and researchers must always rely on their own experience and knowledge in evaluating and using any information, methods, compounds or experiments described herein. In using such information or methods they should be mindful of their own safety and the safety of others, including parties for whom they have a professional responsibility.

With respect to any drug or pharmaceutical products identified, readers are advised to check the most current information provided (i) on procedures featured or (ii) by the manufacturer of each product to be administered, to verify the recommended dose or formula, the method and duration of administration and contraindications. It is the responsibility of practitioners, relying on their own experience and knowledge of their patients, to make diagnoses, to determine dosages and the best treatment for each individual patient and to take all appropriate safety precautions.

To the fullest extent of the law, neither the Publisher nor the authors, contributors or editors, assume any liability for any injury and/or damage to persons or property as a matter of product liability, negligence or otherwise, or from any use or operation of any methods, products, instructions or ideas contained in the material herein.

National Library of Australia Cataloguing-in-Publication Data

---

Ellis, Daniel.

Cases in pre-hospital and retrieval medicine / Daniel Ellis, Matthew Hooper, Neel Bhanderi, Fran Lockie

2nd edition.
978-0-7295-4362-0 (paperback)

Includes index.

Content Strategist: Elizabeth Ryan
Content Project Manager: Shivani Pal
Edited by Jo Crichton
Index by GW Tech
Typeset by GW Tech
Cover and internal design by Gopalakrishnan Venkatraman
Printed in India by Multivista Global Pvt. Ltd.

Contents

CONTENTS

Forewords to the 1st Edition

Pre-hospital care of the injured and ill is a complex and challenging field of medical endeavour. The breadth of clinical presentations encompasses all fields of trauma and acute internal medicine. Ideally, patients should receive the most advanced care possible at the earliest time, integrated with expedient transport to the most appropriate definitive care facility. The ability to deliver this is resource- and system-dependent with unique modifiers including aircraft and road transport logistics, environmental impacts and integration with other responding emergency services.

In this selection of clinical scenarios, Dan Ellis and Matthew Hooper have provided an extensive insight into the challenges that the pre-hospital and retrieval team faces in urban, regional and rural settings. They have drawn on their experience in civilian and military emergency medical services in UK, Australia and internationally, as well as their passion for teaching a generation of clinicians. Each case takes the reader through the mission with exposure to a wealth of clinical, logistic and problem-solving insights. Indeed, the great strength of this text is its artful blending of evidence-based clinical assessment and management with the operational skills and common sense essential for safe and effective participation in these most difficult environments. The question and discussion format lends itself to integration with a clinician training programme, with current literature references included for further study.

This text integrates knowledge of emergency medicine and critical care with a comprehensive exposure to pre-hospital and retrieval protocols and procedures derived from the authors' many years of participation in fixed and rotary wing missions. As such, it is a unique and invaluable reference for all pre-hospital and retrieval clinicians and supporting personnel.

Allan MacKillop, FANZCA FFPMANZCA
Chief Medical Officer
CareFlight Group
Queensland, Australia
12 July 2009

Experience gained at London HEMS and in aeromedical operations in Australia has given the authors unique exposure and experience in the delivery of pre-hospital and retrieval medicine. Their passion and commitment to this complex arena is obvious to those who have worked with them and distilled in this text for those who have not.

Much is written about the theory of pre-hospital medicine but little is based in real-life scenarios, such as those the authors have faced. This book gives the reader a genuine view of the dilemmas and solutions of every day pre-hospital and retrieval care for both the patient and the clinical team.

The style of the text reflects the authors' depth of clinical understanding, their enthusiasm for human factors and the need for a team approach. The commentaries and discussions draw on their real-life experiences and are underwritten by well-chosen references.

The best performing units in the world deliver clinical excellence, not because they provide unique treatments or have access to highly technical equipment but because they deliver the most basic of care in a quality-assured manner with exquisite attention to detail. Such care is exactly what this book expounds.

It is with great pleasure that I commend this book to the pre-hospital and retrieval enthusiast from any background.

Gareth Davies, FRCP FFAEM
Consultant in Emergency Medicine & Pre-hospital Care
Medical Director, London HEMS
London, UK
16 July 2009

Preface

The first edition of *Cases in Pre-Hospital and Retrieval Medicine* was conceived in 2005 and published in 2010. During the last decade, Pre-Hospital and Retrieval medicine (PHRM) has grown into a distinct sub-specialty with wide recognition in several countries across the globe. It is well known that early intervention is key in managing critically ill and injured patients and it has become increasingly apparent that this intervention can and should be commenced before the patient gets to a major hospital. Clinicians working in this challenging environment have therefore further evolved to have specific, early resuscitation, stabilisation and critical care skills. *Cases in Pre-Hospital and Retrieval Medicine* is aimed at these clinicians.

Having worked extensively in the pre-hospital and retrieval environments of Australasia and the United Kingdom we felt that while several textbooks covered the relevant material, none had presented it in such a 'user friendly' case-based format. This particular format allows readers to become more immersed in the unpredictable and challenging pre-hospital and retrieval environments. In addition, we believed it would encourage the sort of lateral thinking required to provide safe, effective and high-level clinical care in such situations.

This book is not a replacement for any of the existing pre-hospital and retrieval texts; rather it is a complement to them. It provides an opportunity to consolidate the many disparate themes of this growing specialty and tie them together in a realistic, recognisable format that has a beginning, middle and end. The discussion presented for each case is not intended to provide a definitive review. Instead, reflection on personal experience and discussion with colleagues is recommended as there may be regional variation in several areas. When used in this way, we hope to have provided a valuable tool for teaching and learning that will appeal to a wide audience.

Both pre-hospital and retrieval medicine are sufficiently distinct from other critical care medical specialties to warrant consideration for independent specialty recognition. Whilst we believe that both fields of practice have enough in common to allow a single area of specialty to develop over time, we have maintained an arbitrary divide between the sections of the book to reflect that some clinicians are involved only in pre-hospital care and others only in medical retrieval. A third section for special circumstances and service development is aimed at highlighting the importance of crew resource management and the developing area of clinical coordination as well as covering medical tasks that remain on the fringe of pre-hospital and retrieval medicine, but which we believe are integral to the specialty. This second edition now includes a fourth section to cover Paediatric and Neonatal Retrieval. Worldwide, this area is rapidly expanding as paediatric and neonatal services become more centralised. At the time of writing this edition, there are not many PHRM textbooks that specifically concentrate on Paediatric and Neonatal Retrieval medicine in case-based format. Paediatric and Neonatal critical care medicine can be of low volume but is a highly specialized area of retrieval medicine. These patients present with wide range of complex pathologies and can take an increased amount of time to resuscitate and stabilise prior to moving from the referring site. The cases in this section therefore highlight this and aim to give the reader some pragmatic key learning points to use in the real-world environment. This is not a textbook for the latest management of emergency medical pathophysiology in itself, nor will it turn the reader into a trauma, intensive care, major incident or extrication specialist. Rather, we have used real emergency medical issues to highlight the role of the pre-hospital and retrieval specialist. This specialist must operate in a complex environment where approaching the scene, liaising with other emergency personnel and maintaining dynamic situational awareness can be at least as important as providing timely and high-level medical interventions.

All of the questions in *Cases in Pre-Hospital and Retrieval Medicine* are drawn from our collective experience over many years as pre-hospital and retrieval doctors and, thus, are based on real cases. We have also utilised the experience of acknowledged colleagues who have provided both images and commentary. On occasion, we have varied the images and the cases to augment key learning points and ensure patient confidentiality. However, we have attempted to always ensure that the reality of each case is reflected in the questions and discussions.

This text has become both a highly regarded tool for education and a ready reference guide for clinicians, especially doctors, working in the out-of-hospital environment. By offering generic but relevant 'real case' discussion, we hope that the book will remain a useful resource for many years to all our colleagues engaged in this exciting and continually evolving specialty. We also envisage that this text will continue to support emerging specialists training for examinations in PHRM as well as our paramedic and nursing colleagues.

Daniel Ellis
Matthew Hooper
Neel Bhanderi
Fran Lockie
Adelaide, South Australia
January 2022

About the authors

Associate Professor Daniel Ellis

MBBS (London), FIMC & DRTM RCSEd, FACEM, FCICM, FRCS(Eng), MRCP(UK), DMCC, GCertCU

Director of Trauma, Royal Adelaide Hospital

Co-Chair, Statewide South Australian State Trauma Service

Consultant in Emergency Medicine, Royal Adelaide Hospital

Pre-Hospital and Retrieval Physician, MedSTAR, Emergency Medical Retrieval Service, Adelaide

Clinical Associate Professor, Faculty of Health and Medical Sciences, Adelaide Medical School, University of Adelaide

Associate Professor, School of Public Health and Tropical Medicine, James Cook University, Queensland

Dan graduated from the medical schools of Guy's and St Thomas' Hospitals (University of London) and directed his initial training towards a career in emergency and critical care medicine. He gained early experience in pre-hospital medicine while working in the ambulance service in Jerusalem and then as a military doctor in Israel. After returning to the United Kingdom, he continued basic and advanced level training in emergency medicine, intensive care medicine and Pre-Hospital and Retrieval Medicine (PHRM).

Dan has worked extensively in PHRM for over 25 years including stints with the London Helicopter Emergency Medical Service (HEMS), the Children's Acute Transport Service (CATS) in London, Essex and Herts Air Ambulance (Medical Lead), Careflight Queensland (Regional Director of Operations and Training) and MedSTAR Emergency Medical Retrieval Service in South Australia, including over 5 years as the MedSTAR Clinical Director. Whilst in London he was an active member of the British Association for Immediate Care (BASICS) in London and was involved in two major incidents, including the terrorist attacks in London on 7 July 2005. He has worked as a Consultant in Emergency, Intensive Care and Pre-hospital and Retrieval Medicine both in the UK and Australia. In 2013, Dan was part of the Australian Medical Assistance Team (AUSMAT) deployed to the Philippines for Typhoon Haiyan. He holds an academic title with the James Cook University teaching the postgraduate educational modules for aeromedical retrieval.

Dan is an examiner for the Diplomas in Immediate Medical Care (DipIMC) and Retrieval and Transfer Medicine (DRTM) at the Royal College of Surgeons of Edinburgh as well as a member of the Court of Examiners for the Diploma in Pre-Hospital and Retrieval Medicine (Conjoint Faculty of Pre-Hospital and Retrieval Medicine, hosted by the Australasian College for Emergency Medicine). He is the current Chair of the PHRM Accreditation Committee. Dan has also spoken at local, national and international conferences on major incidents, pre-hospital and retrieval medicine and critical care and has published widely including chapters in several PHRM textbooks.

Dan is married with two children and currently lives in Adelaide, South Australia.

Associate Professor Matthew Hooper

MBBS (Adelaide), DipIMC & DRTM RCSEd, FACEM, FCICM, PGDipCU, PGDipPM

Founding Director and Senior Consultant, MedSTAR Emergency Medical Retrieval Service, South Australia

Director of Intensive Care – Calvary North Adelaide Hospital

Senior Consultant, Intensive Care - Calvary Adelaide Hospital.

Associate Professor, School of Public Health and Tropical Medicine, James Cook University, Queensland

Squadron Leader, Royal Australian Air Force Specialist Reserve

Matt graduated from the University of Adelaide School of Medicine and subsequently commenced specialist emergency medicine training in South Australia, Western Australia and Queensland. He developed a keen interest in pre-hospital and retrieval medicine during this time, gaining further experience in the United Kingdom initially as a paediatric intensive care retrieval fellow with London's Child Acute Transport Service (CATS) and then as a specialist registrar in pre-hospital trauma care with the London Helicopter Emergency Medical Service (HEMS). In 2002, he was awarded the gold medal by examination for the Diploma in Immediate Medical Care from the Royal College of Surgeons of Edinburgh before returning to Australia to complete Fellowships with both the Australasian College for Emergency Medicine and the Joint Faculty of Intensive Care Medicine.

Prior to returning to Adelaide in 2007, Matt was involved in the redevelopment of retrieval services in Queensland as the Regional Director of Operations and Training for CareFlight Medical Services. He holds an academic title with the James Cook University and has been involved in the development of the postgraduate educational program for aeromedical retrievals.

From late 2007, he led the development and implementation of South Australia's single, integrated emergency medical retrieval service - MedSTAR. He has also held the positions of Medical Donor Advisor for North Queensland, Chief Medical Officer for the South Australian Ambulance Service and Director of Cardiothoracic Intensive Care at the Royal Adelaide Hospital and has worked as an Intensive Care Consultant in Townsville Hospital, Flinders Medical Centre and Calvary Adelaide.

Matt is an examiner for the Diplomas of Retrieval and Transfer Medicine at the Royal College of Surgeons of Edinburgh as well as a member of the Court of Examiners for the Diploma in Pre-Hospital and Retrieval Medicine (Conjoint Faculty of Pre-Hospital and Retrieval Medicine, hosted by the Australasian College for Emergency Medicine). He is also a Squadron Leader with the Royal Australian Airforce Specialist Reserves.

Following a career long interest, he is completing a Masters in Palliative Medicine at Cardiff University.

Matt has two teenage children and lives in Adelaide, South Australia.

Dr Neel Bhanderi

MBBS BSc FACEM
Consultant in Emergency Medicine, Royal Adelaide Hospital
Consultant Pre-Hospital and Retrieval Physician and Head of Unit Education & Training,
    South Australia Ambulance MedSTAR Retrieval Service

Neel trained as an Emergency Physician and worked as a Consultant at St George's Hospital Major Trauma Centre in London for several years. After completing his Fellowship in Emergency Medicine, he worked for Air Ambulance Kent Surrey and Sussex for 15 months in a full-time capacity and continued to work with them on a regular basis for several years whilst working as an Emergency Physician in London.

In 2016, Neel decided to emigrate to Australia where he gained the Fellowship from the Australian College of Emergency Medicine and worked as an Emergency Specialist at the Townsville Hospital in North Queensland. In 2017 he landed his ideal job plan as a Consultant Emergency Physician at the Royal Adelaide Hospital and a Consultant Pre-Hospital and Retrieval Specialist with MedSTAR Emergency Medical Retrieval Service. His interest in teaching led him to become the Head of Unit for Education and Training at MedSTAR in 2021. He is also a member of the Court of Examiners for the Diploma in Pre-Hospital and Retrieval Medicine (Conjoint Faculty of Pre-Hospital and Retrieval Medicine, hosted by the Australasian College for Emergency Medicine).

Neel lives in Adelaide, South Australia with his wife, three children and a cocker-spaniel.

Dr Fran Lockie

MBBS, BSc (hons), MRCPCH, FRACP
Senior consultant in Paediatric Emergency Medicine (PEM), Women's and Children's
    Hospital (WCH), Adelaide
Consultant and Acting Head of Unit MedSTAR Kids, Pre-Hospital and Retrieval Medicine,
    MedSTAR Emergency Medical Retrieval Service.

Dr Francis Lockie is a paediatric emergency specialist and retrieval physician. Early experiences at the Trauma Unit at Cook County Hospital, Chicago and at St Mary's Hospital during the 2005 London bombings reinforced his interest in acute care paediatrics. He trained in London before moving to Sydney to work for NSW paediatric and neonatal transport service (NETS) and complete his training in paediatric emergency medicine. He worked on the faculty at Sydney Children's and British Columbia (BC) Children's Hospitals before moving to Adelaide to take up a combined position in PEM and paediatric & neonatal retrieval. He is interested in emergency airway management and currently chairs the WCH airway safety group. He is an active APLS instructor and enjoys teaching on the annual instructor course in Sri Lanka. Fran deployed to Samoa for the measles crisis with the Australian Medical Assistance Team (AUSMAT) and also runs the safety and quality programme for PED. He lectures nationally and internationally on paediatric emergencies and retrieval.

Fran lives in Adelaide with his wife and three children.

Acknowledgements to the 1st Edition

The authors would like to thank the following colleagues and institutions, without whom the production of this text would not have been possible:

Dr Jane Cocks
Dr Gareth Davies
Dr Tim Harris
Dr David Lockey
Mr David Tingey
Dr David Zideman

Helicopter Emergency Medical Service (HEMS London), UK
The Essex and Herts Air Ambulance Trust, UK
South Australian Retrieval Services (Royal Adelaide Hospital, Flinders Medical Centre, Women's and Children's Hospital)
MedSTAR Emergency Medical Retrieval Service, South Australia
CareFlight Medical Services, Queensland, Australia (Now LifeFlight)

Picture acknowledgments

The pictures in the text belong to the authors unless indicated below:

Section A

1.1   London HEMS
2.8   South Australian Retrieval Services
3.1   London HEMS
6.1   London HEMS
8.1   London HEMS
12.1 London HEMS
20.1 Dr Matt Gunning and Kent, Surrey and Sussex Air Ambulance
20.2 London HEMS
21.1 Dr Zane Perkins
23.1 London HEMS
25.1 CareFlight Medical Services, Queensland (Now LifeFlight)

Section B

26.1 With permission. This image was previously published as Figure 14.1B in Mohr (2004), Stroke: Pathophysiology, Diagnosis, and Management, 4th edition, Churchill Livingstone, Elsevier

Appendix 1
Thoracotomy: London HEMS
Thoracostomy: London HEMS

Acknowledgements to the 2nd Edition

Picture acknowledgements to the 2nd Edition

The pictures in the text belong to the authors unless indicated below:

17   Dr Stephen Hearns

18   Dr Andrew Pearce - MedSTAR Emergency Medical Retrieval Service (SA Ambulance)

27.1 (and Front Cover) Associate Professor William Griggs AM ASM

27.2 RFDS Medi-Jet 24 with people loading – Royal Flying Doctor Service of Australia Central Operations - Dr Mardi Steere

32   Dr Thiru Govindran

33   Dr Stefan Mazur

39   Dr Stefan Mazur

44   Dr Stefan Mazur

54   Dan Martin - RAAF (www.defence.gov.au)

56   Dr James Doube

68   Dr Rebecca Cooksey

Contributors to the 2nd edition

Associate Professor Sam Alfred, MBBS, FACEM, Dip Tox
Pre-Hospital and Retrieval Physician, MedSTAR Emergency Medical Retrieval
  Service
Emergency Medicine Physician, Royal Adelaide Hospital
Clinical Toxicologist, Royal Adelaide Hospital and New South Wales Poisons
  Information Centre

Belinda Amber, BN, GCertPaedCritCare, PGCertAeromedRet, GCertNeonatalICU
Retrieval Nurse Consultant, MedSTAR kids, Rescue Retrieval & Aviation Services,
  South Australia
Executive Officer, South Australian Neonatal Resuscitation Group
Clinical Senior Lecturer, Charles Darwin University, Menzies School of Medicine

Associate Professor Elliot Long, BSc, BMBS, FRACP, PhD, GCertCU
Paediatric Emergency Physician, The Royal Children's Hospital, Melbourne
Clinical Associate Professor, Department of Critical Care, The University of
  Melbourne
Research Fellow, Murdoch Children's Research Institute
Melbourne Children's Clinician Fellow

Dr Elizabeth Bhanderi, BDS, BN (Hons)
General Dentist, Adelaide

Jane Cocks, MBBS, DCH, FRACP, FACEM, FCICM, PGCert Aeromedical
  Retrieval
Paediatric Emergency Physician, Paediatric Emergency Department, The Women's
  and Children's Hospital, North Adelaide

Associate Professor John Craven, BSc (Hons), BMBS, FRACP, FACEM,
  GradDipMedEd
Paediatrician and Emergency Physician
Clinical Director Emergency Department, Mt Barker District Soldiers Memorial
  Hospital, BHFLHN
Associate Professor, Flinders University
Adjunct Associate Professor, Charles Darwin University
Clinical Associate Professor, The University of Adelaide

Dr James Doube, AAM, BSc, BMBS (Hons), FRACGP, FACRRM
Interim Chief Medical Officer, South Australian Ambulance Service
Medical Retrieval Consultant, SAAS-MedSTAR Emergency Medical Retrieval
  Service

Michael Goldblatt, BMBS (Flinders University Adelaide), FANZCA, Diploma
  Clinical Hypnosis
Senior Staff Specialist, Department of Anaesthesia, Flinders Medical Centre
Specialist Anaesthetist, Stace Anaesthetic Services, Adelaide
Director GLO Clinical Hypnosis, Adelaide
Education Faculty (Lecturer and Examiner), South Australian Society of Hypnosis
Member Australian Society of Hypnosis and Australian Society of Psychological
  Medicine

Dr Thiru Govindan, MBBS, FACEM, FRCEM, AFRACMA, AFACHSM, CHM
  Dip*Clin*US, CCPU Dip*Med*Tox
Emergency Physician and Clinical Toxicologist
Senior Consultant and Staff Specialist, Royal Adelaide Hospital
Clinical Senior Lecturer – Acute Care Medicine, University of Adelaide,
  South Australia

Associate Professor William Griggs, AM ASM, MBBS (Adel), PGDipAvMed
  (Otago), MBA (Adel), DUniv h.c. (Adel), FANZCA, FCICM, FPA, FAICD
Commissioner and Chair of Operations Branch, St John Ambulance (SA)
Retired Director of Trauma, Royal Adelaide Hospital
Retired Consultant in Critical Care and Anaesthesia, Royal Adelaide Hospital
Retired Pre-Hospital and Retrieval Physician, MedSTAR, Emergency Medical
  Retrieval Service, Adelaide
Retired State (Disaster) Controller, Health and Medical, SA Health

Dr Richard Harris, SC OAM, BMBS, DA (UK), FANZCA, Dip DHM, Post Grad
  Cert Aeromed, FFEWM, D. Univ (Flind), D. Univ (JCU)
Consultant Anaesthetist, Adelaide, South Australia

Dr Stephen Hearns, MB ChB, FRCEM, FRCS, FRCP, FRGS, DIMC, DRTM
Consultant in Retrieval Medicine, Emergency Medical Retrieval Service
Consultant in Emergency Medicine, NHS Greater Glasgow and Clyde
Director, Core Cognition Ltd

Dr Bron Hennebry, MBChB (Birmingham), MSc (Oxon), FRCPCH(UK), FRACP
Paediatric Retrieval Consultant, MedSTAR, Emergency Medical Retrieval Service,
  Adelaide
Neonatologist, Ashford Hospital, Adelaide
Senior Clinical Lecturer, Adelaide Medical School, University of Adelaide

Associate Professor Ben Lawton, MBChB, BSc (Hons), FRACP, MPH
Deputy Director (Paediatrics) Department of Emergency Medicine, Logan Hospital
Staff Specialist Paediatric Emergency Physician, Queensland Children's Hospital
Associate Professor, School of Medicine, Griffith University

Dr Shona Mair, BSc, MBBS, MPH, FRACP, FCICM
Director, Children's Advice and Transport Coordination Hub (CATCH), Children's
  Health Queensland Hospital and Health Service (CHQHHS)
Paediatric Intensivist, Queensland Children's Hospital (QCH) and Gold Coast
  University Hospital (GCUH)
Paediatric Medical Coordinator, Children's Health Queensland Retrieval Service
  (CHQRS)

Associate Professor Daniel Martin, RN, BN, GCertEmerg, BNPracEmerg, GCertNScRet, PGCertAeromedRet
Director of Nursing, South Australia Ambulance Service, MedSTAR Emergency Medical Retrieval
Associate Professor, School of Public Health and Tropical Medicine, James Cook University, Queensland
Squadron Leader, Health Operational Conversion Unit, Royal Australian Air Force

Dr Adela Matettore, MD, FAAP, FRCPC
Pediatric Critical Care Consultant, BC Children's Hospital
Pediatric Intensive Care Unit Transport Lead, BC Children's Hospital
Clinical Instructor, BC Emergency Health Services
Clinical Assistant Professor, University of British Columbia

Dr Stefan M. Mazur, BPhEd, MB ChB, FACEM, PGCertAME, DipIMC & DRTM (RCSEd), GCertCU
Consultant in Emergency Medicine, Royal Adelaide Hospital
Pre-Hospital and Retrieval Physician, MedSTAR, Emergency Medical Retrieval Service, Adelaide
Associate Professor, School of Public Health and Tropical Medicine, James Cook University, Queensland

Dr Krista Mos, MD (Hons) FCICM Clin DipPallMed
Paediatric Intensivist, Women's and Children's Hospital, Adelaide, South Australia

Sharon Paddock, RN, Dip Nurs, ENB 100 (Intensive Care Nursing), BSc (Hons) (Manc Met), Grad Cert Clin Ed
Retrieval Nurse and Nurse Educator, MedSTAR Emergency Medical Retrieval Service, Rescue Retrieval & Aviation Services, South Australia Ambulance Service, Government of South Australia

Associate Professor Andrew Pearce, BSc (Hons), BMBS, FACEM, PGCERT, Aeromed Retrieval DRTM (RCSEd), GAICD
Director Clinical Services, MedSTAR Emergency Medical Retrieval Service, Adelaide
Senior Consultant in Emergency, Medicine Royal Adelaide Hospital
Associate Professor, School of Public Health, James Cook University, Queensland
Group Captain, RAAF
MCAT Senior Instructor

Dr Cheryl Peters, BN, BSc (Med), MD, FRCPC (Anesthesiology and Critical Care)
Consultant Pediatric Anesthesiologist and Pediatric Intensivist, BC Children's Hospital, Vancouver, British Columbia (BC), Canada
Educator, BC Emergency Health Services
Clinical Assistant Professor, University of British Columbia

Jacintha Pickles, RN, BN, GradDipClinNurs (CritCare Paed), GradDipMidwifery, PGCertAeromedRet
Nurse Consultant, SAAS MedSTAR Emergency Medical Retrieval Service, Adelaide

Marco Pillen, RP, AFACP
Rescue and Retrieval Paramedic, Rescue, Retrieval and Aviation Services, SA Ambulance Service

Mardi Steere, MBBS, MBA, FAAP, FACEP, FRACP
Executive General Manager, Medical and Retrieval Services, Royal Flying Doctor
  Service of Australia, Central Operations
Consultant Paediatric Emergency Physician, Women's and Children's Hospital,
  South Australia
Adjunct Associate Professor, Menzies School of Medicine, Charles Darwin
  University
Courtesy Assistant Professor, Emergency Medicine, University of Florida

Associate Professor Warwick Teague, MBBS (Adelaide), DPhil (Oxford), FRACS,
  FRCSEd, MRCP (UK)
Director of Trauma Services, The Royal Children's Hospital, Melbourne, Australia
Clinical Lead, Burns Service, The Royal Children's Hospital, Melbourne, Australia
Consultant in Paediatric Surgery, The Royal Children's Hospital, Melbourne,
  Australia
Co-group Leader, Surgical Research, Murdoch Children's Research Institute,
  Melbourne, Australia
Associate Professor, Department of Paediatrics, University of Melbourne,
  Melbourne, Australia

Reviewers to the 1st Edition

Scott Devenish, MVEdT, BN, Dip Para Sc, MACAP
Lecturer, Bachelor of Clinical Practice (Paramedic) and Bachelor of Nursing/
Clinical Practice (Paramedic), School of Biomedical Sciences, Charles Sturt
University, Bathurst, Australia

Dr Stephen Hearns, MBChB, FRCS, FCEM, DipIMC
Consultant in Emergency and Retrieval Medicine, NHS Greater Glasgow and Clyde,
UK
Lead Consultant Emergency Medical Retrieval Service

Dr Michael Hill, MBBS, FRACGP, FACRRM, DRANZCOG, DCH, DipAvMed
Senior Medical Officer, Royal Flying Doctor Service of Australia, South Eastern
Section

David Lighton, MEd, BA, CELTA, Certificate Trauma & Assessment, Certificate
Applied Science (AO), MACAP
Senior Lecturer, Paramedicine and Emergency Management, Auckland University of
Technology, Auckland, New Zealand

Dr Bevan Lowe, MBChB, FACEM, Dip Obstet, Dip Sport Med.
Senior Staff Specialist & Emergency Director of Trauma, Division of Emergency
Medicine, Princess Alexandra Hospital, Brisbane
Course Coordinator, Queensland Health Skills Development Centre, Royal Brisbane
& Women's Hospital
Senior Lecturer, School of Medicine, University of Queensland, Australia

Bronwyn Tunnage, MSc, RGN, Advanced Paramedic
Senior Lecturer, Paramedicine and Emergency Management, Auckland University
of Technology, Auckland, New Zealand

Sarah Werner, BHSc (Nursing), PGCertHSc (Resuscitation), Dip Ambulance
(Paramedic)
Lecturer, Paramedicine and Emergency Management, Auckland University of
Technology, Auckland, New Zealand

Dr David Zideman, LVO, QHP(C), BSc, MBBS, FRCA, FIMC
Consultant Anaesthetist, Imperial College Healthcare NHS Trust, London, UK
Honorary Consultant, Helicopter Emergency Medical Service, Royal London
Hospital, London, UK
Chairman, British Association of Immediate Care (BASICS)
Lead Clinician for Emergency Medical Services, 2012 Olympic Games, London, UK

Introduction

Approach to *Cases in Pre-Hospital and Retrieval Medicine*

This case-based book uses real pre-hospital and retrieval situations presented in a question format, followed by an extensive discussion. Each question and discussion consists of approximately 1000–2000 words and is usually illustrated with a photograph. The cases have been arbitrarily divided into those with a predominantly pre-hospital theme, those based around adult retrieval medicine, a section focusing on special circumstances and service development and a fourth section on paediatric and neonatal retrieval. In addition, a series of appendices provides information of use to pre-hospital and retrieval practitioners. Each case can be read as a 'stand-alone' scenario, although each section has a structure that builds on the key concepts discussed in earlier cases. As such, each section is ideally approached in numerical order.

Practical points

This book is primarily designed for the 'hands-on' pre-hospital and retrieval clinician. It is also likely to be of significant interest and use to a broad range of emergency services, aviation and other non-medical personnel. Each question is written with the assumption that a doctor forms part of a highly trained pre-hospital and retrieval medicine (PHRM) team. Although the composition of such teams varies widely internationally, the key learning points for each question are relevant to all professional medical, paramedical and nursing personnel engaged in this challenging and unpredictable area of practice.

Medical practice will also vary regionally. For this reason, this book does not always provide extensive detail regarding precise therapies, clinical guidelines and drug doses. It is not a definitive text on emergency or critical care medicine. Instead, it provides a scenario-based approach to highlight key areas of pre-hospital and retrieval medicine.

Definitions

PHRM refers to a system of specialist clinical practice inclusive of the following.

Clinical coordination

Clinical coordination involves the dedicated multidisciplinary (medical, nursing, paramedical, logistics) coordination system or processes led by appropriately qualified and credentialled specialist medical practitioners in PHRM, offering high-level clinical and logistical advice and decision making. Ideally, clinical coordination should be provided from a dedicated, centralised, operational centre with 24/7 access via a single point of communication.

Clinical coordination commences with a referral, usually from a healthcare facility, incident scene or ambulance service. Planning and intervention priorities for each case must be determined quickly and efficiently via Standard Operating Procedures (SOPs) and can include:
- immediate care or advice
- telemedicine

- need for PHRM team
- urgency of dispatch
- destination planning
- consideration of complex decision making involving logistics, crew configuration and transport platforms
- creation of pre-flight assessment documentation and updates on clinical/logistical considerations during transport.

Operational response

Operational response refers to the dedicated multidisciplinary teams with flexibility to respond to the healthcare facility or incident scene and provide a level of clinical care at least equivalent to the referring facility and preferably enhanced. This team should provide 'point to point' care from referral centre to receiving facility overseen by the Clinical Coordination Centre. The response is further defined by the following sub-categories:

- Pre-hospital task ('primary') – A pre-hospital task is any clinically coordinated task that involves a patient response in the out-of-hospital environment. A patient assessment and/or intervention may occur by the roadside, in a public place or in a private dwelling. It is a location that does not normally have 'medical' personnel on-site to assess and manage the patient. The out-of-hospital environment typically has few, if any, health resources available, such as oxygen, suction and other conventional treatment therapies, although these will arrive with the ambulance/ PHRM service.
- Modified primary – Occurs when, due to time and/or distance, a pre-hospital patient (as defined above) has left the scene of the incident and by the time the PHRM team arrives that patient is in a healthcare environment with minimal health infrastructure (e.g. rural clinic, GP practice, back of an ambulance) and with limited clinician input (e.g. nurse/paramedic only, single-handed GP).
- Retrieval task – A retrieval task is a clinically coordinated interhospital transfer of critically ill or injured patients using specialised PHRM staff, transport platforms and equipment. The scope of these tasks encompasses transfers from (and between) all healthcare facilities with an inpatient capability. Note: non-critical, low-acuity interhospital transfers (by road or air ambulance) are not encompassed within the definition of a PHRM response.

Training and education

PHRM teams must possess a broad understanding of critical care medicine. In addition, PHRM teams require specialist skills and training in pre-hospital and retrieval medicine. This includes but is not limited to how critical care medicine is applied in the PHRM environment, interactions with other emergency services personnel, teamwork and human factors, aviation medicine and specific clinical governance structures. However, training and education in PHRM must also encompass the low-frequency, high-acuity, high-consequence challenges inherent in the PHRM environment.

Clinical governance

In addition to specialist medical practitioner-led clinical oversight, PHRM services must also utilise a dedicated multifaceted clinical governance framework. This should encompass multidisciplinary audit, morbidity and mortality reviews, risk management, training and education, competency and credentialling and research. These facets must be specifically designed for the pre-hospital and retrieval environment and ideally delivered by specialists in PHRM. Clinical governance also extends to operational performance; i.e. response times, online service availability, etc.

For the purposes of this book, the PHRM team will always have a dedicated person tasking them and acting as the communications hub throughout the mission. For ease of reference, this person is referred to as the coordinator/clinical coordinator and the organisation in which they work will be the tasking agency/coordination centre.

Sample question format

Most cases in this book follow a consistent format.

Incident

This section presents a brief synopsis of the task for which the PHRM team has been activated. This may range from the pre-hospital mechanism of injury through to the presenting patient illness, physiological parameters and location. The information available during the early stages of pre-hospital and retrieval tasking is often sparse. To provide the reader with a sense of realism, this is reflected in the information made available in the synopsis. In some cases, further information or images may be made available as the reader progresses through the question. This aims to improve the fidelity of the question.

Relevant information

This section is usually divided into four sub-headings:

1. PHRM team transport options: a description of the transport resources available on the day. Options may include aircraft (rotary-wing and fixed-wing), land ambulances or a combination of these resources. As airframes may differ across jurisdictions, specifications will only be provided when relevant to the question.

2. Additional resources: in most pre-hospital and retrieval environments, other resources will be available. In the pre-hospital environment, this will include a mixture of Fire & Rescue, Police and Ambulance Service teams. In the retrieval environment it will usually refer to resources available at the local medical facility.

3. Retrieval options/destination: regional resources and geography play a major role in the clinical and logistical decision making required of the coordinator and PHRM team. If indicated, details of nearby hospitals and their facilities will be provided to allow the reader to decide which facility is most appropriate. This may involve bypassing the nearest hospital for one better able to manage the patient's acute or ongoing care. In cases where the receiving hospital is predetermined, information regarding flight times and aircraft endurance are supplied when relevant.

4. Other: key information not included under the above headings can be given in this section. For example, the weather often plays a key role in the pre-hospital and retrieval environment. Additionally, the time of day and traffic conditions may be relevant points for consideration.

Questions and discussion

Questions, answers and discussion will be structured to lead the reader through key learning points in a realistic fashion. Subsequent cases will introduce new material while reinforcing key topics and themes (e.g. scene safety or aviation physiology) introduced previously. Where appropriate, references to other cases are given to allow similar themes to be further explored.

Key points

A summary of the key learning objectives will feature at the end of most cases. In addition, references and an additional reading list have been added where relevant.

Glossary and key to cases

A glossary of definitions has also been included to clarify terminology (e.g. what is meant by the term 'regional hospital'). The glossary also includes a list of common acronyms used in the text.

A full list of key topics covered in specific cases can be found at the end of the book. This provides for rapid reference or review of specific topics.

SECTION A

Pre-hospital theme

Foreword to the Pre-Hospital Section

One of the problems of writing a successful book is that all too soon an updated version is demanded. Dr's Ellis, Hooper, Bhanderi and Lockie have risen to the challenge and once again delivered a valuable resource which can be used by a diverse range of clinicians to educate, review and stimulate. An overwhelming amount of clinical information is now instantly available online on almost any subject and it can be difficult to focus on what really improves practice. The format of this book provides an excellent way of using common and less common case presentations to explain the background knowledge, decision making, clinical and system factors which need to be applied to deliver the best outcomes in the pre-hospital phase of care. The authors use clear scenarios reinforced with questions, photographs and diagrams to transport the reader to the roadside and effectively remind them of previous cases or challenges that have yet to be encountered. Those in training will benefit from the extensive practical range of material that is relevant to pre-hospital services world-wide and those who train will value the excellent opportunities that the text provides to guide case -based discussions.

The authors are to be congratulated for communicating their longstanding energy and pursuit of high quality clinical care to our pre-hospital and retrieval community with this excellent educational resource.

Professor David Lockey
MB BS MD(Res) FFICM FIMC RCS(Ed) FRCA FFSEM
Consultant, Pre-hospital Emergency Medicine, London's Air Ambulance & National Director, Emergency Medical and Retrieval Service Wales, UK
Gibson Chair & Immediate Past Chair, Faculty of Pre-hospital Care, Royal College of Surgeons of Edinburgh, UK

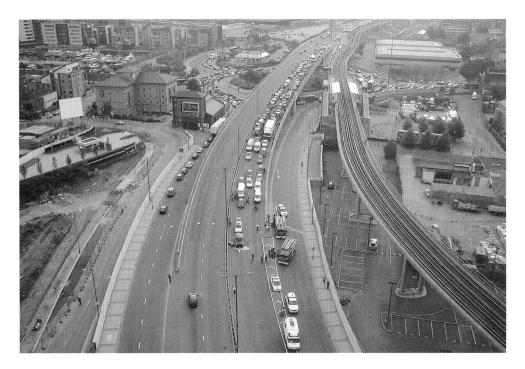

Incident

A car has collided with a motorcycle 15 minutes ago at an estimated combined speed of 80 km/h (53 mph). The motorcyclist is trapped under the car.

Relevant information

- **PHRM team transport options:** Rotary-wing aircraft.
- **Additional resources:** One land ambulance. Two ambulance response vehicles. Police and Fire & Rescue services.
- **Retrieval options:** Regional hospital 15 minutes by road. Major trauma hospital 30 minutes by air.
- **Other:** Friday 17:20 hours.

Question 1.1

Outline in detail your approach to the scene.

Discussion 1.1

In brief, the approach to the scene offers an opportunity to:
- Identify the potential hazards
- Briefly 'read' the likely mechanism
- Identify the patient numbers, distribution and acuity of injury
- Commence formulating a pre-hospital plan.

Scene assessment is critical to ensuring team, scene and, ultimately, patient safety. It begins as soon as the details of the task become available. Available and relevant further information may be forwarded to the team en route by the tasking agency.

Arrival by air

Approaching the scene from the air offers considerable advantages over a road response. The entire Helicopter Emergency Medical Service (HEMS) crew (of which the pre-hospital and retrieval medicine (PHRM) team are an integral component) should utilise this opportunity to study the incident scene from above and ensure all potential aviation hazards are communicated clearly and succinctly. This should be done by referencing a clock face (where the nose of the aircraft is at 12 o'clock) and using the terms 'high' or 'low' to point out hazards. Landing site selection is at the discretion of the pilot(s), who is ultimately responsible for aircraft safety. A landing site may be pre-arranged with on-scene emergency services to facilitate landing, but the final decision always rests with the pilot(s).

Key points (note many of these in the above scene) to look out for from the air in the HEMS environment are detailed utilising a 'HEMS' acronym in the box below.

Key points to note in the HEMS environment

H   **Hazards**
- Aviation (power lines, wires, fences, trees, light posts, towers and loose objects) and drones.
- Scene (moving vehicles, open roads, fire hazards and scene topography including height risks).

E   **Emergency services on scene**
- Ambulance resources (may alter what is taken from the aircraft, e.g. additional oxygen, splints or other equipment).
- Other services (particularly note the absence of Fire and Rescue and/or Police, thus requiring additional team vigilance).

M   **Mechanism**
- Deformation, debris spread, tyre marks, distance between involved vehicles, vehicular mass and speed limit of road.

S   **Scene geography**
- Number and position(s) of potential casualties. The distance and location of the patient(s) in relation to the vehicle
- Areas for safe access, on scene assessment, procedures and egress.

In any pre-hospital emergency situation, scene safety is the primary concern and, as detailed above, plans for approaching the scene should be made on, or prior to, landing. The PHRM team should adopt the 'safe self, safe team, safe scene, safe patient' approach.

Arrival by road

The PHRM team will regularly arrive at a scene by land vehicle, usually driven by one of the team. Advanced driving using emergency lights and sirens is a complex skill that requires training and regular review by a qualified instructor. On arrival at the scene, ensure the sirens are switched off promptly (when safe to do so) to avoid disrupting teams already on the scene. Park close to the scene but do not obstruct the access or egress of other emergency service vehicles. Try to park in the 'fend off' position (at an angle to the scene) to improve safety in the event of oncoming traffic striking the rear of your vehicle. Consider leaving the keys within the vehicle and leave the emergency lights on if yours is the first vehicle on the scene, but bear in mind that the vehicle battery could be exhausted if the scene time is prolonged or if the team escorts the patient to hospital in a different vehicle. Take all the necessary equipment initially as returning to the vehicle may become difficult if the scene becomes more complicated.

Personal and team safety

The PHRM team should arrive at the scene together and be adequately attired. Each member requires appropriate personal protective equipment (PPE). The team must be adequately trained and governed to ensure they are able to account for themselves in the pre-hospital environment (See appendix 3).

Scene safety

Following vehicle accidents, such as the one above, the Fire & Rescue Service are the lead safety authority and must be consulted first for advice on scene safety. Identify the Fire & Rescue team leader (either by uniform/helmet markings or by direct questioning) and specifically ask whether or not the scene is safe to enter. If these personnel have deemed the scene unsafe, the PHRM team should not proceed under any circumstances. For incidents involving violent crime and/or assault, the Police will be in charge of the scene and should similarly be approached and questioned about scene safety. It is common for the Police to set up a rendezvous point (RVP) away from the primary incident where medical teams and other services can gather. This enables the Police to make the scene safe prior to the arrival of additional medical resources. Again, the PHRM team should not proceed to the scene before it has been declared safe to do so.

Standing back from the scene may be harder than it seems, particularly if seriously injured patients, especially children, are visible. However, even in these circumstances, the PHRM team should inform the Fire & Rescue or Police service team leader that they are ready to enter the scene on their instruction. They should then stand back until the scene is declared safe. Experienced and adequately trained PHRM teams should be able to make suggestions to the relevant team leader (e.g. information obtained during aerial scene assessment) and make a balanced risk benefit analysis regarding scene safety. Similarly, if the PHRM team are the first to arrive on the scene (i.e. before the Fire & Rescue or Police services), then they will need to make an independent assessment of scene safety. Actively developing personal and team situational awareness is critical in such circumstances.

For a road vehicle crash, one such assessment would be:

Scan the scene and consider verbalising hazards to your fellow team members, as you approach to observe:
- Traffic flow
- Scene topography
- Fallen power lines
- Smoke.

Stop about 5 metres from the scene and analyse what you perceive in depth, e.g.
- Liquid on the floor
- The smell of petrol

- The stability of the vehicle or other structures
- Key personnel including injured person(s).

Ensure appropriate resources are en route.

- Communicate with tasking agency/other services.

Enter the scene with caution.

- Reassess the scene frequently.

Other incident scenes may require a level of assessment beyond even the most experienced PHRM team (e.g. building collapses, terror attacks) and, in such circumstances, the best response will be to make a cursory inspection and wait for expert support. Entering an unsafe scene to look for injured people must be avoided. Patients who are clearly visible within the scene and who appear in extremis pose a particular problem. The PHRM team leader should weigh up the risk–benefit of emergency ('crash') extrication versus waiting for expert help to arrive (see Case 4).

When the fire service or Police arrive, the PHRM team leader should hand over the scene assessment and formal scene control.

It is important to note that safety takes absolute priority and forensic evidence does not. The PHRM team should not be prevented from entering a safe scene simply to preserve evidence. Even if the victim is presumed to be deceased, the PHRM team should usually be allowed access to confirm death. It is the responsibility of the PHRM team to make every effort to preserve the scene for the Police and nothing should be moved unless necessary to save life or limb.

Patient safety

The assessment of patient safety overlaps significantly with the assessment of scene safety, but is included to encourage the team to focus on the patient and the immediate environment. Removing the patient from danger to a safe area of the scene with improved patient access is both a priority and the first step in any therapeutic intervention.

Key points

- A 'safe' approach is critical:
  - Safe self and team.
  - Safe scene.
  - Safe patient.
- Scene assessment from the air offers many advantages.
- Adequate PPE is a mandatory requirement.
- Liaise early with the lead scene safety authority.

Additional reading

Calland V. Safety at scene: a manual for paramedics and immediate care doctors. Mosby, 2001.

Nutbeam T, Boylan M. (Eds) ABC of pre-hospital emergency medicine. Wiley Blackwell, 2013.

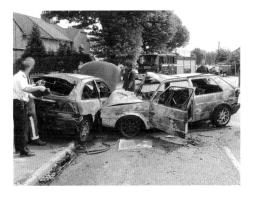

Image A

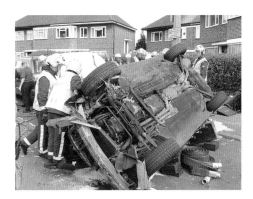

Image B

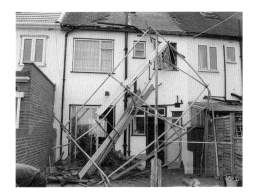

Image C

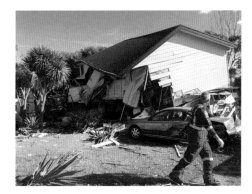

Image D

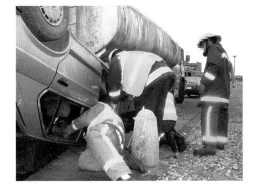

Image E

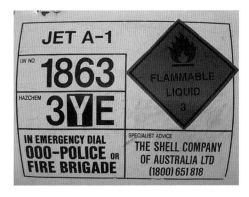

Image F

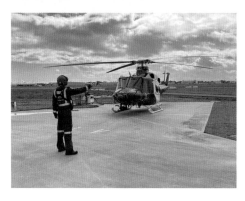

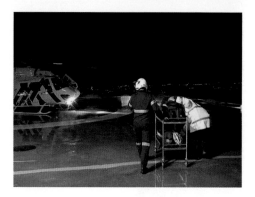

Image G   Image H

Question 2.1

Describe the scene in each of the images A–H, giving the relevant safety information that is specific to each.

Discussion 2.1

Vehicle crash: car versus car (Image A)

The key concern here is fire. The Fire & Rescue Service is in attendance and there are several people on the scene. The casual appearance of the attending personnel at this scene does not make the safety aspects any less important and other emergency services (in this case the Police service) close to the scene do not necessarily mean that the scene is safe. In addition, the fact that other emergency services have removed parts of their PPE should not encourage the PHRM team to do likewise. The Fire & Rescue team leader should be found, and scene safety verified before approaching the vehicles.

At the scene, careful attention is required to vehicles that may be hot to touch. A build-up of noxious fumes is also possible within the vehicles. A smoldering vehicle may reignite without warning and a safe distance should be kept from the scene after the initial assessment has been carried out.

Be wary of other traffic passing by. Drivers will be looking at the incident and there is the risk of being hit by another vehicle. Ensure the Police service has closed both lanes of the road if you plan to spend time near the vehicles (e.g. for extrication).

Vehicle crash: partial rollover (Image B)

Vehicle stability is a problem here and the PHRM team will need to discuss with the Fire & Rescue Service the best way of stabilising the vehicle considering the occupant's condition. Plastic blocks and wedges can be used to minimise movement, and, on occasion, a chain can be used to hold the car in position. The stabilisation will need to be more secure if the PHRM team is planning to access the vehicle and treat the patient inside.

Hydraulic cutters used by Fire & Rescue pose a risk to the trapped patient and the rescue teams. These pieces of equipment are large and cumbersome. Each individual on the scene is responsible for keeping themselves clear of the cutting tools and the associated hydraulic lines. A designated person should ensure the patient is not injured by the tools or shrapnel from their use. Specially designed hard plastic boards positioned between the tool and the patient offer reasonable protection ('hard protection'). Cut surfaces may be dangerously sharp and should be appropriately covered. The Fire &

Rescue Service will carry a variety of different-sized covers specially designed for this purpose ('soft protection').

The picture below shows the lamp post directly above this incident (also visible in the background of the initial picture). This highlights the importance of the visual sweep when approaching the scene, remembering that hazards can be in any direction.

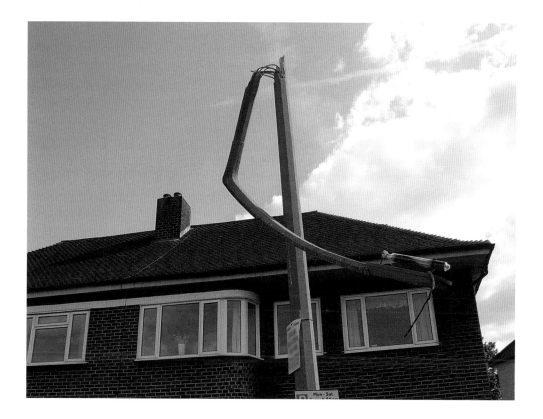

Scaffold collapse (Image C)

The whole scene looks highly unstable. The twisted scaffold poles appear under some tension. Roof tiles have collapsed onto the scene. The structural integrity of the building cannot be assumed from this picture (e.g. why was the scaffold put up in the first place?). In the absence of structural engineers, immediate advice would need to be taken from the Fire & Rescue Service. In this type of incident, it is possible that the Fire & Rescue Service has not been called and, ideally, no one should enter the scene until they arrive. In such circumstances, urgent removal of seriously injured patients from under the rubble may be considered. However, a prompt risk–benefit analysis would be required, and any patient would almost certainly require an emergency ('crash') extrication (see Case 4). Complex building collapses may require specialist rescue teams.

Vehicle crash: car struck building (Image D)

First impressions again relate to structural damage to a building; however, the damaged car in the foreground does not match the apparent energy transfer required to cause such damage. Closer inspection reveals a 5-ton truck embedded in the house – likely now to be the main source of support for the building. The safest option here, after consulting with the Fire & Rescue Service, would be to urgently assess, and, if required, extricate any patients from the truck to continue treatment in a different location. Remember that someone may have been injured in the building. The Fire & Rescue Service should ensure that the building is safe to enter before assessing whether there are any victims inside.

Vehicle crash: car versus truck (Image E)

The essential point to note in this image is that the truck is, in fact, a tanker. It should not be assumed that emergency services on-scene are aware of this fact. The PHRM team must ensure that this critical observation is shared with the Fire & Rescue Service. No question or comment should be considered 'too obvious' in the pre-hospital environment. The potential for this crash to become a major incident needs to be addressed and the Police service should also be consulted in order to create a wide cordon. Always remember to check the hazard plate on any tanker to confirm the nature of the contents. If the contents are toxic, then the team should consider declaring 'major incident standby' (see Case 23) and requesting specialist 'hazardous incident' teams. The nature of the entrapment in this scene is complex and careful thought should be given to an emergency ('crash') extrication and relocation to a safer site.

The hazard plate (Image F)

All tankers should carry information about their contents. The information should be on a hazard plate on the outside of the tanker as shown in the picture. There may be more information in the driver's cab (perhaps in the glove compartment or door pocket). This information will have phone numbers to call in the event of an incident. There are some simple rules for hazard plates, but probably the most important thing to look for on the plate is the letter 'E' after a numerical code. The presence of this letter signifies dangerous cargo, which means the team should evacuate the scene immediately pending the arrival of the Fire & Rescue Service. There may be a need for advanced PPE and breathing apparatus, or an extensive evacuation may be required. A useful aide memoire is 'if E is on the hazard plate, always think Evacuate'.

The plate in the picture shows the warning for a flammable substance as well as having an E on it. In this instance, the name of the chemical (aviation fuel, Jet A-1) is on the plate as well as emergency contact numbers.

Approaching the helicopter with rotors running (Images G and H)

The PHRM team must be familiar with helicopter safety issues. These may vary slightly depending on the type of helicopter, but some generic rules are always applicable. Before approaching any helicopter, ensure that you are appropriately attired and that clothing or equipment is securely in place. Ear protection must be worn when the rotors are running. Helicopters must be approached from the front. As outlined in Case 1, the nose of the aircraft is classically described as the 12 o'clock position on the clock face. The aircraft should be approached between the '10 and 2 o'clock' positions. The rear of the aircraft is dangerous because of the tail rotor, engine exhaust and the lack of pilot visibility. If the aircraft is on a slope, approach from the side with the most clearance between the rotor blades and the ground. Walk towards the aircraft and stop well outside the rotor disc. Make visual contact with the pilot and wait for a thumb-up signal. Respond with a thumb-up in return and walk steadily to the aircraft. Never approach without receiving this signal. Upon reaching the aircraft, if not already wearing a helmet (in which case, ear protection must be worn), don the appropriate helmet to allow communication with the pilots, as required. If you need to leave the rotor disc for any reason, you must again obtain a thumb-up from the pilot. More information regarding other rotary wing aviation issues is discussed in Case 48.

Note the additional safety concerns in image H: it is night, it has been raining and the equipment is relatively unsecured on a mobile wheeled trolley (about to be rolled under the rotor disc on an elevated rooftop helipad). Where possible, all equipment (and personnel) should be secured on board the aircraft prior to engine start.

Key points

- Scene safety is paramount, and each pre-hospital scene is unique.
- Actively developing personal and team situational awareness is critical.
- Do not assume that even the most obvious hazards have been noted by other emergency services or other members of your PHRM team.
- Even when performing relatively routine and 'straightforward' activities, ensure situational and hazard awareness is maintained.

Additional reading

Advanced Life Support Group (ALSG). Major incident medical management and support (MIMMS), 3rd edn. Blackwell Publishing, 2012.

Calland V. Safety at scene: a manual for paramedics and immediate care doctors. Mosby, 2001.

Nutbeam T, Boylan M. (Eds) ABC of pre-hospital emergency medicine. Wiley Blackwell, 2013.

CASE 3

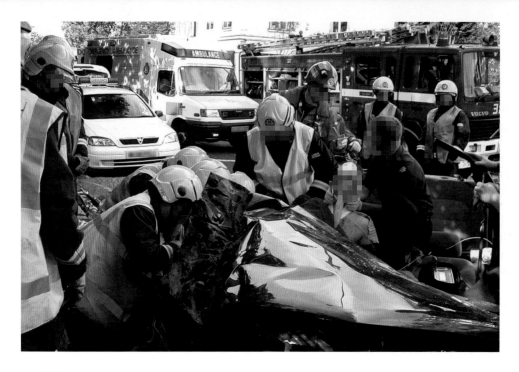

Incident

A car has collided with a bus 30 minutes ago at an estimated combined speed of 80 km/h (53 mph). The driver of the car is trapped and combative.

Relevant information

- **PHRM team transport options:** Rotary-wing aircraft.
- **Additional resources:** One land ambulance. One ambulance response vehicle. Fire & Rescue and Police services.
- **Retrieval options:** Regional hospital 15 minutes by road. Major trauma hospital 30 minutes by air.
- **Other:** Ambient conditions: Clear 12°C (54°F).

Question 3.1

Summarise your pre-hospital plan.

Clinical information

On-scene, the lead paramedic hands over the following clinical information:

- P 105.
- SBP 100 mmHg.
- Clear airway.
- RR 20.
- GCS 12 (E3, V4, M5).
- Oxygen mask and cervical collar in situ.
- The patient is trapped by his legs.

Question 3.2

Assuming the scene is safe, who do you approach first and why?

Question 3.3

Explain the terms 'relative' and 'actual entrapment'.

Discussion 3.1

A pre-hospital plan is a continuously evolving dynamic plan of action that the members of the PHRM team will make as soon as they are activated, using the information given by the tasking agency. In many cases, this initial information is vague or incomplete, which reflects the problems experienced when receiving early phone calls about an incident. Although making a plan prior to arrival with limited information has drawbacks, there are clear benefits in arriving at the incident with a strategy for scene and patient management already in place. The plan often develops as the team travels to the scene and therefore valuable time en route should not be wasted.

When at the scene, the PHRM team must have the skill to listen to all members of the emergency services and weigh up their suggestions as part of the overall plan. This may be difficult in the noisy, high-pressure environment of the pre-hospital arena. However, the PHRM team has overall clinical responsibility for the patient and, as such, key medical decisions should go through them.

A generic pre-hospital plan could be:

The scene

- A safe approach (self, team, scene and others).

The patient

- Likely requirements would be a need for extrication, assessment and stabilisation.

The destination

- Triage options.
- Transport platform options.

When applying a generic plan to this scenario, there should be both pre-arrival and on-arrival considerations:

Pre-arrival

- The **scene** is of a vehicle accident with patient entrapment. The PHRM team can therefore expect a busy scene with multiple emergency services personnel and vehicles. PPE, including safety helmets, will be required (see Appendix 3).
- The **patient** is combative, which suggests serious pathology. In addition, time has moved on from the initial report and the PHRM team should be expecting an unstable patient.
- Early **destination** options can be considered. The mechanism (bus versus car) and initial report suggest major trauma which will influence the PHRM team or tasking agency's decision on the nearest suitable hospital for the patient. It can also factor in time of day (e.g. rush hour) and weather, etc. In addition, the team should consider drawing up appropriate drugs if not already pre-drawn (e.g. for rapid-sequence intubation) if any additional time is available.

13

On arrival

Once the PHRM team arrives on scene, more content and structure may be added to the plan or a complete revision may be required. Key elements of this dynamic plan must be communicated between PHRM team members and relevant on-scene emergency services personnel.

A typical extension to such a plan for this scenario after the initial assessment could be:

The scene

- Safe self, team in adequate PPE.
- Safe scene – safety issues addressed with the Fire and Rescue service as required.
- Continuous scene reassessment.

The patient

- Conduct a rapid but thorough primary survey on the entrapped patient to identify any life-threatening injuries and to ensure the feet are not trapped under any pedals, which would prevent an extrication.
- Plan initially to perform a controlled extrication but ensure the time-critical nature of the extrication is well understood. Give a clear time frame to the Fire & Rescue Service personnel and advise them that the plan may change if there is a delay (e.g. beyond 10 minutes) in extrication or further patient deterioration.
- Stabilisation: preparations for patient assessment and likely therapeutic requirements (including pre-hospital anaesthesia) may require the functional division of the PHRM team during the extrication. A safe area of the scene, allowing 360° patient access, should be preselected for this purpose.

The destination

- Once the patient is assessed and any required on-scene interventions have been performed, the patient will require rapid transport to a major trauma hospital. Transport times and platform options should be considered early. An early 'sit-rep' can allow the tasking agency to contact the receiving hospital. This can facilitate having a specialist surgeon; for example, a neurosurgeon, to be present as part of the trauma team on the arrival of the PHRM team.

Note how the plan is full of 'ifs and maybes', reflecting the inherent flexibility of the plan. This, in turn, reflects the unpredictable nature of pre-hospital and retrieval medicine. By having a pre-hospital plan, the team can add structure to their actions and, in doing so, develop a shared mental model inherent in teams that function in such high-acuity, high-consequence environments (see Case 11). Actions are much easier and often performed much more quickly if there is a beginning, middle and end for the plan. Don't forget to share your plan with the entire team (including air crew where relevant), all relevant emergency services on-scene as well as the tasking agency.

Discussion 3.2

After the Fire & Rescue team leader (see Case 1), the Ambulance Service personnel looking after the patient should be approached. If at all possible, this should be before the PHRM team speaks to or assesses the patient. This is essential for several reasons:

- The ambulance team may have been on-scene for some time and can give you a precise summary of the situation, including the changing clinical picture over time.

- It is important to know the state of the patient when the first Ambulance Service personnel arrived and also to know which drugs, fluids and treatments have been administered.
- There may be other patients in other vehicles that you are unaware of.
- Professional courtesy to pre-hospital multidisciplinary colleagues.

Discussion 3.3

Relative entrapment is a situation in which the patient is trapped because of their injuries (e.g. a broken leg with disabling pain), their location (e.g. a cave), or the ambient environment (e.g. a blizzard). If it were not for these factors, they would not require help to extricate.

Actual entrapment occurs when patients are physically held in a location by the structure itself. For example, a major vehicle deformation with cabin intrusion, or a building collapse.

Key points

- The pre-hospital plan is both a shared PHRM team mental model and a structure to help rapid integration of the team into an already busy scene.
- Close liaison with other emergency services already on the scene will assist in delivering coordinated pre-hospital patient care.
- When planning to extricate a trapped patient, establish whether they are relatively or actually entrapped.

Additional reading

Calland V. Safety at scene: a manual for paramedics and immediate care doctors. Mosby, 2001.

Hearns S. Peak performance under pressure: lessons from a helicopter rescue doctor. Class Publishing, 2019.

International Fire Service Training Association. Principles of vehicle extrication, 4th edn. IFSTA, 2017.

CASE 4

Incident

The patient from Case 3 has deteriorated. You are told he is still trapped in the sitting position. However, the vehicle's roof has been removed. The patient's lower leg has an open fracture but appears to be free in the foot well.

Clinical information

- P 150.
- SBP 60 mmHg.
- RR 5 and grunting.
- GCS 6 (E1, V2, M3).
- Oxygen saturation (SaO_2) 80% on high-flow oxygen.

Question 4.1

What are the principles of safe patient extrication?

Question 4.2

How does this deterioration change your management?

Discussion 4.1

The aim is to remove the patient from the vehicle as safely and as quickly as possible while minimising excessive handling and repeated transfers. The key determinant in this plan (apart from safety) is the condition of the patient. Excessive focus on spinal immobilisation can be unwarranted and may contribute to delays to definitive care. While historically the focus has been on spinal protection, there is a growing awareness of the benefits in reducing clot disruption, pain exacerbation and inflammatory response by gentle handling at this stage. Clearly, unstable patients will need rapid extrication (see below) but the ability to predict which patients are unsuitable for a more methodical extrication due to the anticipated clinical course is more challenging. It may be better to decide on a more expeditious extrication plan earlier rather than have an emergency ('crash') extrication situation develop 30 minutes later.

Fire & Rescue will have access to the specialised equipment required in these scenarios. Without good teamwork between the services, the extrication will be significantly hindered.

General principles of extrication
(refer also to Additional Reading below)
Make a plan with the Fire & Rescue Service and ensure the scene is safe.

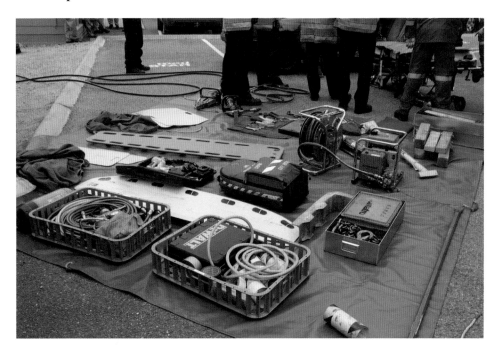

Reduce the risk of fire.
- Switch the ignition off.
- Move onlookers away.
- Cover any obvious leaks with sand.
- Disconnect the battery.

Consider other hazards.
- Airbag safety.
- Seatbelt pre-tensioners.
- Automatic roll bars.
- Leaking fluids (fuel, oil, brake fluid and battery acid).

Stabilise the vehicle.
- Check that the handbrake is on.
- Use 'blocks and chocks'.

Manage any glass.

When deploying specialised cutting tools:
- Ensure safety of the teams.
- Ensure safety of the patient (hard and soft protection; see Case 2).
- Cover all sharp or jagged areas.

Check the side entry.
- Remove the door (it may open in the usual fashion).
- Remove the entire side of the vehicle ('B' post removal or 'rip').

Check the top entry.
- Remove the roof (flap backwards, forwards or to the side).

Disimpact the vehicle around the patient.
- Use chains, winches and other vehicles (Wik et al 2004).
- Use the 'dash roll'.
- Adjust and/or remove the seat (it may slide back in the usual fashion).
- Clear the foot well (remove the pedal, cut the 'A' post).
- Remove the steering wheel and column.

Remove the patient.
- Use an extrication board or other device.
- Employ a multi-service team to help with patient movement.

Special situations.
- Every crash is unique as the location and deformity of the vehicle will always generate slightly different problems.
- The team will also need an approach to issues such as the upside-down car, the heavy goods vehicle and multi-vehicle incidents.

Discussion 4.2

This significant deterioration places the team at a crucial crossroad. Delays to patient extrication will almost certainly lead to progressive clinical deterioration. After attempting to exclude obvious life-threatening pathology such as airway obstruction or tension pneumothorax, two options remain: attempt aggressive medical management in the vehicle or emergency extrication. In order to make this decision, the team will need to stop and reassess the patient's degree of entrapment, together with the Fire & Rescue team leader and the local ambulance team. There are very few situations in which the entrapment is so absolute that aggressive extrication attempts will fail. At the scene, there may be resistance from the Fire & Rescue Service, in particular, to hurry the process for fear that the spine may be jeopardised. The PHRM team needs to take the lead here and voice with clarity that the patient is peri-arrest and unless extrication occurs within the next few minutes the patient may die. It is important to stress 'death' in this situation (provided that is your genuine clinical assessment). Asking the Fire & Rescue team leader how they would get the patient out if the vehicle suddenly caught fire is another way of explaining the gravity of the situation and may generate new ideas.

The process of emergency ('crash') extrication

- Gain everyone's attention – suggest a 'team time out' (this is easier said than done; use a loud, clear voice).
- Clearly explain to all members of the emergency services that an emergency extrication is about to take place. Briefly explain what it means and why it is required.
- Decide on the best extrication option (i.e. straight up using an extrication board if the roof is off, or rotate to the side and out the side door using an extrication board, etc.).
- Attach a rescue team member to each shoulder, each side of the pelvis and as much of the legs as possible.
- A dedicated person should control the head and spinal column.

- Plan for another team of rescue workers to take over the patient halfway through the manoeuvre, as the physical position of the rescuers may make it impossible to continue past a certain point. This is especially relevant for the person responsible for the head.
- Perform the manoeuvre avoiding unnecessary patient movements and preferably directly to a patient transport stretcher. The patient may clinically deteriorate on extrication as the tamponade effect of the dashboard on the pelvis and lower limbs has been removed. This can be mitigated by setting up a clear, safe place to where the patient will be extricated ('a pit stop'). Roles and tasks can be allocated to paramedic colleagues; for example, an immediate application of a pelvic binder and traction splints on extrication.

On the rare occasion when extrication is not possible, the PHRM team will need to consider aggressive medical management in the vehicle. This should be considered only as a last resort for the following reasons:

- Scene time will increase.
- The procedural environment will be unfamiliar, making procedures more difficult.
- A critical patient will still require close monitoring, which will be difficult in this environment.
- Invasive devices placed (e.g. a tracheal tube) are at risk of dislodgement during extrication.
- Seriously injured patients can deteriorate precipitously, especially after pre-hospital anaesthesia. The options for further management in this situation are severely restricted.

The airway needs particular care in these and other situations in which the patient is not in the standard supine position. The sitting patient is reasonably straightforward to intubate, although due consideration to aspiration must be given. Other more complex patient positions must be approached with great caution. Heroic attempts at invasive airway management with limited access (e.g. when the patient is upside down) should not be attempted unless absolutely unavoidable. Consider the laryngeal mask airway as a temporising measure. On rare occasions, a primary surgical airway is required.

Key points

- Extrication techniques and timeframes predominantly depend on the patient's condition.
- Highly unstable patients should undergo emergency ('crash') extrication.

Reference

Wik L, Hansen TB, Kjensli K, Steen PA. Rapid extrication from a car wreck. Injury 2004; 35:739–745.

Additional reading

Calland V. Safety at scene: a manual for paramedics and immediate care doctors. Mosby, 2001.
International Fire Service Training Association. Principles of vehicle extrication, 4th edn. IFSTA, 2017.
Nutbeam T, Boylan M. (Eds) ABC of pre-hospital emergency medicine. Wilcy Blackwell, 2013.

CASE 5

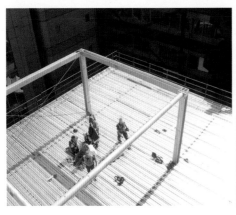 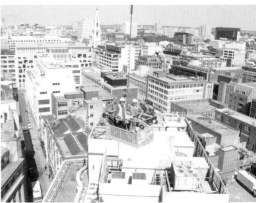

Incident

A 45-year-old male construction worker on a building site has been struck on the head by a scaffold pole. The patient is confused and combative, and access to the scene is by crane only.

Relevant information

- **PHRM team transport options:** Rotary-wing aircraft landing site 1 km (0.6 miles) away.
- **Additional resources:** One land ambulance. Police service.
- **Retrieval options:** Major trauma hospital 25 minutes by road.
- **Other:** Senior construction-site personnel available on-scene.

Question 5.1

What is your initial pre-hospital plan?

Question 5.2

Briefly describe your approach to this particular scene.

Clinical information

- P 110.
- BP 140/80 mmHg.
- GCS 13 (E4, V4, M5).
- Confused and combative.

Question 5.3

Discuss the different options for managing this patient's airway, highlighting the 'pros and cons'. Give your final decision.

Question 5.4

How will you retrieve this patient to the receiving hospital?

Discussion 5.1

Scene

Note that this is an atypical scene. The risks of working at height should be considered.

Patient

Getting a confused and combative adult male off a roof will be challenging. The requirement for pre-hospital anaesthesia is a distinct possibility.

Destination

This should be to a major trauma centre. The PHRM team should prepare for an extended scene time.

Discussion 5.2

There are clear safety implications for the PHRM team in this scenario. Locate the most senior construction site personnel available. Confirm that the only way to access the patient is via the crane (e.g. ask questions, such as *Are there stairs or a builder's elevator on the side of the building? How safe is the location of the patient –near the edge, on a weak floor, etc.? What extra PPE is required – are fall-arrest harnesses appropriate?*).

Remember scene safety is the responsibility of every member of the PHRM team. If the scene is too unsafe for the team to enter, the patient will have to be brought to the team by alternative means, in the safest way possible. You can assist in this process by offering verbal advice as required. If time allows, the Fire & Rescue service may be called to assist in planning a more formal extrication.

Discussion 5.3

The different options in this patient's case relate to whether or not rapid-sequence intubation (RSI) is appropriate. Pre-hospital RSI is a difficult and complex procedure, even for the skilled practitioner. Correct patient selection is paramount. Suggested indications for pre-hospital RSI are outlined in the box below.

Suggested indications for pre-hospital RSI
• Actual or impending airway compromise. • Ventilatory failure. • Safe facilitation of procedural requirement. • Unconsciousness. • Unmanageable or severely agitated patients after head injury. • Anticipated clinical course. • Humanitarian indications. • Flight or pre-hospital safety issues.

Always perform an on-scene risk–benefit analysis on each case considered for pre-hospital RSI. Points to consider in such an analysis include:

- PHRM team skills, experience and training.

- Available skilled assistance (ideally pre-hospital RSI should not be a solo procedure).
- Anticipated airway difficulty.
- Proximity to hospital and required transport times.
- Patient acuity and physiologic instability.
- Mode of transport (road transport may allow more flexibility).

A sensible risk–benefit analysis will prevent pre-hospital RSI from becoming 'mandatory' for certain groups of patients. While the performance of pre-hospital RSI should be standardised (see Case 6), the risk–benefit decision making should remain dynamic. In broad terms, pre-hospital RSI should be viewed as a three-stage procedure with each stage carrying equal importance. If the PHRM team lacks the skills required for any stage, then pre-hospital RSI should be reconsidered.

Three stages of pre-hospital RSI

Stage 1: Patient selection.
Stage 2: Technical challenge of drug-assisted tracheal tube placement.
Stage 3: Continued initial management of the critically injured ventilated patient.

In this particular case, there are other issues that need to be considered.

In favour of RSI

- Safety: The crane basket seems to be the only way down. It is not acceptable to place the safety of the patient and the team in jeopardy by trying to move a combative patient in this way. The patient is unlikely to be rational or cooperative, and a struggle in the crane basket could be disastrous. In addition to the crane issue, the patient has either a road or helicopter trip ahead before arriving at the receiving hospital.
- Patient: In the PHRM trauma environment, an adult with a GCS of 13 or 14 following head injury has a significant chance of intracranial pathology (Ellis et al 2007). Early control of the airway and ventilation will facilitate improved cerebral protection and avoid common secondary insults. On arrival at the trauma hospital, the patient will require trauma imaging, which may require anaesthesia.

Against RSI

- Safety: Moving the patient following RSI is going to be considerably more difficult due to the high level of monitoring required. Will the immobilised, ventilated patient and all the monitoring, oxygen and other equipment fit in the crane basket? In addition, a member of the PHRM team will need to travel with the patient as well as all the pre-hospital equipment.
- Patient: In view of the patient's precarious location, is a safe pre-hospital RSI technically possible? (Can 360-degree access be obtained in this situation?)

Bottom line

- The risk–benefit approach illustrated above should be performed for each patient to be sure that the PHRM team has fully analysed each case on its merits. In this case, the patient should be anaesthetised where he is and then evacuated from the roof.
- Any service that performs pre-hospital RSI should have audit and clinical governance processes and structures specifically to examine failed intubation rate, number of attempts, oxygen saturations and other measures of dynamic physiologic stability before, during and after the procedure. This will ensure the risks of RSI do not outweigh the benefits at each instance (Davis 2008).

Discussion 5.4

Roof to ground

In transferring the patient from the roof to the ground, the general rules for transporting the ventilated patient apply (see Case 26). In this instance, a member of the PHRM team must remain with the patient at all times. It is unlikely that there will be absolutely no room for anyone but the patient in the crane basket. However, if the team members found themselves in such a position, other options may be available, such as a vertical-winch rescue, utilising an appropriate rotary-wing aircraft (see Case 49) or advanced roping vertical-rescue techniques. If these options are not available, the PHRM team could consider splitting up after the RSI and having one member on the ground and the other on the roof. In this setting, the patient must be adequately secured and packaged with optimised physiology on the transport ventilator. Lowering of the basket should be as swift as practicable. Communication should occur between the team by radio or mobile phone.

Ground to hospital

This patient should go by road to the major trauma hospital. The helicopter is 1 km (0.6 miles) away from the building site and, in either case, the patient will need to be packaged in an ambulance. Driving this distance and then transferring the patient to the helicopter, repackaging and flying to the trauma hospital is unlikely to be quicker than simply going straight from the building site by road.

Do not forget to communicate your decision with the pilots and the tasking agency.

Key points

- All medical interventions in the pre-hospital environment are relatively high risk and require careful risk–benefit analysis.
- The performance of pre-hospital RSI is a three-stage procedure.
- Patients requiring complex extrication and pre-hospital RSI pose specific challenges.

References

Davis DP. Early ventilation in traumatic brain injury. Resuscitation 2008; 76(3):333–340.

Ellis DY, Davies GE, Pearn J, Lockey D. Prehospital rapid-sequence intubation of patients with trauma with a Glasgow Coma Score of 13 or 14 and the subsequent incidence of intracranial pathology. Emerg Med J 2007; 24(2):139–141.

Additional reading

Gravesteijn BY, Sewalt CA, Ercole A et al. Variation in the practice of tracheal intubation in Europe after traumatic brain injury: a prospective cohort study. Anaesthesia 2020; 75(1):45–53

Lockey DJ, Wislon M. Editorial: Early airway management of patients with severe head injury: opportunities missed? Anaesthesia 2020; 75:7–10.

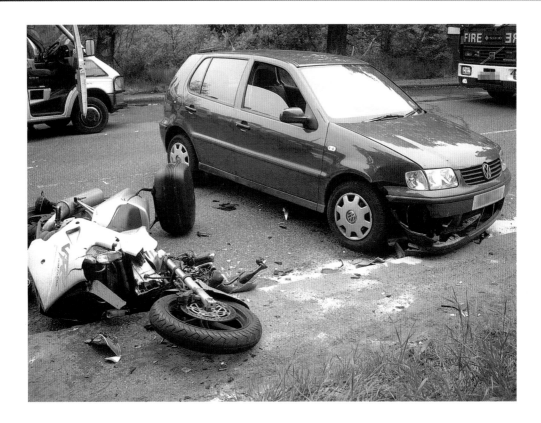

Incident

A 48-year-old male motorcyclist has collided with a car and is reported to be 'unconscious'.

Relevant information

- **PHRM team transport options:** Rotary-wing aircraft – landing site less than 200 m (600 ft) from the incident.
- **Additional resources:** One land ambulance. Police service. Fire and Rescue Service.
- **Retrieval options:** Major trauma hospital 30 minutes by road or 10 minutes by air.
- **Other:** Monday 08:00 hours. Ambient conditions: Clear 2°C (36°F).

Question 6.1

Using the information available so far, outline your pre-hospital plan prior to arrival on the scene?

Clinical information

- P 115.
- BP 150/90 mmHg.
- GCS 6 (E1, V2, M3).

Question 6.2

Describe the key steps required in the performance of a pre-hospital RSI.

Discussion 6.1

Scene safety involves considering all the issues and potential hazards involved in such an incident (see Case 1). Also, in this case, you need to factor in the near-freezing temperature. The patient is reportedly 'unconscious', meaning that the requirement for pre-hospital anaesthesia is very likely. Patient selection for RSI has been addressed in Case 5. A few seconds with the patient (GCS 6) should provide adequate assessment to confirm this requirement. Given the mechanism, vehicle deformation, possible multi-injuries and current patient condition, definitive care will require transport to a major trauma hospital. In view of predicted transport times, the proximity of a landing site to the incident and time of day, air transport is appropriate.

Discussion 6.2

In comparison with the in-hospital environment, pre-hospital airway management is more complex. Challenges in a pre-hospital and retrieval setting include the following.

- Non-fasted, awake or combative patients.
- Airway trauma.
- Unpredicted difficult anatomy.
- Blood, vomit and debris in the upper airway.
- Difficult access to the patient.
- Extreme environmental challenges (ambient light, noise and temperature).
- Logistic challenges associated with the required patient transport.
- Extreme acuity of injury or illness.
- Limited equipment and monitoring.
- Lack of back-up.

The PHRM team should, therefore, work on the principle that *every* pre-hospital airway will be difficult. When performing pre-hospital RSI, all efforts should be made to optimise the first attempt's success. Key considerations to this approach are outlined below.

Checklist

The use of checklists in medicine has become ubiquitous in recent years and highlights the importance of systems to manage high-acuity, high-risk interventions in a challenging environment. Pre-hospital RSI is such an intervention, and use of a team checklist is mandatory. Even in emergent situations, a checklist should be utilised and many services have both a 'standard' checklist and an 'emergent' checklist to cater for all situations. An example of RSI checklists can be found in Appendix 1.1.2.

Location

The patient should be moved to a safe area of the scene with 360-degree access obtained wherever possible. A few minutes spent creating space before RSI will be rewarded if or when difficulties are encountered. In addition, the patient should be positioned on a stretcher wherever possible. Likewise, environmental factors need to be taken into account. Shelter from sunlight, heat, cold, wind or rain can be achieved by moving the patient into the transport vehicle. However (dependent on vehicle configuration and size), this may compromise the 360-degree access. Other emergency services can help by holding up tarpaulins or blankets to shield patients from the elements as well as from onlookers. Be aware that sun glare may affect laryngeal view as the operator's eyes pass from the bright sunlight to a larynx lit only by the relatively poor artificial light of the laryngoscope. Likewise, the screen of a video laryngoscope may also be susceptible to bright light or glare.

Patient preparation

Assessment for predictors of airway difficulty should occur during this phase. The 4 Ds, while not representing an exhaustive list, will assist in this regard.

Distortion
- Airway trauma.
- Airway foreign bodies.

Disproportion
- Short thyromental distance.
- Small jaw.
- Short neck.
- Truncal obesity.
- Pregnancy.

Dysmobility
- Neck movements.
- Mouth opening and jaw protrusion.
- Tongue mobility.

Dentition
- Prominent upper dentition.
- Dentures.

In addition, an appreciation of the patient's physiologic reserve is required. Critical illness and injury will lead to reductions in physiologic capacity, leading to precipitous deterioration soon after anaesthesia. Minor difficulties in airway management can be compounded by hypoxia and hypotension in the patient with limited physiological reserve. Opportunities to improve physiological stability include splinting of fractures, haemorrhage control, judicious volume resuscitation, and airway opening with assisted ventilation.

Equipment access and 'kit dump'

The suggested contents of the pre-hospital airway bag and drugs for RSI can be found in Appendix 2.1. Equipment should be checked and readily accessible before the procedure begins. This can be achieved in two ways. See picture on next page for a standardised 'kit dump', which often uses a disposable template or a customised RSI pack that replicates a kit dump when opened. High-quality suction, a bougie and the ability to check for end tidal carbon dioxide ($ETCO_2$) are essential in the pre-hospital environment. Basic (e.g. oropharyngeal and/or nasopharyngeal airways) and rescue airway (e.g. laryngeal mask airway (LMA)) devices should be instantly available.

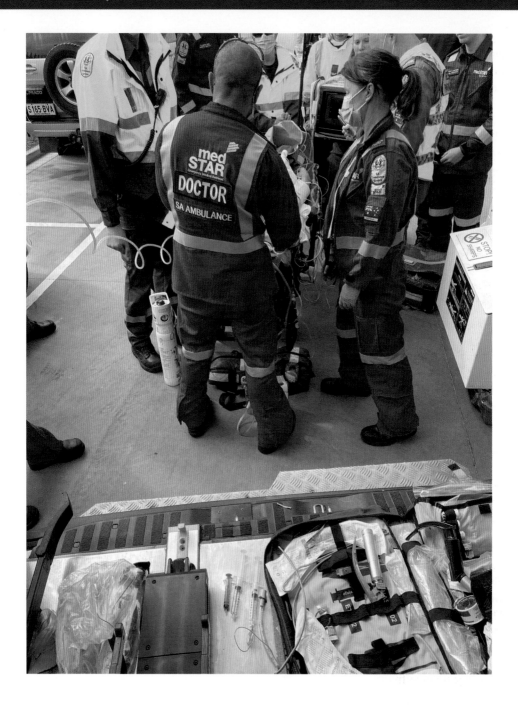

Team development

Pre-hospital RSI is ideally a four-person job. In general, the lead airway clinician and airway assistant should be the generic PHRM team. The other roles can be shared among the other emergency services personnel on the scene, preferably within the Ambulance Service. It is possible that the ambulance personnel on the scene have not participated in emergency drug-assisted intubation before. Each role should be succinctly but accurately explained to the designated person. A few minutes spent creating a shared mental model could prevent a serious complication later. The role of various personnel involved in pre-hospital RSI are:

1. Lead airway clinician: Operator

Leads the RSI and performs laryngoscopy and intubation.

2. Assistant 1: Airway assistant

The *sole* job of the airway assistant is to ensure equipment is checked and readily accessible and to assist the lead airway clinician during the procedure. It is crucial that the airway assistant is not distracted by other tasks.

3. Assistant 2: In-line cervical immobilisation

If a cervical collar has been applied, it should be released during the preparation phase and, from below on the patient's left side, gloved palms should be placed on either side of the patient's head to restrict movement. Small anterior flexion or extension movements that facilitate swift tracheal intubation are acceptable (Austin 2014).

4. Assistant 3: Delivery of anaesthetic drugs

The choice of agent and/or dose for safe and effective anaesthetic induction in the pre-hospital setting is variable. Physiologically unstable, critically injured patients will not tolerate standard doses of induction agents, and modifications are frequently required. Ketamine (0.1–1.5 mg/kg) is the induction agent of choice in pre-hospital trauma with the consideration of adjunctive opiates (e.g. Fentanyl). Rocuronium is the RSI muscle relaxant of choice for pre-hospital anaesthesia.

An adequate dose of rocuronium (1.5–2 mg/kg) is indicated to maximise onset and effect. An alternative agent for muscle relaxation is succinylcholine (2 mg/kg). A modified approach using a muscle relaxant without any induction agent is infrequently indicated in profoundly shocked unconscious trauma patients. All drugs should be pre-drawn and clearly labelled. Any instructions given to a third party when delivering such drugs should be clear.

Laryngeal manipulation and Cricoid pressure

Laryngeal manipulation or 'Backwards Upwards, Right and Pressure' (BURP) is distinct to cricoid pressure and may be performed by the airway assistant or by the airway clinician with the right hand, while continuing with laryngoscopy with the left. The latter is termed 'bimanual laryngoscopy'. Cricoid pressure is variably applied in modern airway management. If applied, the removal of cricoid pressure should be an immediate consideration if there is any difficulty intubating or ventilating the patient (White et al 2020). For inexperienced assistants, both BURP and cricoid pressure may require guidance from the lead airway clinician.

Checklist run through

At this point, running through the RSI checklist using challenge and response is required even if the checklist has been used to facilitate the set-up. In this way, the checklist facilitates the sharing of a clear mental model and plan. Visual cross-checking by both team members while running through the checklist is vital to ensure no equipment is missing.

Confirmation of tracheal intubation

Confirmation includes (but is not limited to) direct visualisation (tracheal tube passing through cords), auscultation in both axillae and over stomach and confirmation of $ETCO_2$ by continuous waveform capnography. Additional tools include in-line single-use colorimetric $ETCO_2$ detection devices.

Maintenance of anaesthesia and ongoing timely care

The period of time immediately following pre-hospital RSI should be used productively. There is risk of a 'therapeutic vacuum' during this phase with time passing during which patients do not receive meaningful interventions. This translates into a longer on-scene time, and delays to definitive care. The therapeutic vacuum is commonly experienced following critical interventions or during handover of care. Methods to minimise the therapeutic vacuum include parallel processing of required interventions (e.g. splinting, packaging, loading) and continuous verbalisation of the pre-hospital plan with reference to timeliness. The time elapsed from the start (decision to commence RSI) to the finish (the securing of the tracheal tube and maintenance of anaesthesia) should not, in most cases, exceed 10 minutes.

Unless there is a clear contraindication, cautious titration of intravenous sedation and analgesia (via constant intravenous infusion whenever possible) should be used. Regional variation will dictate the specific practice adopted. If ongoing muscle relaxation is indicated, frequent assessment should be made to avoid awareness, particularly with extracranial trauma and burns. Ketamine may be of assistance in this setting (see Case 20).

Failed intubation drill

The PHRM team should have a thorough understanding of a failed intubation drill. A plan for the response to a failed intubation must be discussed during the preparation phase. When faced with an unstable, hypoxic, multiply injured and apnoeic patient who is unable to be ventilated by either a bag valve mask (BVM) device or LMA (i.e. a 'can't intubate, can't oxygenate' situation), there should be no hesitation to proceed immediately to a surgical airway.

A suggested RSI algorithm and surgical airway technique can be found in Appendix 1.1

Key points

- Pre-hospital RSI should not be a 'solo' procedure.
- Checklist use is mandatory
- Preparation is the key to success.
- Always consider the failed intubation scenario.
- Be aware of the therapeutic vacuum.

References

Austin N. Airway management in cervical spine injury. Int J Crit Illn Inj Sci. 2014 Jan-Mar; 4(1):50–56.

White L, Thang C, Hodsdon A, et al. Cricoid pressure during intubation: a systematic review and meta-analysis of randomised controlled trials. Heart Lung. 2020 Mar–Apr; 49(2):175–180. doi: 10.1016/j.hrtlng.2019.10.001. Epub 2019 Nov 2. PMID: 31685271.

Additional reading

Burtenshaw A, Benger J, Nolan J (Eds). Emergency airway management, 2nd ed. Cambridge University Press, 2015.

Gawande A. The checklist manifesto. Picador, 2011.

Hearns S. Peak performance under pressure: lessons from a helicopter rescue doctor. Core Cognition, 2019.

Levitan RM, Kinkle WC. Pocket guide to intubation, 2nd ed. Airway Cam Technologies, 2007.

Lockey DJ, Crewdson K, Davies G et al. Safer pre-hospital anaesthesia 2017: Association of Anaesthetists of Great Britain and Ireland. Anaesthesia 2017 Mar; 72(3):379–390.

Incident

A 43-year-old woman has slipped from a crowded platform and fallen into the path of an incoming train at an underground station. She has been dragged under the first carriage and now lies between the rails 5 to 10 metres into the single exiting tunnel. Initial Ambulance and Fire & Rescue Service crews on the scene have ensured that the scene is safe and you are able to confirm this with the line controller (see Case 13). The first paramedic on the scene is with the patient and reports the following clinical information.

Clinical information

- Alert with a clear airway but laboured breathing.
- Weak radial pulse (58 beats per minute).
- Crush injury to pelvis and bilateral open femoral fractures.
- Partial amputation just below right knee.
- Not physically trapped, but in severe pain.

He has had two unsuccessful attempts at gaining intravenous access.

In addition to your standard pre-hospital equipment, the items shown in the photographs are available to you.

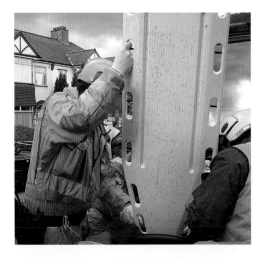

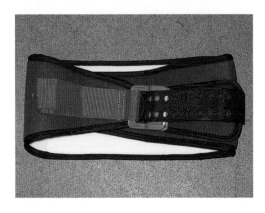

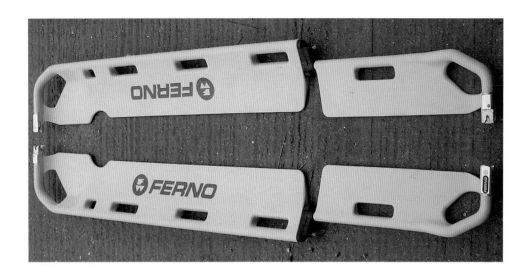

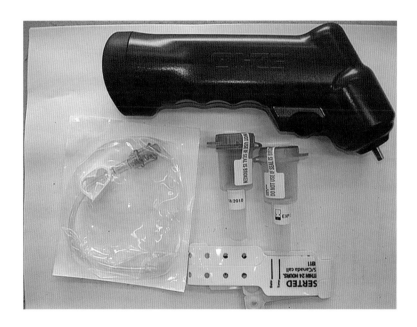

33

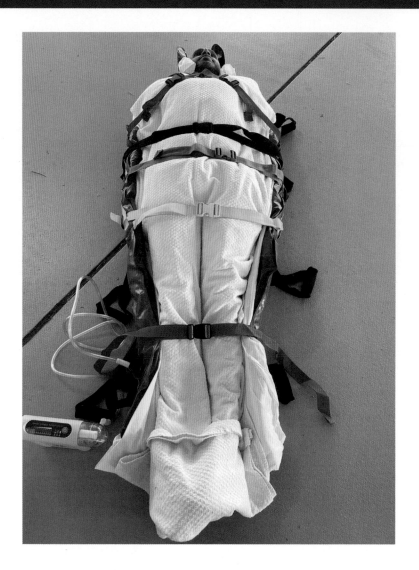

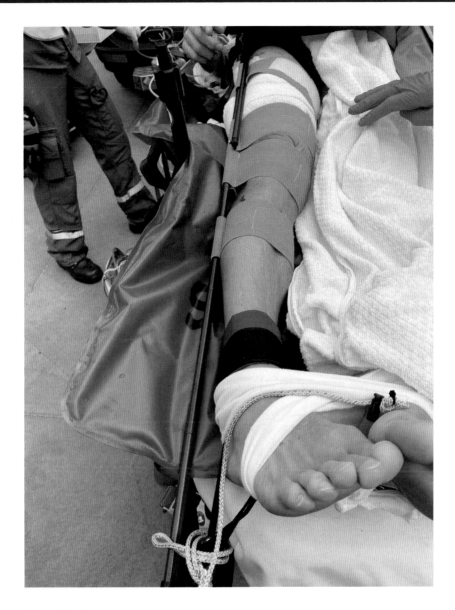

Question 7.1

For each of the devices illustrated, outline briefly how they are used.

Question 7.2

What are the benefits and limitations of each device in the management of pre-hospital trauma?

Question 7.3

How will you utilise this equipment in the management of this case? You may select all, none or some of the equipment available. Are any pieces of equipment contraindicated?

Discussion 7.1

Extrication board

Used for removing patients from confined or difficult access areas. Frequently used for facilitating extrication from a motor vehicle (rear, vertical or seated rotation and side door egress) by sliding the patient onto the device. This piece of equipment is also useful, with the patient supine upon it, in extrication over uneven or rough terrain, such as through tunnels or collapsed structures where lighter devices (e.g. Sked or Chrysalis rescue stretchers) are not available.

Pelvic splint

Applied when there is a confirmed or suspected pelvic fracture. Requires planning for application (i.e. at the time of patient packaging) and must be placed in alignment with the greater trochanter on each side. Many pelvic splints are single use and have a force/tension measurement capacity. There is a risk of posterior displacement of a pelvic fracture by over-tightening the binder. The ankles should be bound together using a triangular bandage utilising a figure-of-eight method.

Scoop stretcher

Drawn out to length and divided into left and right sections by lock release at head and foot ends. Placed one side at a time under the patient with gentle (20 degrees) log roll following exposure and clothes removal. The head and foot end are then locked and secured. Some PHRM services, where transport times to hospitals are short, will advocate leaving the patient on a scoop stretcher and placing it on a vacuum mattress (not removing the air). This minimises handling of the patient and prevents clot disruption. However, on longer transfers, the scoop stretcher can cause pressure injuries.

Intraosseous access device

Used to assist the placement of an intraosseous (IO) cannula by providing battery-powered, high-speed drilling of bevelled, hollow, drill-tipped needles. Provides secure, controlled vascular access via the IO route to patients of all ages in emergency situations when vascular access is challenging or impossible. The intraosseous space allows drugs and fluids to reach the central circulation as IO vascular flow continues, even in shocked states. For sites of IO access see Appendix 1.2.3.

Femoral traction splint

Used in the stabilisation and reduction of femoral shaft fractures. Ankle harnesses and straps attached to the distal traction component allow for measurable dynamic traction to the femur as required. Elastic leg straps are then applied in order to minimise mid and lower limb movement. Peripheral pulses should be checked and marked before and after application.

Vacuum mattress

An adjunct to the packaging process, the vacuum mattress offers the ability to immobilise the patient and assists in transfer to and from stretchers and hospital trolleys.

The patient is placed on a sheet on top of the mattress, which is then moulded around the patient. Air is removed from the mattress utilising suction, preserving the mattress shape and providing ongoing support.

Discussion 7.2

Benefits and limitations of pre-hospital trauma devices

	Benefits	Limitations
Extrication board	Common Tough Slides easily facilitating extrication Has handles for rope and/or strap attachment Low profile Various lengths	May result in poor spinal column position and midline pressure. Incompletely limits patient movement during carriage. Minimal/no lateral support. Size and/or weight may limit storage in aircraft. Lateral slide removal to a stretcher or hospital bed may result in significant spinal column movement.
Pelvic splint	Splints and supports pelvic bony fracture segments Reduces pelvic potential volume for haemorrhage in 'open book'-type pelvic fractures	May be harmful if incorrectly applied. May further displace lateral compression pelvic fractures. Access to groin limited when applied.
Scoop stretcher	Adjustable in length Facilitates transport of the supine patient with minimal movements Avoids central spinal column pressure and allows natural position Facilitates any additional transfers (road to stretcher, stretcher to hospital bed, etc.) with minimal patient movement	Size and/or weight may limit storage in aircraft. Does not limit patient movement during transport when used in isolation. Older devices may not be radiolucent. Not ideal for very tall, short or obese patients.
Intraosseous access device	Rapid, secure access to the central circulation either primarily or as a 'rescue' access device Robust and compact Variable insertion points offer flexibility when patient access is limited (see Appendix 1.2.3) Paediatric, adult and bariatric needles available Drill offers minimal lateral movement on insertion and, therefore, reduces bone damage Can be inserted in conscious patients with minimal discomfort	May be used in preference to simpler and cheaper techniques (given ease of insertion). Flow rates for volume resuscitation are far less than large-bore peripheral intravenous access. Fluid extravasation through insertion site or occult adjacent fractures may occur. Administration of blood leads to haemolysis. Infection risk increases if not removed within 24 hours.

Continued

Benefits and limitations of pre-hospital trauma devices—cont'd

	Benefits	Limitations
Vacuum mattress	Provides additional splintage and immobilisation of fractures Minimises patient movement and subsequent clot disruption Aids in patient transfers Reduces heat loss	Bulky and heavy. Limits access to patient. May obscure visual identification of significant haemorrhage. Effectiveness may be impacted by altitude. Potential for puncture, damage or valve failure.
Femoral traction device	Lightweight Easy to apply Variable length to suit patient Access to groin maintained Variable (and measurable) traction load	Requires an intact ankle/lower tibia and fibula. Removal at receiving hospital not always possible – PHRM team may need to reclaim device at a later time. Separate bindings may be misplaced. Overhang may impede aircraft or ambulance loading.

Discussion 7.3

The patient requires rapid extrication to facilitate assessment, stabilisation and timely transfer to a major trauma hospital. The plan should be to move her to the train platform in the first instance. Although not physically trapped, her location in the tunnel, injury complex (including potential pelvic and/or spinal cord disruption) and analgesic requirements will make extrication challenging.

An extrication board (or similar sliding rescue litter) will allow the patient to be moved out along the tracks under the train. A rope or pulley device and assistance from on-scene emergency service personnel may assist here. Adequate analgesia is mandatory and, in the absence of a swiftly inserted intravenous line, an intraosseous cannula should be placed to allow analgesic titration (e.g. ketamine and/or opiates). Prolonged attempts at gaining intravenous access in cramped and difficult circumstances should be avoided. With significant lower-limb and pelvic injuries, the proximal humerus will be the intraosseous insertion site of choice (see Appendix 1.2.3). Fluid resuscitation can be delayed until the patient is extricated and a more thorough assessment of her injuries and pre-hospital fluid requirements are made. The findings on further assessment will guide any necessary interventions and the method for pre-hospital splinting and packaging.

Application of a pelvic binder is required early following removal of all clothing (see Case 8). A femoral traction splint should be applied on the left leg. The presence of a partial amputation on the right side, limits options for right femoral fracture stabilisation. Simple anatomical alignment using simple splints (e.g. a box splint) may be all that is feasible. A scoop stretcher will then allow transfer to a vacuum mattress facilitating transfer to hospital with minimal patient movement.

Key point

- Appropriate and timely selection and application of available pre-hospital equipment will facilitate patient assessment, treatment and transfer.

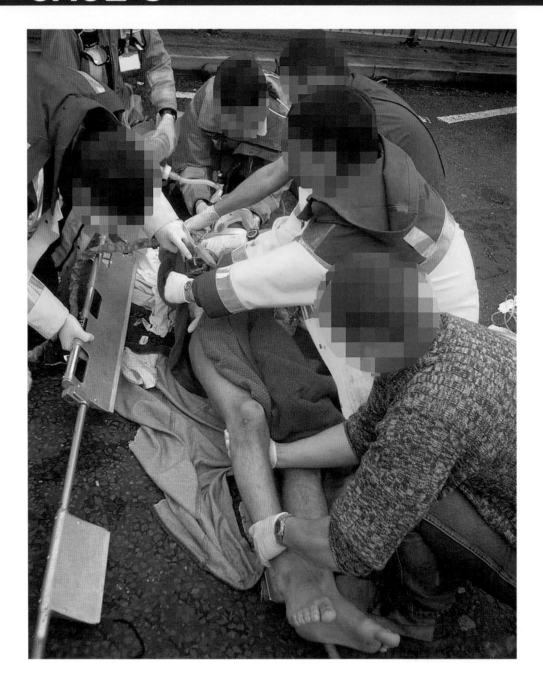

Incident

A 21-year-old male passenger has been involved in a side impact collision with another vehicle. He was initially trapped and unconscious but has since been extricated.

Relevant information

- **PHRM team transport options:** Rotary-wing aircraft.
- **Additional resources:** One land ambulance. Police and Fire & Rescue services.
- **Retrieval options:** Major trauma hospital 15 minutes by road.
- **Other:** RSI has been performed by the PHRM team due to unconsciousness; the patient is otherwise physiologically stable.

Question 8.1

How will you package this patient?

Discussion 8.1

Packaging the patient depends on the mode of transport and nature of injury. Primary trauma patients should be managed in a similar fashion whatever the mode of transport to enhance operational consistency. Minor differences in packaging will be inevitable due to the variable design of ambulances, rotary-wing and fixed-wing aircraft. Even within helicopters, there are multiple design differences that will affect packaging. However, the basic principles should be unchanged.

The main aim of packaging is to minimise repeated disruption of tissue injury. This will reduce clot disturbance, blood loss and inflammatory cytokine release. Good packaging will also reduce pain and the need for excessive pharmacologic analgesia as well as facilitate improved patient flow and early assessment and intervention on reception at the receiving facility.

Extrication boards, scoop stretchers and vacuum mattresses

Further to the discussion in Case 7, such devices are often referred to as 'spinal boards', but the name 'extrication board' better explains the role of this device. It is an invaluable tool for removing trapped patients from vehicles while reducing avoidable patient movement. However, the board is hard, and the supine patient can experience pain and early pressure necrosis after even a short period of time. A better device for transfer is the vacuum mattress. Patients found on extrication boards should be resuscitated in situ but should be transferred to a vacuum mattress (ideally using a scoop stretcher) for all but the shortest of journeys.

Clothing

As a general rule, all clothing should be removed as part of the assessment and packaging process. Using a high-quality pair of trauma shears, cuts should be made up each arm and leg, across the waist and in a 'Y' pattern across the chest. Careful attention to removal of clothes initially will save time and effort later.

Log roll

A log roll is not mandatory in the pre-hospital environment as part of the effort to minimise movement. Often, a partial log roll (to 20 degrees) is performed to put the patient on a scoop stretcher, and, at this point, a cursory examination of the back may be appropriate. Penetrating disease is a notable exception as the patient should be fully log rolled (to 90 degrees) to inspect for further entry/exit wounds (see Case 16). Remember to tell the receiving hospital team whether or not a log roll has been performed.

The supine patient

The majority of patients will be supine. Take a handover from Ambulance Service personnel and assess the patient. Then decide which pre-hospital interventions are required, including vascular access, advanced airway management and the reduction of fractures. In this case, the patient is supine, anaesthetised and has a cervical collar in situ. Management of the spine in the pre-hospital environment has changed markedly over recent years. A lack of evidence behind cervical spine collars has resulted in a reduction in their use. Current practice instead focuses on manual immobilisation techniques and minimising excessive patient movement.

The next step is to 'scoop' the patient to a vacuum mattress placed on a transport stretcher.

- Split the scoop, draw out to length and place either side of the patient.
- Maintain manual in-line cervical immobilisation.
- Perform a partial log roll (to 20 degrees), assess the patient's back and remove any debris. Push any clothing that cannot be easily removed to the far side of the patient.
- Put half of the scoop under the patient, skin to scoop. A pelvic splint, if appropriate, can be placed at this point.
- Lower the patient onto the scoop, have the team swap sides and perform a log roll the other way, to 20 degrees only.
- Remove the remaining clothing and insert the other half of the scoop, again skin to scoop.
- Clip the top and bottom together then lower the patient. Ensure that no patient anatomy is trapped by the closed blades of the scoop.
- Immobilisation of head and spine on the scoop stretcher or vacuum mattress will vary with local practice.
- Lift the patient (one person on each corner), remove any clothing hanging underneath the scoop and place onto a vacuum mattress or similar, and then the ambulance/helicopter stretcher.
- Ensure the intravenous site is accessible (use extension tubing if necessary). Full monitoring should be in place. Make sure the patient is kept warm by using blankets, including chemical heating blankets, where appropriate.

Patients lying in the lateral position

- Take extra time to adequately assess the airway.
- Cut and remove the clothing and assess the patient's back.
- Lie half the scoop next to the patient.
- Log roll the patient onto one half of a scoop stretcher.
- Continue as for the supine patient.

Prone patients

- Careful airway assessment: if the airway is obstructed or ventilation is inadequate, the patient will need to be promptly but cautiously log rolled supine.
- Even if ventilation is satisfactory, the patient will still require log roll to the supine position. In order to minimise unnecessary patient movements, this can be done by cautiously log rolling the patient to 90 degrees, placing an intact scoop stretcher at the patients back and completing the log roll to the supine position with the patient ending up on the scoop stretcher.

Sometimes the position of the patient makes packaging difficult, and some degree of movement is inevitable. The PHRM team must accept this, but should try to get the balance between minimal patient movement and timely evacuation. As a general rule, thorough patient packaging should take no longer than five minutes.

Patients who require complex extrications (e.g. vertical lifts in confined spaces) pose major logistical problems, especially if they have been anaesthetised. A scoop stretcher is unlikely to suffice in these situations and the team should liaise closely with the on-scene Fire & Rescue service personnel. Specialist stretchers (e.g. Neil Robertson, Sked or Chrysalis stretcher) should be used.

Head-injured patients, especially those who have been anaesthetised, should have the cervical collar loosened, if applied. This, together with a slight head up-tilt, can facilitate cerebral venous drainage and may attenuate raised intracranial pressure in transit.

Note that, in this case, a 'lay person' is assisting the PHRM team in packaging the patient. The decision to use external help rests with the PHRM team leader and a non-critical role should be given to such personnel. PPE (in this case gloves) must be offered and used.

Key points
• Good patient packaging represents a pre-hospital therapeutic process and facilitates improved reception at the receiving facility.
• Thorough explanation of packaging procedures and good clear instructions to all members of the team will save time and reduce complications.

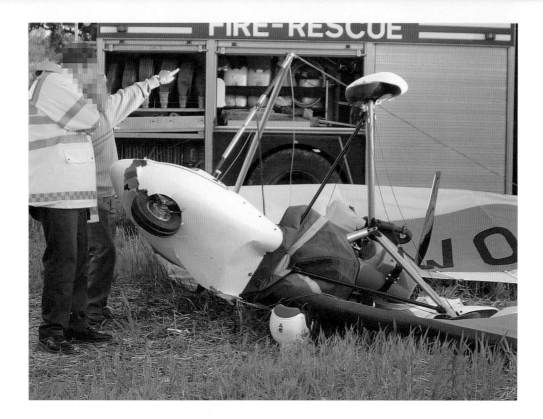

Incident

A microlight aircraft has landed heavily. The ambulance crew on the scene has requested assistance via the tasking agency.

An aircraft rigging wire has struck the pilot across the anterior neck and he now complains of difficulty breathing. In addition, he remains trapped by the lower limbs within the damaged aircraft. The patient's right leg has sustained a compound fracture.

He is alert but anxious and tachypnoeic with an RR of 28. All other vital signs are currently within normal limits.

Relevant information

- **PHRM team transport options:** Rotary-wing aircraft.
- **Additional resources:** Two land ambulances. Fire & Rescue Service.
- **Retrieval options:** Major trauma hospital 15 minutes by air, 40 minutes by road.
- **Other:** The scene has been declared safe by the Fire & Rescue Service.

Question 9.1

What is your initial pre-hospital plan prior to arrival?

On arrival, you find the patient anxious but lucid. He has just been freed from the wreckage. He complains of severe anterior neck pain and is spitting out bloody saliva.

His voice is hoarse. He remains tachypnoeic with a rate of 30 breaths per minute. Examination reveals an acutely tender anterior neck. There is slight crepitus over the laryngeal structures. There is a compound fracture of the right tibia and fibula with good distal perfusion. No other injuries are detected.

Question 9.2

What is your initial management and how will you transport?

Question 9.3

Describe how you will notify the receiving hospital of your planned arrival.

Discussion 9.1

Scene

The safety of the scene should be reconfirmed with the on-scene Fire and Rescue service personnel on arrival.

Patient

The airway is of concern due to the mechanism and clinical information. Advanced airway management, if required, is likely to be problematic.

Destination

Already established pending decision on transport platform.

Discussion 9.2

The main issue here is airway management in the presence of major laryngeal trauma. The initial concern that the airway is not secure is justified, but attempting to secure the airway in this scenario could be disastrous. At present the PHRM team has a stable self-ventilating patient and a 40 minute road trip to a major trauma hospital. It is highly likely that the hospital will have fibre-optic equipment, senior anaesthetic personnel and possibly ear, nose and throat (ENT) specialist assistance on-site. The PHRM team should package the patient for road transport to the major trauma hospital as rapidly as possible. At the same time, prepare the drugs and equipment for RSI and have the front-of-neck access kit to hand. Contact the tasking agency and ask that they check the availability of a senior anaesthetist and ENT surgeons at the receiving hospital.

Attempts to secure the airway in this instance are complicated, mainly due to the unpredictability of airway damage. For example, following anaesthetic induction, there may be a Grade I Cormack and Lehane view, but damage distal to the cords may prevent the passage of the tracheal tube. Repeated attempts to pass the tracheal tube may further damage the airway, rendering ventilation by any modality difficult or impossible. Abnormal anatomy secondary to trauma may make emergency cricothyrotomy impossible and, in any case, the obstruction may be distal to the cricothyroid membrane.

If at all possible, the patient should be transported by road. The cabin of a helicopter is not the place for assessing the deteriorating airway. In the event of a major deterioration, the PHRM team should consider the following approach:

- Bag valve mask until arrival.
- RSI without BURP or cricoid pressure (laryngeal trauma is a relative contraindication) and using a smaller-sized tracheal tube (e.g. size 6).

- Laryngeal mask ventilation.
- If the external anatomy looks excellent, consider a primary surgical airway without muscle relaxation.

Discussion 9.3

En route, the PHRM team must put in a pre-alert call containing relevant information to the receiving hospital. This can be done via the tasking agency using a multiagency radio network or voice/video-conference call. Delegation of this pre-alert call to the tasking agency should be avoided as there is a risk of a breakdown in the chain of accurate information sharing. The pre-alert call must identify the urgent clinical issues. Do not be drawn into a lengthy discussion about other clinical issues (e.g. intravenous access, minor injuries, bed availability, etc.). Use a method that is familiar to both the PHRM team and the receiving team, and that follows a standardised template; for example, ISBAR. The following is an example template.

- Introduction: who you are.
- Situation: patient's main injuries only.
- Background: patient's sex, age and mechanism of injury.
- Assessment: ventilated or not, the immediate needs.
- Recommendations: what response you require (trauma team and, in this case, ENT/anaesthetics).
- How long you will be (estimated time of arrival).

Deliver the message concisely and clearly. Do not be vague (e.g. asking for a senior ENT doctor to be available could imply anything from available at home to currently in theatre). The pre-alert call should take no longer than 30 seconds. Consider rehearsing the pre-alert call and the handover with your team member while en route to the hospital. The aim of this is to ensure the call and handover will be concise and will contain the relevant details. For example:

> 'This is Dr Smith on the pre-hospital response team.
>
> 'We are en route to you with a 21-year-old male who has been involved in a light aircraft crash. He appears to have a fractured larynx with airway compromise. He is currently self-ventilating.
>
> 'We require a trauma response and a senior ENT doctor immediately available in the resuscitation room. We will be with you in 15 (one five) minutes.'

Confirm that the message has been received. The PHRM team must always find time for the pre-alert phone call. Sometimes, with a time-critical patient, it is difficult to allocate time for this. However, the extra time taken to ensure a good trauma team response will improve the reception at the receiving facility.

Key points

- Always perform a risk–benefit analysis for pre-hospital RSI.
- Every primary patient transfer to hospital should be preceded by a pre-alert phone call.

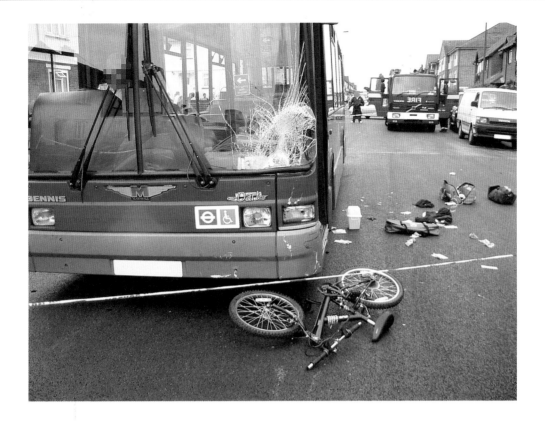

Incident

An 8-year-old male cyclist has been struck by a bus. The cyclist was not wearing a helmet. Although initially 'unconscious', he is now reported to be 'confused'.

Relevant information

- **PHRM team transport options:** Rotary-wing aircraft.
- **Additional resources:** One road ambulance and crew. Police and Fire & Rescue services.
- **Retrieval options:** Regional hospital (no neurosurgery) 5 minutes by road. Major trauma hospital 30 minutes by air.
- **Other:** Flight time to scene less than 15 minutes.

Question 10.1

Using the information so far available, outline your pre-hospital plan prior to arrival on-scene?

Question 10.2

Comment on the picture of the above scene.

On arrival, the patient's GCS is 11 (E3, V4, M4). A 'large' forehead laceration has been dressed by the paramedic on-scene.

Clinical information

- P 95.
- BP 110/75 mmHg.
- SaO$_2$ 97% on high-flow oxygen.
- Combative and pushing the oxygen mask away.

Question 10.3

Outline your initial management.

In preparing the patient for transport, you remove the loosely placed head bandage to reveal an extensive de-gloving soft-tissue injury over the right side of the face and scalp. Immediately post-RSI, the child's heart rate increases to 200 beats per minute and no radial pulse can be felt. Two minutes post-RSI, a review reveals the following.

Clinical information

- P 133.
- BP 70/50 mmHg.
- SaO$_2$ 90% with hand ventilation via a self-inflating bag valve mask device.
- ETCO$_2$ 22 mmHg (3 kPa).
- Right pupil fixed and dilated.
- Left pupil small and reactive.

Question 10.4

Outline your response to this situation.

Discussion 10.1

In this scenario, the key aspect of the pre-hospital plan is the age of the patient. The PHRM team should utilise the response time to prepare adequately. The mechanism sounds significant and severe injuries are likely. As a team, calculations should be made and recorded regarding potential drug, fluid and equipment requirements. PHRM services should consider the use of digital technology to assist with paediatric dose and equipment calculations. Particular attention should be given to preparing for potential pre-hospital anaesthesia. If not already done so, drugs should be drawn and labelled clearly. Early triage possibilities, given the patient's age and potential injuries, should also be considered.

Discussion 10.2

The scene has been cordoned and the road appears to be closed. The stability of the bus is unclear and a driver sits at the wheel. Clarification should be sought from on-scene senior Fire & Rescue personnel regarding scene safety. The patient has presumably been removed to an open and safe area of the scene following initial interventions. There is evidence of a significant mechanism of injury. There is damage to both the bicycle and the corner of the tempered glass window of the bus. The position and appearance of the windscreen damage would suggest impact with the right side of the child's unprotected head. There is also damage to the front left-hand side of the bus lower down. There are faint tyre skid marks visible for some distance behind the bus, suggesting at least moderate speed at impact.

Discussion 10.3

Significant mechanism should always be assumed to be associated with significant injury until proven otherwise. This is even more important when early activation and short response times are considered. The classic signs of severe injury are often subtle and difficult to detect at such an early stage in the pre-hospital environment. 'Reading the scene' can, however, provide valuable information regarding the mechanism and potential injuries, including their severity.

The child's conscious state is at best fluctuant and at worst deteriorating. Given both the clinical information and the scene assessment, a severe head injury is likely, despite the relatively high-scoring GCS. Furthermore, this combative patient requires definitive assessment and management that is unlikely to be available at the nearest hospital. A 30-minute flight is required, and pre-hospital anaesthesia is indicated.

The driver should be escorted from the bus and briefly assessed. Psychological support is often required following such incidents and, whenever possible, the driver's contact details and local family doctor should be recorded.

Discussion 10.4

The appearance of such a significant scalp and facial injury is often visually alarming. However, the appearance of a number of insults leading to secondary brain injury is of far greater significance. The child is hypotensive, tachycardic, hypoxaemic and hypo-capnoeic. Furthermore, there is now a potential lateralising neurological sign. A rapid assessment is required aimed at identifying causes of secondary brain injury correctable with pre-hospital intervention. Time spent on-scene to ensure such correction is time well spent, although the focus should always be on swift transport to definitive care.

There is desaturation and a low $ETCO_2$ so a rapid assessment of the airway is required. If the $ETCO_2$ waveform analysis is consistent and the child is ventilating, it is unlikely that the tracheal tube has significantly dislodged. However, displacement to either of the main stem bronchi or to the pharynx is possible and the pre-calculated length of the tracheal tube at the teeth should be confirmed. A quick reassessment of oxygen flow should confirm maximum fractional inspired oxygen is administered. Rapid assessment of the chest is also required with simultaneous administration of bolus fluids to address potential hypovolaemia. Auscultation of the chest should be performed but is not always of additional benefit in this environment. Palpating the chest and looking across the patient's chest wall from the patient's feet will give the most information regarding potential thoracic pathology. If available and if the PHRM team are adequately trained, point-of-care ultrasound is of benefit in patient assessment. If there are clear signs of an expanding pleural collection or if there is an ongoing volume-resistant shocked state without obvious cause, formal pleural decompression is required (see Case 15).

The low SaO_2 and $ETCO_2$ may simply be surrogate markers of poor tissue perfusion and low cardiac output. If the $ETCO_2$ remains low, despite improved haemodynamics, airway and ventilatory equipment and ventilatory technique should be reassessed. Early correct sizing of the paediatric tracheal tube should avoid large air leaks that may be associated with persistently high $ETCO_2$. Some services still use uncuffed tracheal tubes for paediatric intubation but access to an appropriately sized cuffed tracheal tube may help in this situation (see Case 59). If possible, a paediatric self-inflating bag should be used. Check for depth and rate of positive pressure ventilation and adjust accordingly, aiming for normocapnoea ($ETCO_2$ between 30 and 35 mmHg [4.0 and 4.5 kPa]). Ongoing hypoxaemia, despite high fractional inspired oxygen delivery and the above measures, may imply worsening lung contusion.

With resolution of the patient's cardiorespiratory instability, check the pupil size and reaction again. A persistent fixed dilated right pupil implies intracranial haemorrhage. Infrequently, direct ocular trauma can be associated with pupillary dysfunction. Depending on local practice, the use of a bolus hypertonic solution in this setting may be considered.

Finally, the wound should be re-covered with a sterile dressing. Unless there are issues with haemorrhage control from this wound, tight-pressure bandaging should be avoided.

Remember to notify the tasking agency and ensure a pre-alert call is made.

Key points

- Preparation before arrival on the scene is essential, especially for paediatric cases.
- Clinical and situational distractions are commonly encountered in the pre-hospital environment.
- Avoidance of secondary insults in acute severe brain injury is a core function of pre-hospital critical care.

Additional reading

Burns BJ, Watterson JB, Ware S, et al. Analysis of out-of-hospital pediatric intubation by an Australian helicopter emergency medical service. Ann Emerg Med 2017 Dec; 70(6): 773–782. Epub 2017 April 29.

The Brain Trauma Foundation: www.braintrauma.org.

Incident

This case refers to the incident in Case 10.

Following uneventful transport and handover to the trauma service at the major trauma centre, the team in Case 10 returns to base. A hot debrief occurs, during which the rapid sequence intubation is discussed. The team paramedic questions why the doctor requested such a large dose of ketamine, at which point it becomes clear that the child received 140 mg of ketamine instead of 40 mg. The paramedic, who had only recently completed training and is new to the PHRM team had been checking the second suction unit at the time of the drug discussion felt certain he heard the doctor request 140 mg.

As a team you discuss why miscommunication occurred in this case.

Question 11.1

What factors compromised communication in this case and how could they be improved?

Discussion 11.1

Communication is one of the most common causes of medical error. It is a particular challenge in high-pressure situations.

When he was informed about the required drug doses, the paramedic was engaged in checking a suction unit. This resulted in what is termed 'divided attention'. He was attempting to both listen to the doctor and carry out the device check. Unfortunately, none of us can effectively and safely carry out two tasks simultaneously. This will have contributed to his misinterpreting the required drug dose.

We can also become task fixated on a procedure or a problem which compromises our physical ability to hear, and reduces our peripheral vision. This is an evolved response to help protect us from physical attack.

Related to this, and a particular issue in high-pressure pre-hospital situations, is the problem created by distractions. These might include monitor alarms sounding or being interrupted by another member of the team. Distractions cause us to refocus our attention from the person communicating with us.

Individuals operating in high-pressure situations should be aware of their inability to multitask and the effects of task fixation and distraction. It is safer and more effective to undertake two tasks in a serial manner. Focus on and complete one task before moving on to the second.

Focused attention would have reduced the chance of this error occurring. As the drug doses were a critical piece of information, the doctor should have ensured that he had the full attention of the paramedic and that he was actively listening. Simply using someone's name, putting your hand on their shoulder and obtaining eye contact is enough to achieve focused attention prior to the transmission of information.

Repetition is a useful tool for the passage of critical information. The doctor should ideally have stated: 'forty – four zero – milligrams of ketamine'. This would have significantly reduced the chance of misinterpretation.

Closed-loop communication is commonly used in aviation and during radio transmissions. It is also a technique which can be employed during high-stakes team communication. The person receiving the information reads the information back to the person providing it, and, in turn, the person passing on the information confirms that the recipient has received the information correctly.

Commonly in pre-hospital care we are under time pressure. Limited time compromises our ability to accurately pass and receive information. In normal circumstances, if we felt unsure about what someone had said to us, we would ask them to repeat it or to clarify what was meant. If time is limited, we can feel there isn't time to obtain clarification, resulting in misinterpreted information.

A perception of a command gradient may also have played a part in this case. It is possible that the paramedic interpreted the ketamine dose as 140 mg and thought this to be an excessive amount for an 8-year-old child. However, as a new member of the team, he may have felt inhibited from questioning the doctor. This could be because he felt the doctor unlikely to be making a drug error or because, prior to the event, the doctor had not appeared approachable or open.

In high-pressure, high-stakes situations where critical information is being communicated, it is beneficial to avoid command gradients by engendering a culture of a flat hierarchy. In these situations, all members of the team are actively encouraged to speak up if they have ideas or concerns. In pre-hospital teams, this should be emphasised during pre-shift briefings, post-mission debriefs and during drilling and simulation training.

This case represents an adverse outcome that should be recorded and reviewed according to the service's clinical governance framework (see Case 52).

Key points

- Communication in high-pressure situations is a common cause of medical error.
- Task fixation and distraction can impair the PHRM team's performance when carrying out high-consequence tasks.
- Focused attention, repetition and closed-loop communications can help improve communications and performance.

Additional Reading

Hearns S. Peak performance under pressure: lessons from a helicopter rescue doctor. Core Cognition, 2019.

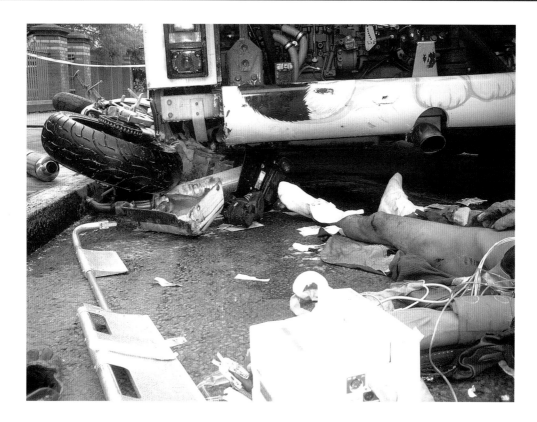

Incident

A 24-year-old male motorcyclist has collided with a bus. He was briefly trapped and has burns to his lower limbs. He is conscious but hypotensive (SBP 80 mmHg).

Relevant information

- **PHRM team transport options:** Rapid response road vehicle.
- **Additional resources:** One land ambulance and crew. Police and Fire & Rescue services.
- **Retrieval options:** Regional hospital 5 minutes by road. Major trauma hospital 30 minutes by road.
- **Other:** Raining.

Question 12.1

What is your pre-hospital plan prior to arrival?

Question 12.2

Comment on the picture of the above scene.

On arrival, the patient is pale and quiet. Initial observations on handover from the paramedic follow.

Clinical information

- P 105.
- BP 75/40 mmHg.
- SaO_2 96%.
- GCS 14 (E3, V5, M6).

A brief clinical examination reveals a clear airway with no respiratory compromise. The abdomen is generally tender. Both legs are externally rotated. There are deep partial thickness burns to both feet. The patient is able to move all four limbs. There is no evidence of long bone fracture or overt haemorrhage.

Question 12.3

Outline your initial assessment and management.

Question 12.4

How will you manage the patient's hypotension?

Discussion 12.1

Potential hazards should be considered. In the absence of further information, fire should be considered a risk to the PHRM team whenever burns are reported. The patient is hypotensive following a significant mechanism of injury. The focus should, therefore, be on rapid assessment, preservation of blood volume, careful packaging and swift movement to definitive care. Patients with multiple injuries displaying pre-hospital physiological instability are best managed in a major trauma hospital, which is the destination of choice in this instance. A high degree of suspicion should apply to the patient with a significant mechanism of injury regardless of the initial findings.

Discussion 12.2

The scene has been cordoned. The stability of the bus is unclear. Furthermore, the bus engine cover has been removed and there is evidence of recent use of a fire extinguisher. Clarification should be sought from on-scene senior Fire and Rescue service personnel regarding scene safety. A motorcycle has come to rest between the underside of the bus and the road kerb. There is significant damage to both the motorcycle and the rear of the bus. The patient lies supine in close proximity to the incident. Initial monitoring, exposure and lower limb wound care has commenced. Both lower limbs are somewhat externally rotated, raising the suspicion of a pelvic ring disruption.

Discussion 12.2

The initial assessment in the pre-hospital environment should be swift and structured. Conscious patients may assist in identifying injury patterns on direct questioning. See box below:

Rapid screening tool for Pre-hospital clinical assessment
Direct questions (if responsive) • Where do you hurt? • Where else do you hurt? • Does your breathing feel normal? • Can you move your fingers and toes and stick your tongue out? **Examination** • Complete visual survey preferably with clothing removed • Palpation of chest wall and abdomen • Assessment of peripheries

The initial assessment confirms that the patient is hypotensive. Without evidence of an obvious non-haemorrhagic cause for hypotension, it should be assumed that the patient has an occult haemorrhagic threat. Scene time should be minimised and swift movement to a major trauma hospital is appropriate. To facilitate further safe assessment, packaging and transport, the patient will need to be moved. It is important to remember that the process of pre-hospital packaging is, in itself, a therapeutic process. The brief amount of time taken to cut the clothes properly, stabilise a suspected pelvic fracture, gently perform a partial log roll and scoop the patient onto a vacuum mattress for transfer to the ambulance stretcher is time well spent (see Case 8). Local practice will guide the specifics of the packaging process. However, the emphasis should be on gentle handling, early splinting, preservation of blood volume, adequate analgesia and swift transfer.

Whenever possible, it is important to avoid excessive truncal movements. This includes avoiding a 'full' log roll to 90 degrees and any 'springing' or repeated examination of the pelvis. Clot disruption, haemorrhage and aggravated inflammatory cytokine generation may be minimised in this way.

The patient displays enough signs of a potential pelvic fracture, in addition to a significant mechanism of injury. A properly applied pelvic splint will minimise any potential fracture segment movement and reduce the volume associated with a potential 'open book' type pelvic ring disruption. Such injuries are relatively common when the anterior pelvis strikes the flared fuel tank of a large motorcycle.

High-flow oxygen should be administered, and secure large-bore intravenous access established (preferably above the diaphragm when abdominopelvic disruption is suspected). The performance of a pre-hospital-focused abdominal ultrasound scan in trauma (FAST) may reveal free intraperitoneal fluid, but will not alter the pre-hospital management or triage decision in this instance (see Case 39). The results of a pre-hospital FAST scan should be made clear during the pre-alert call and at handover to the receiving facility.

Discussion 12.4

A state of reduced organ perfusion should be confirmed. Combined pre-hospital assessment of pulse (quality and rate), skin colour and capillary refill, level of consciousness and serial non-invasive blood-pressure monitoring will assist in this regard. Pre-hospital invasive arterial pressure monitoring may be useful but should not delay transfer to definitive care.

In the absence of a closed head injury and, given the patient's age and current compensation (as evidenced by the level of consciousness), immediate volume resuscitation may not be required. Large volume rapid intravenous resuscitation prior to haemostasis may risk aggravated haemorrhage, soft clot dissolution, and dilution/dysfunction of clotting factors. While it is broadly accepted that, following traumatic haemorrhage, circulating volume should be restored in hypovolaemic patients, there is ongoing controversy as to resuscitative timing, volume and measured resuscitation end-points in this group. Therapeutic decisions are made more complex when longer pre-hospital transport times are considered.

Volume replacement in trauma should be warmed blood and blood products. The carriage of blood is commonplace in many PHRM services, although the carriage of blood products is more challenging. (See Case 28). If blood is unavailable, judicious crystalloid is the fluid of choice.

Most major trauma hospitals will have access to a 'massive transfusion pack' which can be activated upon request (e.g. pre-alert notification) from the PHRM team. Damage control resuscitation is an emerging concept in the early care of major trauma patients (Leibner at al 2020).

Consider the following guidance:

- All haemodynamically unstable trauma patients should be rapidly assessed for non-haemorrhagic causes contributing to a shocked state (e.g. tension pneumothoraces). These should be dealt with as a matter of priority.
- Attention should be paid to haemorrhage control, fracture immobilisation and careful assessment and packaging.
- Whenever possible, all haemodynamically unstable trauma patients should be transported swiftly to the nearest major trauma facility.
- If intravenous fluids are considered appropriate, the initial fluid choice should be blood.
- Administration of tranexamic acid (TXA) is indicated in patients within 3 hours of injury (Roberts et al 2013)

Suggested target end-points of resuscitation are as below:

- In the absence of a closed head injury or a peri-arrest/arrest situation, a large-bore intravenous line should be inserted, and small volumes (250 mL) of bolus blood or crystalloid should be infused slowly to either maintain a response to voice, a radial pulse or an SBP of 80–90 mmHg.
- In the presence of a closed head injury **and** extracranial injury, in which ongoing bleeding is likely and the patient is haemodynamically unstable, a target SBP of 100–120 mmHg is advised. Hypotension is a well-accepted significant secondary insult in traumatic brain injury and must be avoided.
- In the setting of an isolated closed head injury, a Mean Arterial Pressure (MAP) of approximately 80 mmHg is targeted (in longer-distance or inter-facility transfers, vasoactive agents may be required).

In this case, minimal or low-volume blood or crystalloid resuscitation utilising meaningful resuscitation end-points (the maintenance of a response to voice or a palpable radial pulse) and an SBP of 80–90 mmHg is appropriate. Early communication, as well as a focused and thorough patient handover to the destination major trauma hospital, will assist in ensuring optimal patient reception, early definitive investigation and improved clinical outcomes in this high-mortality patient group.

Key points

- Critical assessment of the hypotensive pre-hospital patient will direct appropriate further therapy.
- Different patients may require variable therapeutic interventions in keeping with their underlying injury.
- With all trauma patients, the focus should be on gentle handling, early splinting, preservation of blood volume, adequate analgesia and swift transfer.
- Consider pre-hospital blood transfusion and TXA.

References

Leibner E, Andreae M, Galvagno SM, Scalea T. Damage control resuscitation. Clin Exp Emerg Med. 2020 Mar; 7(1):5–13. doi: 10.15441/ceem.19.089. Epub 2020 Mar 31.

Roberts I, Shakur H, Coats T, et al. The CRASH-2 trial: a randomised controlled trial and economic evaluation of the effects of tranexamic acid on death, vascular occlusive events and transfusion requirement in bleeding trauma patients. Health Technol Assess. 2013 Mar; 17(10):1–79.

Additional reading

Revell M, Porter K, Greaves I. Fluid resuscitation in prehospital trauma care; a consensus view. Emerg Med J 2002; 19(6):494–498.

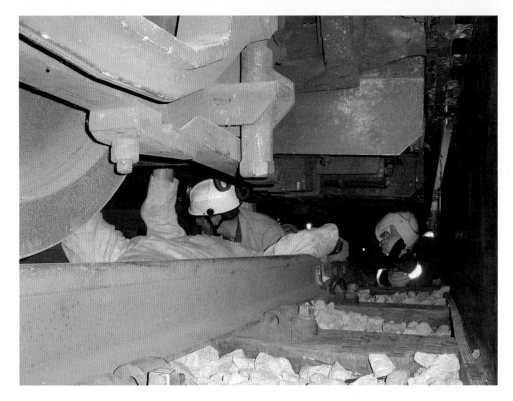

Incident

A 27-year-old female has been struck by an underground electric train. The tasking agency advises that the patient is trapped by her legs but is communicating.

Relevant information

- **PHRM team transport options:** Rotary-wing aircraft.
- **Additional resources:** Landing site less than 200 m (656 feet) from entrance to scene. One land ambulance, Police service, underground train service personnel (including specialist rescue team) and Fire & Rescue Service.
- **Retrieval options:** Major trauma hospital 30 minutes by air.
- **Other:** Patient location is 35 m (115 ft) underground at a metropolitan commuter train station. Ambient tunnel temperature is 29°C (84°F).

Question 13.1

What is your initial pre-hospital plan?

Question 13.2

Describe the arrival and scene management for a case like this.

After successful extrication from under the train, injuries are assessed as:
- Haemopneumothorax on the right side
- Extensive bruising over the right upper quadrant

- Fractured pelvis
- Traumatic brain injury.

The patient has undergone pre-hospital RSI.

Clinical information

- P 105.
- BP 100/60 mmHg.

A right simple thoracostomy has been performed (see Case 15) and large-bore intravenous access established. The patient has received 750 mL of fluid.

Ten minutes into the flight home you notice the $ETCO_2$ trace halves in size and the reading decreases from 35 to 15 mmHg (4.5 to 2.0 kPa).

Question 13.3

Comment on the use of end-tidal carbon dioxide monitoring in the pre-hospital arena and discuss your actions in this instance.

Discussion 13.1

This is a high-risk tasking, particularly because of the presence of trains and electric current. Therefore, the PHRM team should use full PPE throughout the rescue. Significant injuries should be anticipated in rail incidents, regardless of initial clinical signs. Extra equipment (specifically additional oxygen) should be taken to the scene if the incident is underground, as returning to the surface will be difficult during the rescue. Communications are also very restricted underground, meaning communication with the tasking agency may prove impossible throughout the tasking. In this incident, the nearest hospital also happens to be the most appropriate facility for this patient.

Discussion 13.2

Many different teams will be activated to such an incident and the scene is likely to be busy. Scene control is vital for the efficient extrication of the patient. The PHRM team should liaise early with key representatives from each of the other services on-scene. Safety is paramount in this scenario and there are two main areas of concern: electric current and train movement.

Electric current

The energy in electrified train tracks can be lethal. It is therefore imperative that the power has been switched off. In most systems, there will be a 'line controller' (or equivalent) responsible for the trains on that section of the line. The line controller may be in a control room remote from the scene but within telephone contact. It is vital that the PHRM team confirms that the power is off with the line controller directly. If the incident is in a station, there may be a tunnel phone directly to the line controller. The PHRM team must not assume that the scene is safe simply because other services are already on the tracks. Ensuring the line controller is aware of the incident also reduces the risk that the power will be switched back on before the rescue is complete. The PHRM team must avoid any temptation to assess the patient before ensuring the scene is safe.

As a back-up to switching off the power, electric trains may also carry circuit breakers, which are long metal rods that clip between the electrified tracks and short circuit the system, thus removing any residual charge in the live rails. One device should be placed on the tracks at each end of the train. If the power is inadvertently reconnected, these devices should ensure that the area of the rescue is isolated. The PHRM team must visualise these devices at both ends of the train before entering the track area.

Train movement

Electric trains can move large distances even with the power off, so the team must also contact the controller specifically to request a cessation of all train movements. This is also important when there are other train tracks running parallel to the incident site.

Extrication

Removing the patient from under the train is hot, dirty and difficult. The PHRM team should split up so only one member is beneath the train at any given time. If present, a rail specialist rescue team should be closely consulted, as they will know what is possible and in what time frame. There are very limited options if the patient is absolutely trapped. There is a facility to jack up the train but, in a tunnel, this may only gain you a few centimetres (see below) and takes considerable time. Sometimes, the train will need to be moved to facilitate extrication. In these situations, the entire system will need to be powered up again. Under such circumstances, the team should ensure the patient is as stable as possible but must not be under the train when the system is powered up and the train moving. This applies even if the patient is ventilated. Bear in mind that, once the system is powered up, the PHRM team may not have access to the patient again for up to 20 minutes. Ensure that there is adequate oxygen and battery power to last for this time period. After the train has been moved, the team must repeat the process of contacting the line controller and placing the circuit breakers before moving onto the tracks again.

Once the patient has been extricated, stabilise and securely package them on the train platform as the journey back to the transport platform as the journey out of the train station may involve stairs or other obstacles.

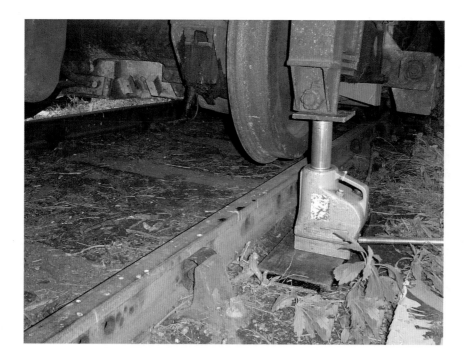

Other issues

Try to find time to speak to the driver of the train. It will have been a traumatic experience for them. Also consider passengers, as the rescue process may have resulted in prolonged confinement on trains with no power for some hours. This is compounded when the network is underground, and passengers may need to be evacuated from trains or tunnels. These passengers may themselves require some attention (dehydration, psychological support). In the underground environment, careful attention should be paid to team and self-management with adequate hydration and rest breaks provided.

Discussion 13.3

Qualitative end-tidal carbon dioxide ($ETCO_2$) is a key monitoring tool in the pre-hospital environment. Potential uses of $ETCO_2$ monitoring include:

- Initial confirmation of tracheal tube placement
- Breath-by-breath respiratory rate (including self-ventilating patients with awake capnography
- Estimation of arterial carbon dioxide tension
- Early notification of tracheal tube dislodgement or ventilator circuit disconnection
- Changes in cardiac output
- Cardiac arrest prognosis
- Assessment of air flow limitation such as bronchospasm.

The sudden decrease in $ETCO_2$ described will need to be addressed immediately. In the back of a helicopter, assessment and treatment options are limited. Deciding to land for clinical reassessment is not usually an option due to both landing site availability and the unavoidable delay associated with finding a safe landing site. In this instance, the PHRM team should:

- Notify the pilot(s) that there is a medical problem with the patient and ask permission to go 'off harness' and move about the cabin
- Look for clues
- Assess the tracheal tube for displacement and check cuff inflation
- Assess for adequate ventilation and airway pressures (Is the chest rising symmetrically? Is the ventilator functioning?) and remove from the ventilator and hand-ventilate if in any doubt
- Confirm a low output state
- Re-measure the blood pressure
- Palpate the rate, rhythm and quality of the peripheral pulse
- Look at the $ETCO_2$ trace and determine whether it is:
  - Improving
  - Static
  - Deteriorating
  - Variable
  - Displaying recognisable patterns (e.g. bronchospasm)
- Attend to the following issues:
  - The chest injury is a major concern. Reinsert a sterile gloved finger into the thoracostomy site to ensure patency.

- In the absence of a pre-departure formal thoracostomy, and with a high index of suspicion of an expanding pleural collection, a needle decompression or simple thoracostomy (if space allows) should be performed in flight (see Case 15).
- Give a 250–500 mL fluid challenge.
- As soon as the helicopter is shut down at the destination, do a swift reassessment before unloading. Auscultation may now be feasible.
- Highlight the recent physiologic instability to the receiving team when handing over.

Key points

- Incidents involving train systems require special safety considerations.
- Continuous monitoring of $ETCO_2$ is standard in the pre-hospital and retrieval environments.

Additional reading

Intensive Care Society. Capnography in the critically ill. Online. Available: https://ics.ac.uk/ICS/ICS/Guidelines/Guidelines_pg2.aspx

Nutbeam,T, Boylan M (Eds). ABC of pre-hospital emergency medicine. Wiley Blackwell, 2013

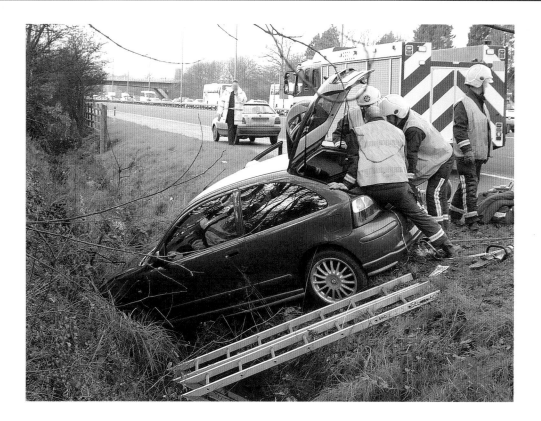

Incident

A 45-year-old male has been involved in a single-vehicle accident. The tasking agency reports that the patient is 'unconscious'.

Relevant information

- **PHRM team transport options:** Rotary-wing aircraft.
- **Additional resources:** One land ambulance. Police and Fire & Rescue services.
- **Retrieval options:** Regional hospital 5 minutes by road. Major trauma hospital 35 minutes by air.
- **Other:** Weather clear 25°C (77°F).

Question 14.1

Comment on the picture of the above scene.

On arrival, you liaise with the on-scene Fire & Rescue Service who are planning to remove the car roof in order to perform a controlled extrication. They are concerned about a potential spinal injury following the collision.

You make a brief assessment of the scene and then receive a handover from the on-scene paramedic who has just instituted continuous non-invasive monitoring. You are informed that, on arrival of the Ambulance Service, the patient had a partially obstructed airway with trismus and was tachypnoeic. At that time, the patient had a

GCS of 7 (E1, V2, M4) with a clear airway. A cervical collar has been fitted and high-flow oxygen applied via a face mask. The vehicle airbags have not deployed. The Fire & Rescue Service are continuing with the planned extrication.

You request a break in the extrication process to make a more detailed clinical assessment of the patient.

Clinical information

- P 94.
- BP 125/70 mmHg.
- GCS 12 (E3, V4, M5).
- Clear airway.
- No respiratory compromise.
- Well perfused but sweaty.
- Not in obvious pain.
- No external injury apparent.

Question 14.2

Outline your initial assessment and management.

Question 14.3

To which hospital should the patient be transported?

Discussion 14.1

The vehicle has left the road and ended up in a ditch. There are several points to note in this scene:

- Scene safety: the road has been closed, which is important for this complex scenario. The Fire & Rescue Service are on-scene but there may be other issues (e.g. is there any water or fluids leaking into the ditch? Has the car been turned off and are the keys out of the ignition?).
- Note the ladders across the ditch to facilitate 360-degree access to the vehicle.
- Vehicle stability is an issue and the Fire & Rescue Service need to work out the best way of stabilising the car to prevent both major and minor shifts of position.
- The vehicle appears minimally damaged (despite having left an apparent high-speed road).
- The driver remains in the vehicle and a paramedic has entered and sits adjacent to the patient.

Discussion 14.2

There is incongruity between the clinical presentation of the patient and the information obtained from 'reading the scene'. The mechanism of injury appears to be relatively minor. There is minimal vehicle damage, no cabin intrusion and the driver's airbag has not deployed. Despite these findings, the initial GCS for the patient was very low. This can be the picture of an occult medical presentation.

While a high index of suspicion should always be maintained when assessing patients in the pre-hospital environment (particularly the elderly), low-energy mechanisms are not usually associated with significant injuries. In this case, the improvement in the GCS over a short period of time, and the absence of other physiologic instability or obvious injury, should all lead the PHRM team to consider an acute medical presentation.

Undeployed airbags pose a significant threat to the patient and to emergency services personnel. The neutralisation of all airbags by the Fire & Rescue Service is increasingly impractical given the manufacturer variability in location and complexity.

To ensure safety, the PHRM team must discuss the scene in detail with the Fire & Rescue Service team leader. This is particularly important in this case as vehicle stability seems precarious. Putting weight on one side of the car (e.g. to examine the patient) could lead to significant movement, which could affect the patient or trap or injure a member of the emergency services team.

The clinical assessment should look for potential non-traumatic causes of an altered level of consciousness. A 'Medic Alert' bracelet (or similar) alerting the PHRM team to chronic medical conditions (such as diabetes, significant heart disease or seizure disorder) should be looked for. In the absence of clues, the team should work through common medical conditions that may predispose to sudden loss of consciousness (see the table below).

Common medical conditions that may predispose to sudden loss of consciousness	
Cause	Notes
Metabolic	Hypoglycaemia must be looked for and corrected if necessary.
Neurological	Although an unexpected finding in this age group, focal neurology suggestive of stroke should be identified.
	Similarly, hippus (fluctuations in pupillary size), nystagmus, and cyclical stereotypical motor manifestations may arouse suspicion of ongoing non-convulsive seizure activity. Spontaneous intracranial haemorrhage can also present in this fashion.
Cardiac	An ongoing disturbance in cardiac rate or rhythm can be excluded both clinically and by the application of a monitor.
	Myocardial perfusion problems are common and may be evidenced by performing a 12-lead electrocardiogram.
Drugs	Drugs and alcohol are a common cause of altered mental state. Assess the patient for the smell of alcohol.
	The pupils may also point towards drugs of abuse. Withdrawal as a precipitant of seizure activity or another acute medical event is also possible.

A controlled and prolonged extrication is not warranted in this case. If physically plausible and safe to do, a simple seated rotation and side extrication utilising an extrication board is adequate. The rationale for this change to the current plan should be diplomatically voiced to all on-scene personnel. It is worth asking the Fire Incident

Commander on-scene not only what their extrication plans are, including if a rapid extrication is needed, but also the estimated time it will take to perform these, remembering that these times may end up being prolonged.

Discussion 14.3

Findings consistent with a medical cause for the patient's condition or ongoing clinical improvement should reassure the PHRM team that major trauma is an unlikely diagnosis. With the exception of specialist medical services (such as coronary angioplasty or specialist stroke services), the nearest regional hospital is a suitable triage decision. Most hospitals will have access to a CT scanner but this should be checked if any doubt exists.

The tasking agency should be informed and the receiving facility alerted.

Key points
• Single vehicle, low-speed incidents with profound alterations in patient physiology are frequently associated with occult medical conditions.
• Liaison with senior on-scene emergency services personnel is critical to good pre-hospital communication and patient care.

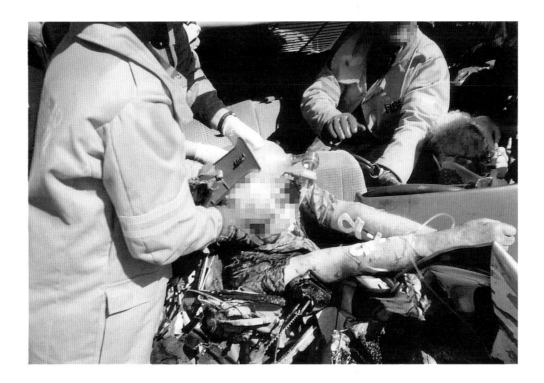

Incident

Multiple vehicles have collided at high speed. The tasking agency reports one patient is dead on-scene. Two patients are said to be trapped.

Relevant information

- **PHRM team transport options:** Rotary-wing aircraft with dual stretcher capacity. Paramedic-staffed air ambulance aircraft (single-stretcher capacity) on-scene.
- **Additional resources:** Two land ambulances. Fire & Rescue and Police services.
- **Retrieval options:** Regional hospital 25 minutes by air. Major trauma hospital 1 hour and 15 minutes by air.
- **Other:** Ambient conditions: Dry, 38°C (100°F).

Question 15.1

Using the information available so far, outline your pre-hospital plan prior to arrival on the scene.

On arrival, you receive a handover from the on-scene flight paramedic. Two vehicles have collided head-on at high speed 35 minutes ago. The driver of one vehicle is deceased. The second vehicle contains two elderly occupants. The driver is trapped and, although he initially responded to voice, he has become unresponsive with increasing respiratory distress. He was intubated (without drug assistance) just prior to your arrival following near respiratory arrest. A weak pulse has been palpable at the wrist. Needle decompression has been attempted on the patient's left side. The front seat passenger is alert, complaining of neck pain and unable to move her hands or lower limbs despite no physical entrapment.

Question 15.2

Comment on the picture of the scene and list, in broad terms, possible life-threatening, traumatic thoracic injuries manageable in the field.

Question 15.3

Outline your immediate approach to the scene.

Question 15.4

Describe the assessment of blunt chest trauma in the pre-hospital and transport environment.

Question 15.5

Outline three relevant pre-hospital chest-trauma interventions. For each, outline advantages and disadvantages.

Discussion 15.1

Your pre-hospital plan should include issues relating to team and scene safety, utilisation of on-scene resources (including an additional rotary-wing aircraft with experienced crew) and the required transport time to hospital, particularly for the nearest major trauma hospital. En route, the PHRM team should also reflect on the number of patients and the predicted severity of injury of the survivors given the known mechanism and reported death on-scene. Time en route should, therefore, be spent discussing a safe-scene approach, preparing for the management of likely severe injuries (including the drawing-up and labelling of appropriate drugs), and potential patient triage decisions.

Discussion 15.2

The image shows only the cabin space of one vehicle with two elderly patients still in the vehicle. There is a marked cabin intrusion about the driver's side, consistent with physical entrapment and suggestive of major truncal injury. Fire & Rescue Service personnel are in attendance. The vehicle has been partially dismantled including incomplete roof removal. It is not clear if the vehicle is stable. A deployed airbag is not visible. There are multiple sharp and exposed metal surfaces. Blood is evident about the driver who has a tracheal tube and bilateral intravenous cannulae secured in place. Assisted ventilation is being performed. The front-seat passenger has had a cervical collar and mask oxygen applied.

Relevant and manageable thoracic threats to life include pleural collections (simple, tension, open or large forms of haemopneumothorax) and large flail segments. Uncontrollable pleural haemorrhage or cardiac tamponade from cardiac or major vessel disruption requires aggressive surgical intervention. This is rarely deliverable in the pre-hospital environment. Unlike penetrating disease (see Case 16), outcomes from pre-hospital resuscitative thoracotomy following blunt trauma are universally poor.

Discussion 15.3

Immediately seek out the senior Fire & Rescue Service officer and confirm that the scene is safe, the vehicle is stable and there are no undeployed airbags. From the received handover, it is clear that the driver requires immediate intervention. However, given the additional patients, the PHRM team should consider splitting up in order to further assess the scene (see Case 21).

Rapidly assess the driver's tracheal tube position (clinically and with capnography), and ensure adequate ventilation is occurring with high-flow oxygen. Assess for any signs of spontaneous respiratory effort and confirm that a peripheral pulse is palpable. Look swiftly but carefully at the nature of the patient's entrapment and liaise with on-scene emergency service personnel regarding the current plan. Inform them that the patient requires rapid removal from the vehicle for him to have any chance of survival (see Case 4 for information on 'crash' extrication). Where possible, extricate the patient immediately to a safe area of the scene and continue simultaneous assessment and resuscitation. Note that, on extrication, clinical deterioration is likely. This may be caused by the release of toxic metabolites from ischaemic compartments, or by the loss of tissue, bony fracture, and vascular compartment external resistance. If a delay in rapid extrication is anticipated, and a state of near or actual cardiac arrest is confirmed, reversible causes of cardiac arrest must be addressed (see Case 19); for example, commence intravenous fluid or blood resuscitation, attach continuous ECG monitoring for rhythm analysis and perform bilateral chest decompression (see below).

The front-seat passenger has a cervical cord injury until proven otherwise and will require controlled extrication. Delegate any spare on-scene personnel to manually stabilise the patient's head, in addition to the applied cervical collar, and assist in the extrication process under the direction of a member of the PHRM team or on-scene senior ambulance personnel.

Assessment of the deceased person(s) and confirmation of life extinct should be communicated to the most senior on-scene Police officer. Always carefully assess deceased persons to ensure that weak vital signs have not been overlooked in the high-pressure multi-casualty scene.

Discussion 15.4

Both the assessment and performance of therapeutic interventions for blunt chest trauma may be challenging in the noisy, difficult and often time-pressured pre-hospital environment. Significant limitations to patient access, as with this case, compound such difficulties.

One of the best places to assess patients for blunt chest trauma is from the patient's feet, looking cranially, with the eyes at the level of the exposed chest wall. Asymmetric movement or expansion and subtle flail segments are far easier to see in this position than at the patient's side or from above. In cardiac arrest caused by blunt chest trauma (and when profound entrapment essentially excludes more detailed assessment), pleural collections under tension should be presumed and managed accordingly. Formal thoracostomy may be both diagnostic and therapeutic in this setting (see below).

In less-acute presentations, pneumothoraces can be difficult to diagnose following blunt trauma, particularly when short response times are considered. Latent development of a pneumothorax after a period of positive-pressure ventilation or on ascent to altitude is not uncommon (see Case 38). In this setting, look out for difficulties obtaining an SaO_2 trace, hypotension without apparent cause and, in ventilated patients, high-peak inspiratory pressures. Such findings are also common with worsening lung contusion. Other common clinical findings suggestive of an underlying pneumothorax include surgical emphysema, bony chest wall crepitus, decreased air entry, wheeze, external signs of trauma (with an associated mechanism), and progressive patient dyspnoea and anxiety. On-scene point-of-care ultrasound is an important tool in the assessment of chest trauma and can rapidly demonstrate the presence or absence of pneumothorax or haemothorax, and may decrease the rate of unnecessary invasive pleural decompression (see Case 39) The ultrasound should be performed at several locations on the chest wall.

Discussion 15.5

Needle thoracocentesis (needle decompression)

This refers to the percutaneous placement of a large-bore cannula or a dedicated pleural catheter device usually anteriorly in the second intercostal space or 5th intercostal space in the anterior axillary line.

Advantages and disadvantages of needle thoracocentesis	
Advantages	Disadvantages
<ul><li>Quick.</li><li>Easy to teach and perform.</li><li>Useful in the entrapped or packaged patient where access is difficult and more formal equipment is not immediately to hand.</li></ul>	<ul><li>May give the false impression that 'the problem is sorted'.</li><li>Transiently removes tension. Rarely facilitates lung re-expansion.</li><li>No benefit for large haemothoraces.</li><li>Cannulae may:<ul><li>Become obstructed on insertion</li><li>Dislodge from the pleural space.</li></ul></li><li>Pleural space may not be reached in many patients.</li><li>Iatrogenic lung injury is possible.</li></ul>

Tube thoracocentesis ('chest drain')

Refers to the placement under direct vision of a large-bore (e.g. 28 French gauge for adults) catheter following blunt dissection (thoracostomy), and securing of such a catheter to both the patient's chest wall and to a system facilitating pleural drainage (such as one-way valve devices, drainage bag systems or underwater seal drains). Generally speaking, a chest drain is indicated when there is a pneumothorax in a spontaneously breathing patient, no associated time-critical injuries, long-distance interhospital patient transfers or, in a single-system injury (chest), particularly penetrating injury.

Advantages and disadvantages of tube thoracocentesis

Advantages	Disadvantages

• Formal drainage, including measurement of pleural fluid.
• Ability to add negative pressure to the drainage system.
	• **Time:** even in the most experienced hands, the time taken from start to finish (securing, suturing, dressing and connection of drainage system) can be in excess of 10 minutes per side.
	• Re-tension can occur in the following ways:
	  ○ Lung or clot obstruction of the catheter within the pleural space.
	  ○ Catheter kinking (either within the pleural space or outside it).
	  ○ Large air leaks may rapidly overfill a closed drainage system or overcome one-way valve flow rates.
	• Clinical assessment of the patient who deteriorates in transit can be difficult where re-tension is a differential and where the catheter is secured and the insertion point covered.

Simple thoracostomy (see Appendix 1.3)

Simple thoracostomy involves performance of tube thoracocentesis but without the insertion of the catheter. Focus is on direct digital assessment of lung inflation and the formal removal of pleural collections with or without tension. It is indicated only in patients undergoing positive pressure ventilation where minimising scene time is critical (i.e. uncontrolled haemorrhagic shock or traumatic brain injury). There may also be a benefit in a patient who presents in actual or near-traumatic cardiac arrest or in a persistent shocked state following trauma. Conversion of the simple thoracostomy to a tube thoracocentesis can occur at the hospital.

Advantages and disadvantages of simple thoracostomy

Advantages	Disadvantages
• Fast (under 1 minute bilaterally). • Simple (same incision as for catheter placement). • Lung can be felt and/or seen to be expanded. • If there is deterioration in flight, thoracostomies can simply be 're-fingered' under sterile conditions to assess lung expansion and thus exclude re-tension pneumothorax as a diagnosis. • Avoids re-tension pneumothorax due to system blockage or catheter kinking.	• Creation of a sucking chest wound: this does not happen with positive-pressure ventilation. • Transient blockage whereby the wound acts like a flap valve. Frequent finger sweeps (with sterile gloves) into the pleural space will help to release any air and blood that is accumulating. • Bleeding: can be more than if a catheter is in place. Focus on blunt dissection to minimise this.

Key points
• Exclusion of serious thoracic trauma in the pre-hospital setting can be difficult. • Consider simple thoracostomy for time-critical, mechanically ventilated patients with pleural collections.

Additional reading

Aylwin CJ, et al. Pre-hospital and in-hospital thoracostomy: indications and complications. Ann R Coll Surg Eng 2008; 90(1):54–57.

Deakin CD, Davies G, Wilson A. Simple thoracostomy avoids chest drain insertion in prehospital trauma. J Trauma 1995; 39(2):373–374.

Jodie P, Kerstin H. BET 2: pre-hospital finger thoracostomy in patients with chest trauma. Emerg Med J 2017; 34(6):419.

Nutbeam T, Boylan M (Eds). ABC of pre-hospital emergency medicine. Wiley Blackwell, 2013.

It is a Saturday night at 23:30 hours. The tasking agency has received a call from the Police service. A young male has been assaulted in a hotel toilet and is 'unresponsive'.

Relevant information

- **PHRM team transport options:** Rapid response road vehicle available.
- **Additional resources:** One land ambulance. Large number of Police service personnel.
- **Retrieval options:** Regional hospital 10 minutes by road. Major trauma hospital 25 minutes by road.
- **Other:** Ambient conditions. Heavy rain, 9°C (48°F).

Question 16.1

What is your pre-hospital plan prior to arrival?

On arrival, you are met by a senior Police officer and escorted through into the hotel entrance. Police are attempting to remove a large crowd from the main bar. A number of patrons have bloodstained clothing. You are the focus of verbal abuse as you pass them.

You are directed up a set of stairs to where the patient has been found slumped in a toilet cubicle. As you enter the crowded corridor outside the toilet, an Ambulance Service paramedic appears. She informs you that on her arrival (less than 5 minutes ago), the patient 'appeared drunk', was combative and refusing assistance. At that time, she had been unable to further assess him.

He has since become 'unresponsive'. She has placed a 16-gauge intravenous cannulae in his antecubital fossa and checked his blood glucose level (within normal limits). She is now unable to feel a radial pulse. From the cubicle door, you can see he is taking occasional gasping breaths.

Question 16.2

Outline your initial management.

The Police have rapidly cleared the upper floor of the hotel. The toilet is being cordoned off and Police guard the door. The patient has been removed from the cubicle to a large floor area and his clothes have been cut off. Non-invasive monitoring is in place. A rapid assessment reveals the following clinical information.

Clinical information

- A – Clear.
- B – Apnoeic. Receiving assisted ventilation with bag valve mask device.
- C – Pale. Cold. No central pulse. BP and SaO_2 machines giving error message. Monitor showing sinus bradycardia (55 beats per minute).
- D – Unresponsive to central stimulus.
- E – See picture over the page.

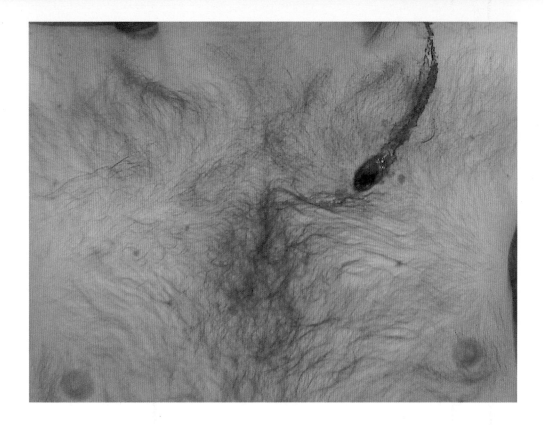

Question 16.3

How will you proceed? Describe the procedure.

A resuscitative thoracotomy reveals a pericardial tamponade. On release, there is spontaneous return of both myocardial contraction and circulation. An apparent right ventricular wound is bleeding minimally. The patient is intubated and ventilated and en route to the ambulance. Contact is made with the receiving trauma hospital and your tasking agency.

Clinical information

- P 105.
- BP 105/64 mmHg.
- ETCO$_2$ 35 mmHg (4.5 kPa).

En route, you notice a return of spontaneous ventilatory effort and occasional coughing. You also notice a moderate amount of blood flowing from the chest wall.

Question 16.4

What will you do now?

Discussion 16.1

You have been tasked to a potentially volatile and unstable scene. The safety of yourself and your team should be your primary concern. The Police service is responsible for scene control in this situation. Plan to liaise with a senior member of the Police before entering the hotel. You must also do your own risk assessment on entering the scene as circumstances may have changed since the Police arrived. If there is no sign of the Police on arrival, urgently contact the tasking agency. A rendezvous point may have been established away from the hotel for incoming emergency service personnel (see Case 1).

PPE is an important consideration. A uniform that clearly identifies the PHRM team as a medical entity may minimise the risks from a hostile crowd. A 'stab vest' offering protection from low-velocity penetrating assault should also be considered in environments where such incidents are common. Universal precautions are mandatory.

You have received minimal clinical information on tasking which is not unusual. An assault is presumed but not proven. The differential diagnosis for a collapsed state of this type includes both traumatic and medical causes (e.g. drug overdose). Pre-arrival triage decisions will be difficult. You should note that both hospitals are some distance by road from the scene and that driving conditions are poor.

Discussion 16.2

Despite the Police presence, the scene remains uncontrolled. Furthermore, the patient is located in a cramped cubicle making meaningful assessment and intervention difficult. There has been a rapid deterioration in the patient's clinical condition. Swift assessment and early intervention are required. To do this, the PHRM team will need to create safe and effective space, communicate clearly and effectively while taking the lead. On entering the scene and walking to the patient, think about the extrication routes available to you. For example, in this instance it will enable you inform the Police service that you will need the corridor, stairs and toilet clear of any non-emergency service personnel. If a brief assessment of the patient confirms that he is pulseless, call for more help and transfer the patient rapidly to a less restricted location, ideally somewhere allowing 360-degree access to the patient. You should now enter into a period of simultaneous assessment and resuscitation.

If the patient remains bradypnoeic, delegate a suitable person to assess and manage the airway and assist with ventilation. Initially, this can be performed by the Ambulance Service and does not necessarily require a PHRM team member. Cut and remove the clothes completely to allow full external examination. Ensure that the intravenous cannula is patent. While non-invasive monitoring is instituted, commence a top-to-toe rapid examination including rapid log roll. Look specifically for any signs of external trauma, overt haemorrhage, recent intravenous drug use or evidence of pre-existing medical illness (a 'Medic Alert' bracelet or similar). Remember to check occult sites (axillae, groin, buttocks, perineum).

Discussion 16.3

There is a penetrating wound over the left anterior chest within the nipple line. The clinical picture is of an obstructed circulation. Pleural or pericardial tamponade are likely. Neck vein distension is an unreliable sign especially in the presence of hypovolaemia. External cardiac compression will be of questionable benefit while mechanical obstruction to cardiac filling and flow remains. Pleural and/or pericardial decompression is required immediately (See also Case 19).

Ensure the patient is intubated or assign a suitable colleague to perform intubation. Drugs are usually not required. If formal thoracostomy equipment is not immediately at hand, thoracic needle decompression of the left chest may be attempted (see Case 15). A formal left-sided thoracostomy should be performed. In the absence of this revealing and reversing a pleural collection under tension (with return of central pulses), immediately perform a formal right-sided thoracostomy. Lung inflation should be assessed bilaterally. If the patient remains in an arrested state, traumatic pericardial tamponade remains the only realistically reversible pathology. In this scenario, on-scene resuscitative thoracotomy is indicated. Needle pericardiocentesis is unlikely to offer effective decompression as pericardial blood can be clotted. The technique for 'clam shell' thoracotomy is briefly described below and in Appendix 1.4.

Clam shell thoracotomy (see also Appendix 1.4)

Prior to starting the procedure, very briefly explain to the emergency services personnel what is about to happen. Extend the thoracostomy incision posteriorly on both sides. Then continue the incision from the left to meet with the right side. If the thoracostomy incisions are not suitably posterior, the chest will incompletely open anteriorly. Use a pair of sterile trauma shears (or similar) to cut through the intercostal tissues and, if possible, through the sternum. The latter may require a Gigli saw. An additional pair of sterile gloved hands will assist in further lifting the anterior chest wall. Rib spreaders, if carried, are ideal.

Identify the major structures. Look specifically for a pericardial tamponade (a dark purple discolouration of the pericardial contents). Use a tissue hook or small pair of curved tissue forceps to 'tent' the pericardium. Make a small incision, then extend the opening as superiorly and inferiorly as possible inferiorly as possible using scissors. A vertical incision reduces the risk of phrenic nerve damage. Remove any clotted blood and assess the myocardium for obvious wounds. A cautiously placed suture, staple or a finger may temporarily stem further cardiac bleeding.

Spontaneous cardiac contractions may occur. If not, immediately commence effective two-handed internal cardiac massage (ICM). Place one palmed hand underneath and the other hand on the anterior surface of the heart. Usually concomitant blood is being given, time each massage to when the heart is felt to be full. Be very cautious not to lift the heart at all from the chest as this will significantly impair great vessel and coronary flow. If the heart appears to be fibrillating, attempt to defibrillate with a finger 'flick' of the myocardium. If not successful, continue effective ICM and prepare to externally defibrillate in the normal manner after releasing the anterior chest wall. Upon restoration of circulatory flow, look again for any overt myocardial or great vessel injury and treat accordingly.

Assess for central or peripheral pulses. The myocardium is likely to be stunned, and low initial blood pressure should be tolerated. If there is good control of any ongoing haemorrhage, judicious volume replacement titrated to a peripheral pulse is recommended.

The chest should rest closed with a sterile dressing placed over it. The patient should be triaged to a major trauma hospital which will require early notification.

Discussion 16.4

The early return of circulation, relative physiologic stability and brain stem activity is encouraging. Any spontaneous respiratory effort through the tracheal tube will, however, be ineffective and the patient will require analgesia, sedation and non-depolarising muscle relaxation.

The thoracotomy technique used in this instance necessarily results in the transection of both internal mammary arteries. These arteries will require clamping following the restoration of circulation. Small sterile curved forceps may be used in this instance.

Key points

- Scenes involving large crowds and serious assaults present very real dangers for the PHRM team and are frequently 'uncontrolled' despite the Police presence.
- Early thoracotomy in appropriately selected patients in cardiac arrest (less than 10 minutes of cardiac arrest with suspected cardiac tamponade) following penetrating trauma can save lives.

Additional reading

Lockey DJ, Davies G. Pre-hospital thoracotomy: a radical resuscitation come of age? Resuscitation 2007; 75(3):394–395.

Lockey DJ, Crewdson K, Davies G. Traumatic cardiac arrest: who are the survivors? Ann Emerg Med 2006; 48(3):240–244.

Teeter W, Haase D. Updates in traumatic cardiac arrest. Emerg Med Clin North Am 2020 Nov; 38(4):891–901.

Wise D, et al. Emergency thoracotomy: 'how to do it'. Emerg Med J 2005; 22(1):22–24.

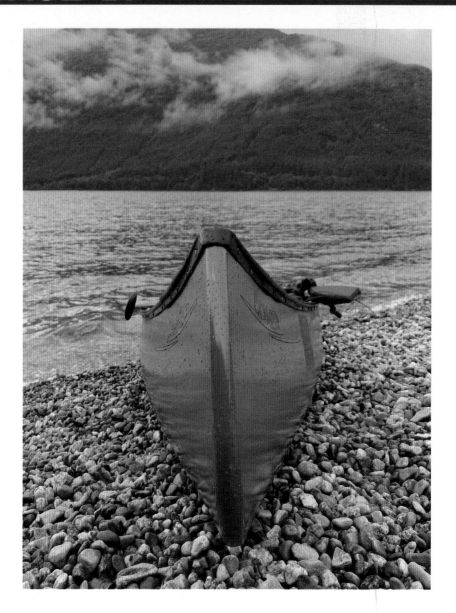

Incident

A male kayaker is in cardiac arrest. Your team is informed that a rescue boat has located the casualty and is bringing him into a marina.

By the time you land and disembark the aircraft, the patient has been removed from the rescue boat. He is on the quayside receiving CPR from the rescue boat crew and two road ambulance paramedics.

The paramedics have inserted a supraglottic airway and have attached a defibrillator. The patient is in asystolic cardiac arrest.

Relevant information

- **PHRM team transport options:** Rotary-wing aircraft.
- **Additional resources:** One road ambulance and crew. Police service. Rescue boat and crew.
- **Retrieval options:** Major trauma hospital 20 minutes by air.
- **Other:** Sea temperature 12°C (54°F). Ambient temperature 9°C (66°F). A mechanical CPR device is available in the rescue boat.

Question 17.1

What are your initial scene and team management priorities?

Question 17.2

What information would you like from the rescuers and bystanders?

Question 17.3

What are your initial actions?

Question 17.4

What are your actions once the mechanical CPR device has been applied?

Question 17.5

The patient's core temperature is 26°C. How does this affect your plan?

Discussion 17.1

Your initial priority is team safety and ensuring an adequate space to work. Frequently, when patients are removed from boats, healthcare providers commence their assessment and treatment immediately adjacent to the water's edge. It is important to ensure that the patient is moved to an area which allows a large team of people 360-degree access for clinical care, and is a sufficient distance from the water to ensure no one is at risk of falling in.

This is an example of a flash team scenario. There will be people from a number of agencies all trying to help the patient. These individuals will have differing levels of medical knowledge and skill and have different mental models of what is happening. It is important to gently but assertively let everyone present know that you will be taking charge of the clinical care of the patient and that you will require their assistance. It is essential to gather as much information from the rescuers and bystanders as possible. It is also important to use the resources available to delegate as many tasks and decisions as possible in order to cognitively offload the main clinical team.

Discussion 17.2

- The time the kayaker entered the water
- Was the casualty's head above the water for all of the period prior to rescue?
- The time the cardiac arrest occurred

- The time he was removed from the water
- The patient's age and past medical history

You are informed that the man was kayaking by himself approximately 4 km offshore. He capsized 3 hours prior to being rescued but was unable to get back into his kayak. He made the phone call to the emergency services but was unable to give coordinates for his location.

The rescue boat commenced a search for him and located him 3 hours after he made his phone call. He was in cardiac arrest at this time. As he was alone it is unknown when he became unconscious or when the cardiac arrest occurred. He was wearing a buoyancy aid and when he was found, his head was above the water.

Discussion 17.3

You should brief the team to achieve a shared mental model and delegate tasks. The team should be told that your priorities are to continue resuscitation efforts, place the casualty on the mechanical CPR device, and to measure his core temperature. Once you have his core temperature, you will be able to make a decision about his chances of survival and whether transferring him for extracorporeal life support (ECLS) may be appropriate.

Chest compressions and ventilation via the supraglottic airway device can be safely delegated to two rescue boat crew members. Confirm that they are competent and confident to do this. One member of the team should be asked to insert a tracheal tube to replace the supraglottic airway. This will allow ventilation at higher airway pressures, if required. Supraglottic airways may also not achieve an adequate seal in cold conditions. Another paramedic should be asked to obtain intravenous access. While they are doing this, they should measure the casualty's blood glucose level.

The team member most familiar with the mechanical CPR device should be asked to prepare it for use. Once this is ready, the team should be briefed to apply the device with a minimal 'off chest' time.

Discussion 17.4

- A large-bore orogastric tube should be inserted and suctioned to remove swallowed sea water from the stomach and air, which may have accumulated during initial ventilation attempts.
- An oesophageal temperature probe should be inserted to measure the core temperature.
- If available, consideration may be made to performing a brief cardiac ultrasound and measuring a potassium level with a near patient testing device.
- If a low blood glucose level is measured, this should be corrected with intravenous glucose.

Discussion 17.5

The patient's core temperature being 26°C could mean two things. The patient may have suffered a cardiac arrest and cooled after the cardiac arrest occurred. It may also mean that the patient cooled prior to cardiac arrest occurring and thus has increased potential for survival following active rewarming.

As the patient's temperature is below 30 degrees, epinephrine should not be administered. Following rewarming, epinephrine can be administered once the core temperature is above 30 degrees but with the interval between doses doubled.

The nearest centre with ECLS capability should be contacted. If they accept the patient, he should be transferred with ongoing CPR.

Any attempts to actively rewarm the patient en route to hospital would be futile and should not be attempted. It is not practical to increase a patient's core temperature in the pre-hospital environment, as the body's specific heat capacity is so great. Attempts at peripheral rewarming run the risk of developing 'afterdrop' – warmer core blood entering newly dilated peripheral vessels and cold limbs, then returning to the core cooler than it was. This can increase the risk of cardiac arrest developing. Attempts should, however, be made to prevent further heat loss by drying the patient and insulating him with dry blankets. The cabin of the aircraft should be warmed to 24°C to 28°C (75°F to 82°F) if possible.

Key points

- Complex multiagency (flash team) scenarios require good communication and assertive leadership.
- Effective delegation will ensure parallel processing of essential tasks.
- Prolonged cardiac arrest associated with hypothermia is a unique and potentially survivable clinical challenge.

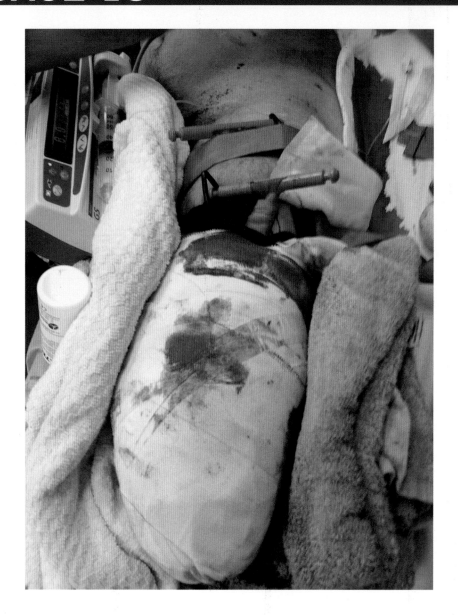

Incident

A 24-year-old male has been involved in a shark attack and has suffered multiple injuries predominantly to his torso and lower limbs.

The incident is 400 km (250 miles) away from the metropolitan area.

Your initial phone call is from the local ambulance resource who informs you that the patient has had his leg 'amputated' and is 'critically unwell'. They are taking the patient to the local hospital.

Clinical information

- P 130.
- BP 80/60 mmHg.
- SaO$_2$ 95% on non rebreathe mask at 15 litres.
- GCS 11 (E2V4M5)

Relevant information

- **PHRM team transport options:** Rotary-wing available. Fixed-wing available. Two stretchers. Land ambulances at both ends of the flight.
- **Additional resources:** Local paramedic-staffed rapid-response vehicle, small country hospital with a GP plus nursing staff.
- **Retrieval options:** Country hospital 20 minutes from landing strip. Major trauma hospital 1 hour and 35 minutes flight from landing strip including 10-minute road leg in metropolitan area.
- **Other:** Ambient temperature is 26°C (79°F), average seasonal sea temperature at incident is 16°C (61°F).

Question 18.1

Assuming you are the clinical coordinator, discuss your options for rendering clinical assistance and logistical support.

The patient has undergone RSI by the local GP. He has received 2 units of O negative blood (exhausting the local supply) and 2 litres of crystalloid. He remains fully packaged in the vacuum mattress which was applied by the local ambulance service.

Clinical observations

- P 150.
- BP 90/60 mmHg.
- SaO$_2$ 95% on FiO$_2$ 0.6.
- ETCO$_2$ 46mmHg (6.13Kpa).

Question 18.2

Assuming you are now the lead clinician on the PHRM team arriving at the country facility, what are your priorities for this case?

Question 18.3

Describe the principles for handing over complex trauma patients to emergency department staff.

Discussion 18.1

The patient has significant injuries to the lower limbs, including an apparent total amputation. He is already in shock. Even with ideal planning and implementation, the PHRM team is more than 2 hours away. On top of that, the PHRM team is mainly a supportive bridge to definitive care, which is likely to be in excess of 4–5 hours away.

Remote assistance of the local team will be key to ensuring early management goals are achieved. The table below highlights potential actions.

Clinical	Logistical

• Time to definitive care
  ○ Where/what is definitive care?
  ○ Parallel processing
  ○ Ability to resuscitate in transit
	• Transport platform (see Case 27)
	  ○ Rotary-wing
	    • Point to point
	    • Need for refuel
	    • Slower in flight
	  ○ Fixed-wing
	    • Secondary transfer
	    • Faster in flight

• Vascular access
  ○ Diameter
  ○ Location
  ○ Number
  ○ Monitoring	

• Volume resuscitation
• Blood products to be taken with PHRM team:
  ○ How many units can be taken?
  ○ Additional blood products available for transport
  ○ Access to Massive Transfusion Packs (MTP) prepared for transport
• Minimal crystalloid
• Preservation of existing volume
• Tourniquets
  ○ Type
  ○ Placement
  ○ Timing
	• Blood options available nearby
	  ○ Red cells at facility
	  ○ Red cells at nearby facilities
	  ○ Blood products nearby
	  ○ Use of ambulance resources to distribute

• Tranexamic acid (TXA) • Haemostatic agents (see Case 28)	
• REBOA as a bridge? (see Case 28)	

	• Patient pick-up from airport
	  ○ Quicker turnaround
	  ○ Risk of clinical deterioration
	• Patient pick-up from facility
	  ○ Slower turnaround
	  ○ Stay in 'place of relative safety'

Clinical	Logistical

• Remote clinical support
   ○ Telemedicine
	• Local support options
	   ○ Special-skill GPs
	   ○ Visiting hospital specialists

• Hypothermia
   ○ Initial patient temperature
   ○ Room temperature in facility
   ○ Cabin temperature on return flight	

	• Early major trauma centre awareness and preparation

Discussion 18.2

The patient remains unstable despite volume replacement. Further injuries should be excluded. The PHRM team deflates the vacuum mattress and gently examines and log rolls the patient to reveal a large quantity of blood in the mattress and the injury shown on the patients left flank in the image below:

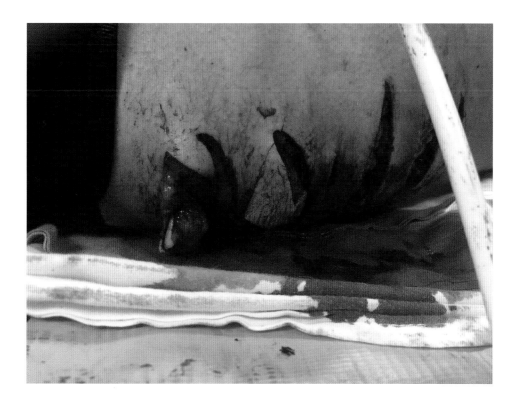

Complete and repeat clinical assessment is important in trauma patients, especially with penetrating disease. Observations made by other providers may not have been handed over or not heard by the receiving team.

The key objective here remains the time to definitive care, and the PHRM team should be aiming for a rapid, safe turnaround time.

Ensuring that ongoing bleeding has been stopped is also a priority. Options for management of the newly discovered flank wounds include direct pressure and pressure dressing, topical haemostatic agents and temporary wound closure (deep suture or staple). The team should be aware that bleeding from this wound may be intraperitoneal and bedside imaging should be utilised (see Case 39).

Ongoing volume replacement, preferably with blood and blood products brought by the PHRM team, may be required, with a focus on minimal volume resuscitation principles (see Case 12).

Adequate analgesia and maintenance of anaesthesia will be important considerations, especially as the team will have several competing requirements during this task and cognitive overload is a possibility (see Case 11).

Adequate and secure large-bore intervenous access is essential, and strong consideration should be given to siting an arterial line for monitoring during the long trip to definitive care. A risk benefit analysis is often required to ensure time at the scene is not unduly extended by this procedure. It is also possible to site arterial access in the fixed wing cabin on the way back.

Communication with the tasking agency throughout will directly benefit patient care by ensuring seamless continuity of care during key interface points. For example, upon landing in the metropolitan area there will be an opportunity for further blood or blood products to be waiting for the team.

Discussion 18.3

An effective handover should provide:

- A synopsis of the patient
- A description of what has been done during the job and why
- An unequivocal transfer of the patient's care to another clinician.

Handover should also be:

- Brief
- Succinct: containing all relevant information
- Clear: the emergency department environment, especially the resuscitation room, is noisy. You must speak loudly and confidently.

The following template is predominantly for the time-critical patient (e.g. trauma). Variations to this approach may be indicated in complex but more stable patients.

Handover can be considered a two-phase process:

Phase 1

En route to hospital

Prepare the handover mentally, writing down key points or using an existing template if available (see Appendix 6) Use the headings in the box below to help.

On arrival

- Locate the team leader (receiving clinician) and make eye contact.
- If the patient requires immediate intervention (e.g. has a dislodged airway, or sudden and rapid physiologic deterioration) then make this clear immediately. Otherwise, state that the patient has 'no immediate needs'. This encourages the receiving team to focus on the handover rather than attempting to search for potential life-threatening pathology.
- Handover should occur either immediately before or immediately after moving the patient across to the hospital stretcher. Local practice will determine which is more appropriate
- Avoid handing over while moving the patient onto the hospital stretcher. The receiving team may not be paying full attention and things will be missed. The PHRM team can then confirm to the entire receiving team that handover will occur.
- The handover should utilise the following structure and overall take less than a minute:
  - Name/age (if known).
  - Brief details of incident (emphasis on mechanism of injury if relevant).
  - Major issues on arrival of the PHRM team.
    - Airway and breathing.
    - Circulation.
    - Conscious state and limb movements.
  - Injuries from 'top to toe'.
  - Interventions.
    - Procedures.
    - Intravenous fluids given.
    - Drugs given (and timing if relevant).
  - Stability during transfer and immediate needs post-handover.
  - Summary: generally only required if the case is very complex.

Example of handover

An example of a succinct yet comprehensive handover would be:

'This is a young (unknown) male who has been attacked by a shark approximately 5 hours ago.

'On arrival of the Ambulance Service, he was GCS 11 (E2V4M5) with a pulse of 130 and an SBP of 80. When we arrived, he had already been intubated and ventilated by the GP at the local clinic with a reported Grade 2 larynx. His injuries from top to toe include penetrating trauma to the lower torso with possible intra-abdominal injury and pelvic involvement identified on log roll. He also has a complete amputation of the right leg above the knee. The amputated limb has not been located. He has 2 tourniquets applied, one above the other on the right limb and no further bleeding is evident.

'He has been sedated on propofol and fentanyl infusions for transport.

'He has 14G cannulae in each antecubital fossae and an arterial line in the left radial artery.

'In total, he has received 5 units of blood, 1 g of TXA and 2500 mL of pre-hospital crystalloid, but remains volume sensitive.'

During handover, mention the following (if applicable):

- Say whether a log roll was done and highlight any findings.
- Tourniquets and tourniquet times.

Immediately after the handover:

- Assist the receiving team in removing the patient from the PHRM team's equipment (e.g. monitors, ventilators, scoop stretcher, etc.)
- Collect all your non-disposable equipment (you may need to exchange splint devices or infusion pumps with the receiving facility).

Leaving the trauma room:

- Inform the team leader that you are leaving the room but will return with completed notes shortly.

There are numerous aide memoires already in existence that can be used to facilitate handover. Examples of two such aide memoires are illustrated below.

Aide memoires used to facilitate handover	
MISTO	**SBARR**
M – mechanism of injury	S – situation
I – injuries sustained	B – background
S – signs and symptoms	A – assessment
T – treatment initiated	R – response
O – other information (e.g. allergies)	R – requirements

Phase 2

Return to the trauma resuscitation bay. Locate the team leader and give them or the scribe a copy of your pre-hospital notes. If electronic patient records are utilised, ensure notes are transferred or printed appropriately. Ask the team leader if they have any other questions for the PHRM team. The PHRM team can address questions now, although they should avoid interfering in patient care at this point.

Key points
• Aim to balance clinical and logistical demands in the PHRM environment.
• Recognise the challenges faced when dealing with complex, unstable patients in remote locations.
• Recognise the inherent value in succinct clinical handover and its importance to high-quality and safe patient care.
• In handing over patient care, be brief, logical and speak with authority and clarity.

Additional reading

Hearns S. Peak performance under pressure: lessons from a helicopter rescue doctor. Core Cognition, 2019.

Wood K, Crouch R, Rowland E, et al. Clinical handovers between prehospital and hospital staff: literature review. Emerg Med J 2015; 32:577–581.

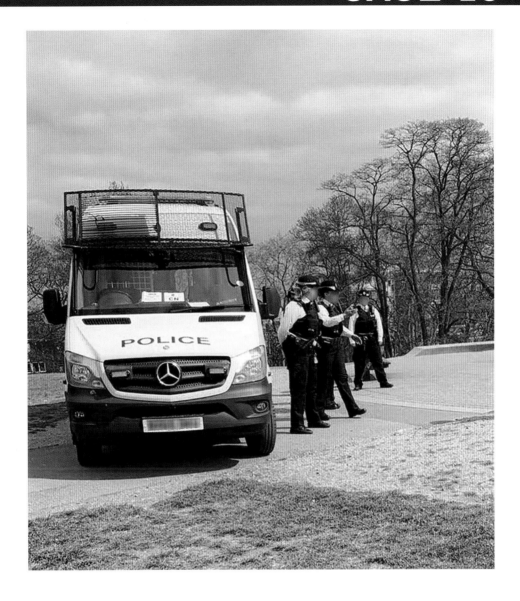

Incident

The PHRM team is asked to provide support to the local Police service for a firearm incident involving suspected terrorists.

Question 19.1

Briefly discuss how you would plan for this.

After 10 minutes, the team is made aware that there has now been an MVA involving a Police officer and the suspects' vehicle. Shortly after, the officer is brought to your location by his colleagues. He is unconscious and his colleagues have started CPR. You are 30 minutes by road from the nearest major trauma hospital.

Question 19.2

Discuss further management.

Discussion 19.1

Such incidents are increasingly common in the urban environment and are rarely planned much in advance. The PHRM team may only have minutes' notice to prepare. Depending on the nature and frequency of the requests, it may be appropriate for the team to be aware of the operation and its location and only attend if an incident occurs. If the Police feel advanced medical attendance is mandatory, they should liaise early with the coordination agency who should ensure that a senior PHRM clinician is part of the decision-making process.

If attending, the PHRM team should make sure that they have an extra layer of PPE in place (e.g. a 'stab vest') and should ask the coordination agency to find details of the emergency services rendezvous point (RVP) (see Case 16). Once at the RVP, the team should stay in contact with the tasking agency and operational Police officers. Listening to a Police radio or shared talk group may help in this regard. In the event of an incident, the PHRM team must not leave the RVP to head to the scene unless the scene is safe and the team has a Police escort. Even then, it is preferable for the casualty to be brought to the RVP if possible.

Discussion 19.2

Scene safety is still paramount, even in the RVP. It may be appropriate to ask an officer if it is safe to treat the patient in the current location or whether you should move somewhere safer. This may delay initial lifesaving interventions from being performed but will enable the PHRM team to subsequently treat the officer in a safer environment. This could be at the back of the ambulance designated to take the team and patient to the major trauma hospital and will allow for a more rapid extrication from the scene. Consider that the officer may be carrying a loaded firearm and other weapons. Never assume these have been made safe and always ask a senior Police officer to remove any weapons prior to treatment.

Initial treatment of the pre-hospital traumatic cardiac arrest is as follows:

- Confirm cardiac arrest and the likelihood of a traumatic aetiology (rather than medical) and note the time. It is important to note that some patients may be in a 'low-flow' state where no pulses are palpable but there is still limited cardiac output. If there has been a confirmed loss of vital signs for longer than 10–15 minutes, the PHRM team can consider stopping resuscitation. The PHRM team should be aware that the assessment of a 'low flow versus no flow' state is challenging in the PHRM environment, especially if the assessment is performed by non-medical personnel. In this highly emotive situation, that will be difficult to do, and it would be justifiable to start resuscitating the officer initially. At this point, the use of POCUS might assist. A single subcostal view can be sought looking for cardiac activity (or tamponade). It is important that this does not delay essential interventions and should happen in parallel with other procedures.
- Simultaneously treat the immediately reversible conditions and start resuscitation. There are several algorithms available that may be useful in these scenarios (Lockey et al 2013, Sherren et al 2013) See below.

- This aspect of treatment is likely to require the assembly of a 'flash team' utilising several existing team members, including from the PHRM team, the Ambulance Service and Police service.
- Team roles should ideally remain within their scope of practice and it may be possible for several interventions to occur at the same time. The PHRM team leader should establish 'expertise, environment, equipment, and elapsed time'.
- Haemorrhage control. Current guidelines recommend the addition of 'catastrophic haemorrhage' ahead of ABC (C-ABC) for traumatic cardiac arrest. In this scenario, there may be the need to splint the legs and bind the pelvis as well as applying direct/indirect pressure or haemostatic gauzes to any open bleeding/junctional wounds.

Airway

- The patient needs a secure airway, and an initial attempt at intubation without drugs should be made. Depending on their scope of practice this can be delegated to one of the local Ambulance Service paramedics. If this is not possible due to the patient gagging or resisting, then the patient may not be in cardiac arrest and rapid-sequence intubation (with a very low dose/no induction agent) may be required. A supraglottic airway (SGA) may be appropriate in the first instance to ensure definitive airway management does not delay other critical interventions. The SGA can be changed to a tracheal tube later as required. Waveform capnography should be initiated at the outset and serial $ETCO_2$ readings following intubation should be noted.

Breathing

- Bilateral simple thoracostomies for potential tension haemo/pneumothoraces should be performed simultaneously by the PHRM team, starting with the most injured side first (see Appendix 1.3). If there are going to be delays in performing the simple thoracostomies (due to personnel or kit issues), then needle decompression may be considered accepting the recognised weaknesses with this technique (e.g. the needle not reaching the pleural space, See Case 15). If performed in traumatic cardiac arrest, needle decompressions should always be considered temporary and should be replaced with simple thoracostomies as soon as practical, assuming the airway has been secured and positive-pressure ventilation initiated.

Circulation

- Apply ECG monitoring and defibrillate as indicated.
- Volume resuscitation with blood components or 500 mL fluid boluses via large-bore IV access or an intraosseous needle.
- Consider thoracotomy. In traumatic cardiac arrests from blunt trauma there is limited evidence to support pre-hospital thoracotomy; however, if ROSC has not been achieved after the above steps have occurred, POCUS (if not already performed) can be used to determine if there is presence of a pericardial effusion. If seen, then a clam shell thoracotomy can be undertaken to not only relieve any tamponade but also to occlude the descending aorta against the thoracic vertebrae (see Case 16 and Appendix 1.4). Volume resuscitation should be continued during the procedure.

- In the absence of cardiac tamponade, thoracotomy would generally not be indicated. However, REBOA can be considered if the PHRM service has an appropriate system in place to deliver this intervention (see Case 28). Similarly, some services also utilise open thoracotomy for proximal hemorrhage control.
- If POCUS reveals cardiac activity but no pericardial effusion, then post resuscitation care can begin, including the administration of vasopressors (e.g. adrenaline), alongside further volume resuscitation. TXA can also be given at this stage.

Reassessment

- Repeat C-ABC approach, look for other injuries, take a brief history from colleagues, and a brief look at the pupils.
- CPR can be started and continued if possible, provided it does not interfere with performing interventions.

Record all interventions

- This is a crime scene and involves a member of the emergency services. The actions of all emergency services personnel, including the PHRM team, will come under subsequent scrutiny and may be the subject of a coronial inquiry. In addition, some emergency services will be utilising 'body cameras' and teams should be aware that footage from these devices will be reviewed.

Plan for early transport from scene

- It is prudent to proceed to the nearest major trauma hospital rapidly, regardless of the response to the above interventions.
- This is a highly charged scenario and the officer's comrades, having carried their wounded colleague (and friend) under great duress to be treated by the PHRM team, will be looking to see that 'everything was done'.
- Even if further resuscitation is ceased en route, it will be beneficial for all involved to move the patient away from the scene.
- Given the nature of the incident and certain post-event scrutiny, this is arguably not the time to pronounce life extinct in the field.
- A sitrep must be given to the tasking agency who should liaise with the receiving major trauma hospital to ensure blood products, a full trauma team and emergency theatre are immediately available.

Stopping resuscitation

- Notwithstanding the above comments relevant to this scenario, as a general rule ongoing resuscitation may be ceased under the following circumstances:
  - Loss of vital signs for longer than 10 minutes
  - Persistent asystole
  - $ETCO_2$ <10 mmHg/1.3 KPa
  - Absence of cardiac motion on ultrasound
  - Discovery of injuries incompatible with life
  - Severe and unsurvivable head injuries (e.g. significant loss of brain matter).

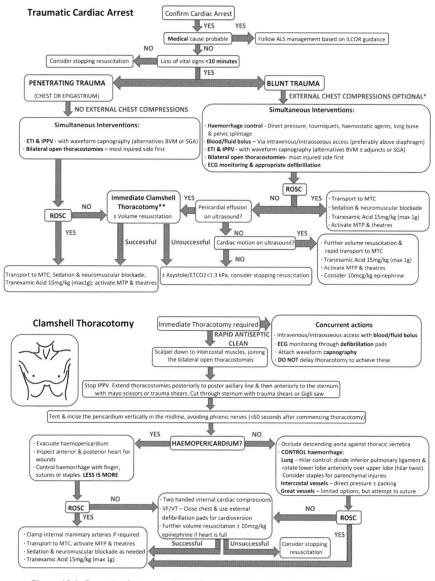

Figure 19.1 Example of a traumatic cardiac arrest algorithm. Source: Sherren et al. 2013

Key points

- Scene safety remains the priority in high-risk environments.
- The structured approach to pre-hospital traumatic cardiac arrest allows for the initial treatment of potentially reversible pathology. The airway may not be the most failed system and thus the 'standard' ABC approach may vary.
- Stopping resuscitation in the field is challenging and may be confrontational especially in key patient groups (e.g. children, emergency services personnel).

References

Lockey DJ, Lyon RM, Davies GE. Development of a simple algorithm to guide the effective management of traumatic cardiac arrest. Resuscitation 2013; 84(6):738–742.

Sherren PB, Reid C, Habig K, Burns BJ. Algorithm for the resuscitation of traumatic cardiac arrest patients in a physician-staffed helicopter emergency medical service. Crit Care 2013; 17(2):308.

Additional reading

France J, Smith J, Jones J, Barnard E. Traumatic cardiac arrest in adults. The Royal College of Emergency Medicine, 2019. Online. Available: RCEM_Traumatic cardiac arrest_ Sept 2019 FINAL.pdf. 18 October 2021. https://rcem.ac.uk/wp-content/uploads/2021/10/RCEM_Traumatic_Cardiac_Arrest_Sept2019_FINAL.pdf

The Royal College of Surgeons of Edinburgh. Concensus statement 2018: management of cardiac arrest. Online. Available: Microsoft Word - TCA submission Oct 2018.docx (rcsed.ac.uk). 18 October 2021. https://fphc.rcsed.ac.uk/media/2577/tca-submission-oct-2018.pdf

Trauma Victoria. Traumatic cardiac arrest. Online. Available: Traumatic Cardiac Arrest-Introduction | Trauma Victoria (reach.vic.gov.au). 18 October 2021. https://trauma.reach.vic.gov.au/guidelines/traumatic-cardiac-arrest/introduction

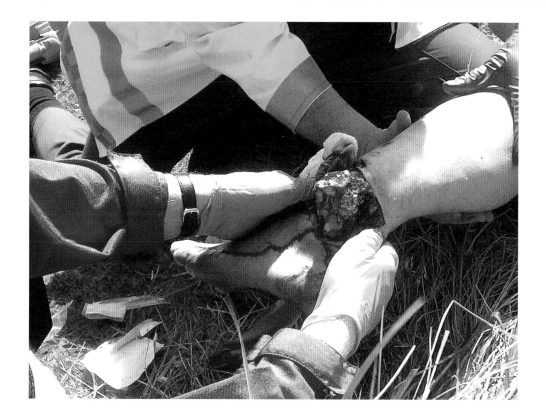

Incident

A cyclist has been hit by a car and has sustained an isolated open fracture dislocation of the ankle.

Clinical information

- P 110.
- BP 150/90 mmHg.
- RR 22.

The foot is dusky and pulseless and the patient is screaming in pain.

Relevant information

- **PHRM team transport options:** Rotary-wing aircraft.
- **Additional resources:** One land ambulance.
- **Retrieval options:** Major trauma hospital 1 hour by air. Regional hospital 15 minutes by air.
- **Other:** Ambient temperature 35°C (95°F).

Question 20.1

How will you go about managing this injury in this environment?

Question 20.2

Given the retrieval options, discuss definitive care for this patient.

Discussion 20.1

This question concerns adequate analgesia but also safe sedation in the pre-hospital environment.

Pain management

Psychological

- Reassurance.
- General patient comfort (ambient temperature protection).
- Explanation – what you are about to do and what to expect.
- Distraction – especially for children but can also be effective for adults.

Non-pharmacological

- Anatomical realignment.
- Splinting techniques.
- Minimising patient movements and handling where possible.
- Covering of open wounds.

Pharmacological

- Oral.
- Inhaled.
- Intramuscular
- Intranasal
- Intravenous
- Regional.

In this instance, it is clear that the patient needs emergency limb re-alignment and plans should be made for this to occur as soon as practicable. In the interim, inhaled analgesic agents, such as Entonox and methoxyflurane, or intranasal agents, such as fentanyl or ketamine, can be administered to the patient.

Preparation for sedation

The patient

- Explain your plan and obtain verbal consent. Complete the primary survey and ensure there are no higher-priority injuries. Make note of any neurovascular deficit in the distal limb. Gain large-bore intravenous access and ensure the patient is adequately positioned in a safe location with 360-degree access.

The team

- Ideally, procedural sedation requires a minimum of two clinicians. One person will need to titrate drugs and continuously assess the patient, while a second person performs the manipulation. In this instance, cervical spine control will be required, as safe clearance of the spine is unlikely given the significant distracting injury. Spinal control should be via manual in-line stabilisation. Ensure that there is a box or vacuum splint available for the realigned limb.

Choice of agent(s)

⦿ The ideal agent for this procedure is ketamine. This drug has a very good safety margin and a proven pre-hospital track record. In addition, it is a potent analgesic which may allow the procedure to be performed under a single agent. Emergence phenomena and occasional hallucinations with severe agitation can limit its use. However, it is significantly harder to rapidly obtain safe levels of sedation and analgesia with other agents such as opiates and benzodiazepines. Non-analgesic sedative/anaesthetic agents causing respiratory depression, such as propofol, should be avoided or used with caution in this setting.

Procedure

Use an initial bolus of 0.5–1 mg per kg of intravenous ketamine. Far smaller doses (0.1–0.2 mg per kg) will usually provide analgesia but inadequate sedation. The PHRM team must have the requisite skills and knowledge to manage an anaesthetised patient should higher sedative doses be used. Some practitioners advocate the addition of 1–2 mg of midazolam (for young adults) to reduce emergence phenomena, but there is little evidence to support this. Ensure the scene is kept relatively calm and quiet as loud or unnecessary noise and inappropriate stimulus can lead to worse emergence phenomena. The patient will normally keep their eyes open and nystagmus is a good early indicator of clinical effect. Gentle movements of the limb should confirm sedation, and manipulation can then occur. The person sedating should observe the patient clinically for chest movement, misting of the mask and signs of inadequate sedation. Awake capnography is strongly recommended in this setting (see below). Once the limb has been manipulated, check distal limb pulses, apply sterile wound dressings and immobilise in a splint. Heavily contaminated wounds should be liberally irrigated with saline, and intravenous antibiotics should be given.

Monitoring

The minimum monitoring requirements are pulse, non-invasive blood pressure and oxygen saturations. Ideally, awake capnography via nasal cannulae should be used for procedural sedation and ensuing transport.

Transfer and handover

Following the procedure, specifically ensure and document the return of distal limb perfusion. Complete the patient packaging process (see Case 8) and transfer to definitive care. Keep the patient monitored until handover.

Give a clear and concise summary of events to the receiving team (see Case 18). Patients recovering from ketamine sedation will have a reduced or altered conscious state and the hospital team may suspect occult head injury unless you explain what the patient was like pre-sedation and what has been done at the scene.

Pitfalls

Most problems will result from inadequate preparation or drug issues. There is an increased clinical risk if you are instructing someone other than a member of the

PHRM team to give drugs, especially sedatives. Clear and concise instructions can help to minimise this risk. It is often clearer if instructions refer to the quantity of liquid in the syringe. For example, say that you want 3 mL given and then point or mark on the syringe to the place where the plunger will be pushed. For once-only drugs, you should discard the surplus drug and ask for the remainder of the syringe to be administered. This will not be practical for drugs that require titration. Another option is to say the dose and quantity of the drug and ask for the drug-giver to repeat that back to you. For example: 'Give 100 mg ketamine, 10 mL'.

Other problems can occur at extremes of age with too much sedative being given. It is worth remembering that while more sedation can be given, excess sedation cannot be removed.

Analgesia only

Many pre-hospital cases will need analgesia but only a few will need sedation. The concept of the pain ladder should be adhered to where possible (starting with simple analgesia and titrating upwards). Ongoing analgesia should be titrated using a self-reported or visual analogue pain scale. There is a role for oral/rectal analgesia and antipyretics especially in the paediatric population. Nitrous oxide and oxygen combined offers excellent analgesia (if regionally available) with the bonus of rapid onset and offset. Methoxyflurane is an alternative inhaled analgesic agent.

As discussed earlier, ketamine is also a useful pre-hospital analgesic agent in lower-dose ranges.

Morphine is a good general analgesic but consideration should be given to newer agents such as fentanyl. Despite requiring more frequent doses, fentanyl acts faster, is more potent and can double as an agent for use in RSI.

Regional blocks

The main regional anaesthetic procedure performed in the pre-hospital environment is the femoral nerve block for proximal and shaft femoral fractures. Many practitioners prefer to reduce the fracture under ketamine, but there is a role for the regional approach either in isolation in patients who are unsuitable for sedation or in whom it is felt emergence phenomena are likely (e.g. co-existing recreational drug use) or as an adjunct procedure following the manipulation. Regional nerve blocks should be performed under aseptic conditions and using ultrasound guidance.

General anaesthesia

Occasionally, the severity of the injuries (see the image on the next page) are such that only general anaesthesia will adequately alleviate the pain. The risks of performing pre-hospital RSI should be balanced against the humanitarian needs of the suffering patient.

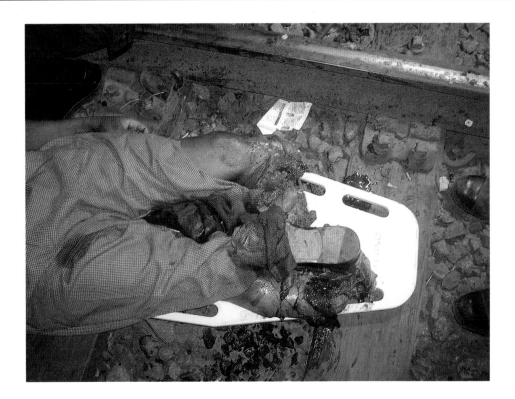

Discussion 20.2

The destination hospital decision will depend on regionally available specialist resources; however, regardless of the additional transport time, if there is any concern about the neurovascular integrity of the foot, a major trauma facility is recommended. These discussions should occur through the clinical coordination centre.

Key points
• Analgesia is a basic requirement for pre-hospital and retrieval medicine.
• Sedation is often required and should be carried out safely and with adequate preparation beforehand.
• In experienced hands, ketamine is an ideal pre-hospital analgesic and sedative agent.

Additional reading

Bredmose PP, Lockey DJ, Grier G, et al. Pre-hospital use of ketamine for analgesia and procedural sedation. Emerg Med J 2009; 26(1):62–64.

Grindlay J, Babl FE. Review article: efficacy and safety of methoxyflurane analgesia in the emergency department and prehospital setting. Emerg Med Australas 2009; 21(1):4–11.

Johnston S, Wilkes GJ, Thompson JA, et al. Inhaled methoxyflurane and intranasal fentanyl for prehospital management of visceral pain in an Australian ambulance service. Emerg Med J 2011; 28(1):57–63.

Mankowitz SL, Regenberg P, Kaldan J, Cole JB. Ketamine for rapid sedation of agitated patients in the prehospital and emergency department settings: a systematic review and proportional meta-analysis. Emerg Med J 2018; 55(5):670–681.

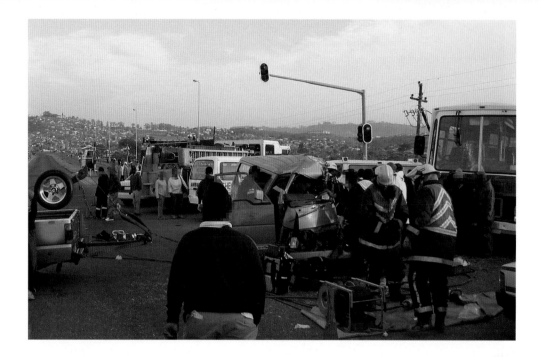

Incident

A van has collided at high speed with a car. The tasking agency reports that there are three severely injured patients including children. All are still in the vehicle and could be trapped. In addition, there is potentially one fatality on the scene.

Relevant information

- **PHRM team transport options:** Rotary-wing aircraft. Maximum of one stretcher case.
- **Additional resources:** Three land ambulances. Police and Fire & Rescue services.
- **Retrieval options:** Major trauma hospital 20 minutes by air. Regional hospital 30 minutes by road.
- **Other:** Rain approaching.

Question 21.1

What is your initial pre-hospital plan?

Question 21.2

Describe your immediate actions on arrival at the scene.

On assessment, there are three patients from the two cars involved in the head-on collision. All have now been extricated from the vehicles.

- Patient 1 is pulseless and apnoeic with a large open skull fracture and extra-cranial brain tissue.
- Patient 2 is a middle-aged female with a rigid abdomen and bruises over the pelvis. She has decreased air entry over the left chest, according to an on-scene paramedic. In addition, her BP is 90 systolic and GCS is 6.

- Patient 3 is 11 years old with closed bilateral femoral fractures who is crying inconsolably. His pulse is said to be 120 beats per minute.
- Patient 4 was in a third vehicle that swerved to miss the accident and mounted the kerb. She is complaining of ankle pain.

Question 21.3

Briefly outline your management and triage/transport decisions for these patients. Which of the patients will you transport by air?

Question 21.4

What is the priority after the job has finished?

Discussion 21.1

Multiple casualties involving children and a lethal mechanism create a highly charged and complicated environment, even for the most experienced PHRM teams. Utilising the time spent en route to scene formulating the pre-hospital plan allows the PHRM team the opportunity to rationalise and mentally prepare for the scene.

Scene safety

With four patients this will be a chaotic scene and patients may be geographically dispersed. Under such pressure, the standard approach to scene safety may have been compromised.

Patients

Four patients may require a temporary team split for initial assessment. Another option is for all PHRM team members to initially assess each patient, which ensures that they all have the same information. Prepare mentally for an injured child, refer to your paediatric resuscitation app or other reference material. Be aware of the reported 'death' on-scene, as the PHRM team will need to confirm this

Destination

There is only capacity for one aeromedical transfer. Inclement weather is approaching rapidly and this may impact on aviation decision making. Slower road transport is another consideration. A regional hospital is available. In consultation with the tasking agency, complex triage decisions will need to occur.

Discussion 21.2

Key elements in the scene approach are:

Scene safety

Confirm with the senior Fire & Rescue Service officer that the scene is safe. Liaise with key emergency service personnel (ideally simultaneously as a team brief) to understand current scene dynamics.

Scene assessment

The PHRM team may need to split up to survey the scene. This is a cursory survey and an attempt to get a brief handover from the on-scene ambulance crews. There may be a senior ambulance officer on-scene (see the team brief above) who can accompany the PHRM team on a brief scene survey. In some ways, this is like a major incident (see Case 23); information must be acquired in order to know the extent of the casualties, share a mental model with others on-scene, and to update your pre-hospital plan. If the team does split, this should be as brief as possible, with a clear plan to remain in contact and regroup following the assessment.

Patient assessment

Your patient assessment should utilise the rapid screening tool (see Case 12), but in these situations when patient numbers begin to exceed team capacity, assessment will become even briefer and more closely mirror the major incident triage sieve (see Cases 23, 43 and Appendix 8). Use of a dedicated multi-casualty patient record can help in these situations. (see Appendix 6.2).

Discussion 21.3

Patient 1 is dead. Although confirming death in the pre-hospital arena can be challenging, this patient has sustained injuries that are not compatible with life. In some jurisdictions, confirmation of death is only possible if there is a cause of death and a certificate, hence the term 'pronounce life extinct' may be used instead. If the PHRM team is certain of death, then the team leader should locate a Police officer and pronounce life extinct in front of the officer, giving the deceased person's details and the pronounced time of death. The PHRM team members should ensure that they obtain the Police officer's details in return and that these are clearly recorded. A formal statement may be required later, so ensure clear and concise notes are taken.

If the PHRM team is not certain that the patient is dead, then basic resuscitative maneouvres should be considered (resources and other demands permitting) until the situation is clarified. This is more straightforward in single-patient scenarios. In the scene described above, spending several minutes resuscitating and reassessing the patient may lead to avoidable deterioration in other time-critical patients who have a much better chance of survival.

Patient 4 was not involved in the primary crash and is essentially physically uninjured. After a rapid assessment of her and her vehicle you may decide to leave her at the scene. Not everyone involved needs ambulance transfer to hospital, especially when resources are stretched (three ambulances, four patients). Under most circumstances, patients left at the scene should be advised to self-present to the local general hospital emergency department (or their general practitioner).

Patient 2 has signs of serious injury and requires prompt assessment and treatment. However, patient 3 (the child) is also seriously injured.

At this point, a brief 'sit-rep' (situation report) should be given to the tasking agency. In PHRM services with established clinical coordination, senior advice may also be available (see Case 22). Giving a 'METHANE' sit-rep to the tasking agency helps it to be structured, detailed and contain all the required information (see Case 23).

On the available evidence, patient 3 is more stable than patient 2. Thus, patient 2 should undergo aeromedical transfer. Despite a logical decision-making process, the final outcome could vary as small changes in this scenario could lead to major changes in the plan; for example:

- What if the scene was more remote and a four-hour road transfer was required to the major trauma hospital? Would this change your plan?

- What if the pilot says they can try to reconfigure the aircraft to accommodate the child? Is this safe and appropriate?
- Should you leave a member of the PHRM team on-scene to stay with the remaining patients? If so, what equipment will be available for each patient?
- If you go by road with both patients to the major trauma hospital, will you be better placed to manage any clinical deterioration that occurs?
- Is 'back-to-back' use of the aircraft an option and, if so, will you split the team, as above?
- What about a 'staged' transport utilising the nearest general hospital? Will this potentially improve or worsen the care for either of these patients?

There is no right answer to this sort of scene, and the PHRM team leader, in consultation with the tasking and coordination centre, will have to carefully weigh their options.

Possibly the best initial approach is for the PHRM team to split. One half should begin to prepare for an RSI on patient 2, utilising other ambulance personnel on-scene. Meanwhile, the other PHRM team member can reassess the child, optimise initial treatment and explain the plan to the ground crew. Moving both patients near to each other within the scene (while maintaining adequate 360-degree patient access) will improve team communications and access to equipment, fluids, drugs and assistance. The child's femoral fractures should be reduced and splinted. However, if a PHRM team member is not going to be accompanying the patient, the ambulance crew may be uncomfortable transporting a sedated child. Return to patient 2, stabilise, package and transfer.

Discussion 21.4

At the conclusion of this task, time should be allocated for a 'hot debrief'. This should be an open forum for all emergency services personnel who wish to attend. Formal psychological support may be provided at this time. Sometimes, individuals involved in this case may be unsure as to why a particular course of action was taken and this can be discussed while the case is still fresh, as part of the hot debrief. This case is also ideal for discussion again at a multidisciplinary audit meeting with other senior pre-hospital medical personnel (see Case 52).

Key points

- Incidents involving multiple patients, particularly those in remote or regional areas, may rapidly overwhelm available pre-hospital resources.
- A 'major incident' type approach and temporary division of the PHRM team may be required.
- Multiagency review of such complex and dynamic tasks is recommended, both as a hot debrief and in a structured audit.

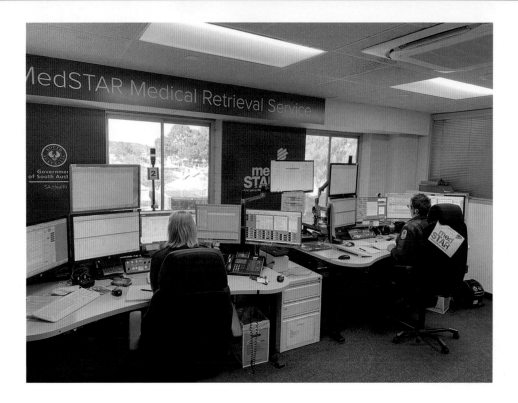

The following questions relate to the tasking and coordination of physician-led PHRM teams (see also Case 42). Tasking and clinical coordination are key aspects of pre-hospital and retrieval medicine. Triage, resource allocation and high-level clinical oversight are core elements to this process.

The following incidents should be considered as being independent of each other for the purposes of this question. In each case, the decision to mobilise, coordinate and support the PHRM team rests solely with you as the clinical coordinator. You have information technology, maps and communications equipment available to you (see picture).

Incident A

The ambulance service has alerted you to an ongoing incident in an urban area of your region. Five minutes previously, multiple calls had been made to the Ambulance Service concerning a motorcyclist who had struck a car at an intersection. The information you have from a member of the public is that the motorcyclist is unconscious.

Incident B

A call is put through to you concerning a shooting incident in a remote village some 50 minutes rotary-wing flight time from the PHRM service base. It is 2 am and raining. A single call was made by a female caller who reports a gunshot and a 'figure lying face down in her garden'. A local ambulance crew has been tasked but will not be on scene for 15 minutes.

Incident C

You are asked by a local ambulance crew on scene to activate the helicopter to a semi-rural property 25 minutes' flight away. A 75-year-old man has collapsed in his living room and cardiopulmonary resuscitation (CPR) is in progress.

Incident D

An ongoing incident has been brought to your attention. A car has been struck by a van on a motorway 25 minutes rotary-wing flight time from the PHRM service base. Information is that one person is dead at the scene and 2 others are trapped one with severe abdominal pain and an SBP of 90 mmHg and the other with a reduced GCS and respiratory distress.

Question 22.1

Discuss key points in the allocation of physician-based PHRM team resources to these incidents.

Discussion 22.1

Incident A

This sounds fairly straightforward and would justify the immediate activation of the PHRM team. A few pointers suggest a significant incident has occurred:
- Multiple phone calls have been made to the emergency services.
- A motorcyclist is involved, suggesting significant mechanism.
- Loss of consciousness has been reported by passers-by.

However, more information should be sought even after activation and, if possible, a call back to one of the people who reported the incident should occur. In this way, it is possible to ask further questions to assess the situation. For example, the motorcyclist may well be awake and alert now. If the witness saw the incident, you can gain valuable information on mechanism. After the conversation, it will be easier to decide whether to continue with the activation or to stand the team down. However, be cautious of altering tasking decisions before the first ambulance resource on-scene provides updated clinical information.

Incident B

The tasking of PHRM teams for pre-hospital incidents is not without risk. The two biggest causes of fatal air medical incidents are night flying and flying in poor weather (Aherne et al 2019, Greene 2009) (see also Case 42). As the clinical coordinator you need to accept responsibility for tasking the aircraft in such conditions and are duty-bound to investigate any potential call-out to ensure air medical tasking is appropriate. Clearly, the final decision concerning flight safety rests with the pilot. If the pilot is aware of the nature of the task (e.g. a 'seriously injured child'), it may impact on their decision making with regards to risk versus benefit.

In this instance, tasking the aircraft 'just in case' is inappropriate. The information in this particular scenario is sufficiently vague to warrant waiting for a situation report (sit-rep) from the local ambulance crew when it arrives. Such decisions should be audited as part of the PHRM service clinical governance framework.

Incident C

The patient in this scenario is currently in circulatory arrest but with attempts at resuscitation in progress. In the absence of a return of spontaneous circulation (ROSC), the chances of the PHRM team value adding to this scenario is slim. Realistically, the helicopter will not be at the scene for over 30 minutes. If the patient is still in cardiac arrest by this time further attempts at resuscitation are likely to be futile. If the patient does have ROSC, there is a reasonable expectation to activate depending on other external factors (weather, resources, etc.).

Activation has been requested by ambulance personnel on-scene. In many PHRM service models, this would lead to automatic activation of a PHRM team. In this case, a direct call to the ambulance team on-scene may provide an opportunity to obtain a clinical update, give clinical advice and explain the rationale for not tasking at this time. You may be able to give advice that may alleviate the concerns of your colleagues. Alternatively, there may be other resources nearby that have extended skills and who could be tasked to assist. It may even be appropriate to decide with the team on-scene when to cease further attempts at CPR. ROSC with evidence of myocardial infarction may lead to the requirement for expedient patient retrieval. Rapid patient movement for urgent percutaneous re-perfusion techniques (such as balloon angioplasty) is increasingly common. If available, mechanical CPR devices may be of benefit to allow transfer to nearby medical facilities.

While not appropriate in this case, in highly evolved PHRM service models with access to staff with the requisite skill mix and equipment, select patient groups may benefit from the pre-hospital establishment of extracorporeal CPR.

Incident D

Physician-based PHRM services should have a system for immediate activation or 'rapid response' of the team on reliable initial information alone. This is particularly important for trauma. In the PHRM environment, information can be variable and inaccurate so there should be the ability to 'stand down' the PHRM team should further relevant information be received. Examples of some immediate activation criteria are detailed below:

- Multiple casualty scenarios.
- Ejection from vehicle in MVA.
- Fatality in same incident.
- Fall from >3 metres.
- Prolonged entrapment.
- Limb amputation.

This incident constitutes an immediate activation. From the initial information, there are two critical patients (at least). Assuming the PHRM team has been activated as an immediate dispatch, there is now the opportunity for additional PHRM resources to attend if available. Some PHRM services will have the ability to add a senior clinician to the response team or send a second team if available. Such taskings should only occur as part of a predefined process led by the clinical coordination team and should not be at the discretion of the operational team or the senior resource.

Key points
• When tasking the PHRM team to a presumed time-critical incident, immediate dispatch may be appropriate, despite incomplete clinical information. • Time of day, weather, type of incident and skills required on-scene are all part of the decision-making process when tasking physician-led teams, especially on aeromedical platforms.

References

Aherne B, Zhang C, Chen W, Newman D. Systems safety risk analysis of fatal night helicopter emergency medical service accidents. Aerosp Med Hum Perform 2019; 90:396–404. doi: 10.3357/AMHP.5180.2019.

Greene J. Rising helicopter crash deaths spur debate over proper use of air transport. Ann Emerg Med 2009; 53(3):15A–17A.

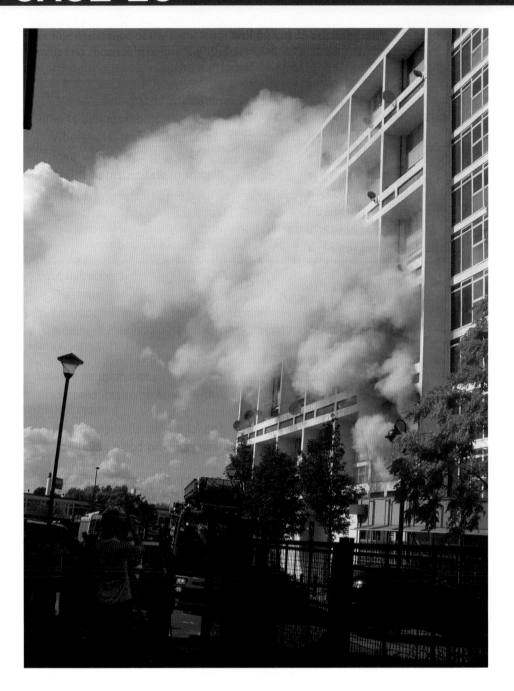

Incident

The tasking agency receives numerous calls reporting multiple explosions in a crowded urban shopping complex and housing development. No other information is available. The PHRM team is activated as part of a multiagency response.

On arrival you are confronted by the image above. You are the first medical team on-scene.

Relevant information

- **PHRM team transport options:** Rotary-wing aircraft.
- **Additional resources:** Initial Fire & Rescue Services only.
- **Retrieval options:** Two major trauma hospitals 10–20 minutes by air. Five regional hospitals at variable distances in the area.
- **Other:** Large urban city, population 4 million.

Question 23.1

How will you deal with this situation?

Question 23.2

What structure will you follow to ensure adequate scene management?

Discussion 23.1

This question concerns the immediate reaction to major incidents. The medical response to major incidents requires a dedicated structured system allowing key participants to operate within a standardised framework. Medical staff who may be involved in major incidents should undertake initial training in this system, followed by regular (e.g. annual) exercises. The Police and Fire & Rescue Service should be aware of what system the medical response will use, to avoid confusion. Major incident medical management and support (MIMMS) is one such method, but there are other systems that can be followed.

In providing rapid response in the urban environment, it is not unusual for the PHRM team to be first on-scene in such an incident and it is likely that the PHRM physician will be the first doctor on-scene. In this situation, the doctor becomes the Medical Incident Commander (MIC), and the paramedic becomes Ambulance Incident Commander (AIC). The team should have tabards labelled MIC and AIC for this purpose. The first teams of the other emergency services (Fire & Rescue and Police) to arrive, will likewise become the respective incident commanders. This nucleus of four constitutes the initial tactical or silver command for the incident and they must remain in contact throughout the incident. As time progresses, it may be appropriate for the initial tactical commanders to be replaced by more experienced personnel.

If arriving by air, the PHRM team has the opportunity to assess the scene from above (see Case 1). Digital photos or even a sketch taken from the air could be useful later.

The scene of a major incident will be stressful and chaotic, and passing accurate information to the clinical coordinator and subsequently to off-site commanders (e.g. Gold) is critical. As first clinician on-scene you will need to pass on what you see to the clinical coordinator in a lucid and cogent fashion. Do not assume that someone else has already done this. The PHRM team leader should radio or telephone the clinical coordinator (or even the emergency services standard number) and state that they are declaring a major incident. This will secure the attention of the call-taker (who should have received training in this area), who can then focus on the situation and should be ready thereafter to receive an information summary. The mnemonic 'METHANE' offers a good method for remembering the initial approach to major incidents (see the box on the next page).

For example:

'Ambulance control, this is team alpha on scene. We are declaring a major incident' (pause)

'Long message to follow' (pause)

'My exact location is the corner of Marble Street and Fitzroy Avenue in the city centre. There has been an explosion in a crowded shopping and residential complex with potential fire and further explosion hazards. Access and egress are currently possible through Fitzroy Avenue. I estimate number of casualties to be over 100 and we require fire, police and bomb squad, and further ambulance assistance. Can you repeat?'

Ensure the information has been taken correctly and that the call-taker has your contact number.

Having the confidence to declare a major incident so early and with incomplete information will not be easy so it is important that PHRM teams are adequately trained in this area. It is better to stand down a major incident declaration later than to delay an appropriate declaration. Declaring a 'major incident standby' (see Case 24) is also an option in this situation.

An initial approach to major incidents (METHANE)

M – major incident–declare.

E – exact location.

T – type of incident.

H – hazards (present and potential).

A – access and egress.

N – number of casualties.

E – emergency response (present and required).

Discussion 23.2

The key now is that the MIC and AIC are able to control the scene. Becoming involved in direct patient care must be avoided as the MIC/AIC need to be overall in command and able to allocate resources as they arrive. This can be challenging, but is imperative if the scene is to remain under control. MIMMS has another mnemonic for the MIC to describe the sequence of events ('CSCATTT').

CSCATTT mnemonic for sequence of events

C – Command and control.

S – Safety.

C – Communications.

A – Assessment of scene.

T – Triage.

T – Treatment.

T – Transfer.

Command and control in a major incident should be 'vertical'. A strategic (gold) command should be set up to deal directly with the tactical (silver) command (i.e. the MIC). In turn, the MIC should allocate forward (bronze) commanders to begin the triage stage of the incident.

Scene safety is paramount, and the MIC must liaise with fire and police services to establish the level of risk. As more ambulance personnel arrive, the AIC can delegate this to a dedicated safety officer. The police will have overall command of the scene, and, at sites of presumed terrorist attacks, it is likely that special police units or the military may be involved. The MIC and the police authorities should work together to balance the potentially competing priorities of the need for medical assessment and treatment versus the broader risks of a dynamic scene and the need to preserve scene evidence.

Communications are critical to successful management of major incidents. Subsequent debriefs of major incidents usually highlight communications as a point of failure. Mobile phones, radios and landlines are all fallible during such events, and due to system overload, many plans will include the use of runners and cyclists, as the most effective means of communications. Using a voice-recording device, app or scribe allows contemporaneous notes to be made. This is important as after a major incident, there will be a detailed examination of decision making. All personnel must try to adhere to the formal reporting/communications mechanisms, even if some aspects seem trivial at the time. It is essential that information is passed up the chain of command (e.g. bronze reports to silver and silver reports to gold).

Assessment of the scene is important for the MIC, and, at this point, they should be getting a better idea of numbers and types of injuries, and assessing the need for more PHRM teams. If the MIC is to request more teams, they should avoid taking them from receiving hospitals. Likewise, requesting resources (e.g. O-negative blood) from receiving hospitals should be avoided.

Tasks for MIC
Make accurate casualty estimates.
Set up a scene plan.
Allocate arriving staff.
Alert potential receiving hospitals (usually via gold command).
Assess requirements for more resources.
Communicate continuously with gold command.
Care for self and team.

Triage is often the defining aspect of medical treatment in major incidents and much emphasis is placed on triaging and labelling the injured. The cornerstones of triage are the triage sieve and, later on, the triage sort. In the urban environment, the casualties may only ever get the triage sieve and it is crucial that triage is repeated to avoid unexpected deterioration later.

An example of a triage sieve, sort and a mock site plan can be found in Appendix 8.

Treatment and transfer are more familiar options for the PHRM team, but limitation of resources may mean that optimal treatment cannot occur for all patients. For example,

111

with four critically injured patients, all needing advanced airway management, it may be better to evacuate all patients immediately rather than trying to stabilise just one, and delay the evacuation of the other casualties. Once additional resources arrive on-scene, there is increased potential for managing multiple critically ill patients and this can occur in a 'casualty clearing station', under the direction of a dedicated casualty clearing doctor.

The role of air medical resources (e.g. helicopters) in such incidents is to support the medical teams, including deployment of additional teams and delivery of supplies. Use of the helicopter for evacuating trauma patients (usually one at a time) is resource intensive and unlikely to be the best use of staff or equipment unless the incident involves long distances or decompensated infrastructure.

Following a major incident, it is important for all team members to debrief. Team members should document their version of events as it is inevitable that later they will be asked to provide detailed statements about the day.

Key points

- Use 'METHANE' to deliver required information in a controlled fashion.
- The 'CSCATTT' highlights the order of actions at a major incident.
- Communications frequently fail at major incidents, so it is important to have a back-up plan.
- PHRM teams who may be involved in major incidents should be familiar with and trained in local major incident response plans.

Additional reading

Advanced Life Support Group. Major Incident Medical Management and Support (MIMMS), 3rd ed. Wiley, 2011.

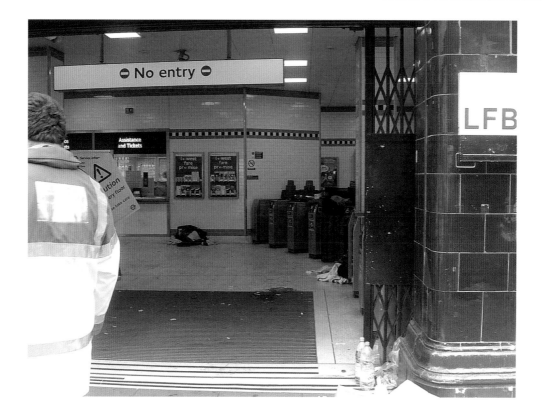

Incident

The tasking agency has received reports of multiple persons collapsed in an underground train station during evening 'rush hour'. No other information is available. The PHRM team is activated as part of a multiagency response.

You are the second clinical team on-scene, a land ambulance having already arrived. A crew member tells you his colleagues went down the escalator 5 minutes ago and reported 'several collapsed persons'. The remaining crewman has called for the Fire & Rescue Service.

Relevant information

- **PHRM team transport options:** Rapid response road vehicle.
- **Additional resources:** Fire & Rescue Service en route. One land ambulance on-scene.
- **Retrieval options:** Three regional hospitals approximately 20 minutes by road.
- **Other:** Monday 17:30. Ambient conditions: Windy 15°C (59°F).

Question 24.1

What are your initial thoughts about this scene?

Question 24.2

After a few minutes, the ambulance officer surfaces and collapses and his colleague runs to help him. What do you do now?

Question 24.3

After the arrival of more resources, what are the key points relevant to the medical management of a chemical incident (or any chemical, biological, radiological, nuclear [CBRN] incident)?

Discussion 24.1

With the information given, the traditional pre-hospital plan stops at safety. Several immediate questions should be considered as outlined below.

Is the scene safe?

This scene cannot be assumed to be safe. There are several warning signs, but most conspicuous is the total absence of people in what should be a busy scene. Where are the commuters, the staff, etc.? Some emergency services have adopted a '3 strikes' rule. This is a technique to alert staff to potential CBRN incidents in public places and applies where there is no obvious cause for the collapsed persons (e.g. trauma):

- One person collapsed – approach as normal.
- Two persons collapsed – approach with extreme caution.
- Three or more persons collapsed – do not approach, return to vehicle and call for assistance.

Should I investigate further?

Entry into such a scene could leave the team contaminated or affected by a potential agent. The safest approach is to speak to the remaining ambulance crewperson and try to get more information. Ask whether they are worried about a CBRN incident and ask if they have notified the Fire & Rescue Service of their concerns. Try to contact their colleague on the radio or mobile phone, or ask ambulance control to try.

Is this a major incident?

This is at least a potential major incident and the local system should have the facility for PHRM teams to declare a 'major incident standby'. As in a declared major incident, the PHRM team leader should give a METHANE report (see Case 23), with appropriate information. This gives the opportunity for the emergency services to prepare for a disaster without mobilising all resources. For example, a gold control room may be activated and the local hospitals would be advised to activate their own major incident standby plans. In addition, there may be local specialist response teams who can be rapidly activated to help with scene assessment.

What do I do now?

If you have declared a major incident standby, then you will have explained your concerns, specifically about CBRN issues. Make sure the call-taker has understood this and that an appropriately equipped rescue team and the Police are on their way. The PHRM team should take an upwind position and await the arrival of the team. Try to prevent anybody else from entering the scene in the meantime.

Discussion 24.2

With this information, the situation has completely changed. Any assumption that this was a routine call-out should now have passed, and the team should declare a major incident, using a METHANE report as previously discussed. Both ambulance crew members are now contaminated and must not be approached without adequate PPE. The PHRM team will need to try and maintain scene control verbally, and should try calling to the ambulance crew members to tell them help is on its way. Any attempt to help your ambulance colleagues will lead to contamination of your team. If this occurs, it will preclude the PHRM team from being an incident resource and will also generate extra patients who will need decontamination and medical assessment by someone else. The situation could rapidly deteriorate if more people begin to surface from the station, and the PHRM team should accept that they may not be able to stop contaminated persons trying to leave the scene. The PHRM team's role until the arrival of Police and CBRN teams is to provide information and communication.

Discussion 24.3

Major incident management

The system for dealing with this incident is similar to a standard major incident (see Case 23) and the CBRN status should not alter the order of the 'CSCATTT'.

Decontamination (see also Appendix 8)

Little treatment is feasible until the patients are decontaminated, so the PHRM team should stand by (or assist, if requested) while the Fire & Rescue teams set up a decontamination zone. Colloquially, the areas are known as 'hot zone' (contaminated), 'warm zone' (part decontamination) and 'cold zone' (fully decontaminated).

It is unusual for any medical team to be required in the 'hot zone' and uncommon for teams to enter the 'warm zone'. Certain PHRM teams, including physician-based teams, should have received specialist training for operations in the 'hot/warm zone'. Even if trained, PHRM teams must not enter without the Fire & Rescue team leader's authorisation. All persons entering these zones require logging in and out, and accurate recording of time spent in the zone. The benefit of entering the contaminated zone in suitable PPE and attempting to treat patients under such imposing physical conditions should be weighed against using this time to prepare a well-organised casualty clearing station in the 'cold zone'.

Treatment

Basic knowledge of the toxicology of chemicals commonly used for military or terrorist activities may give some assistance in identifying the causative agent. For example, patients with seizures, pinpoint pupils and hypersalivation would suggest organophosphate toxicity. In addition, there are commercially available detectors that can identify common agents (and radioactivity) that will almost certainly arrive with the back-up resources. Whatever the causative agent is, it is unlikely that the PHRM team will have enough drugs and equipment to treat more than a handful of patients, and urgent additional supplies would be needed. Many countries have stockpiles of equipment and antidotes for such a disaster. For example, the UK operates a 'pod' system whereby dozens of equipment pods containing antidotes and other medical 'kits' are strategically placed around the country.

A full debrief should occur after such an incident and accurate documentation is essential.

Key points
• The principles of major incident management do not change in CBRN events.
• Scene control is difficult and the PHRM team must liaise promptly with the Police, Fire & Rescue Service and local specialist response teams.
• Entry into the hot and warm zones must be strictly controlled. Medical personnel are rarely required to enter.

Additional reading

Advanced Life Support Group. Major Incident Medical Management and Support (MIMMS), 3rd ed. Wiley, 2011.

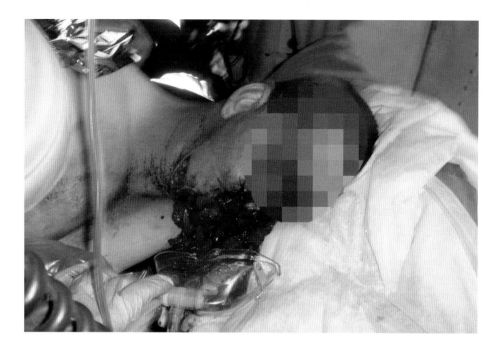

Incident

A 30-year-old male has sustained a self-inflicted shotgun wound to the face on a remote rural property.

Relevant information

- **PHRM team transport options:** Fixed-wing turbo prop aircraft. Two-stretcher capacity.
- **Additional resources:** Nil.
- **Retrieval options:** Major trauma hospital (nearest facility) 2 hours and 15 minutes by air (including additional road transfer).
- **Other:** Dirt landing strip 1 km (0.6 miles) from patient location.

Question 25.1

What factors will you consider when deciding on a retrieval plan of care?

Clinical information

Clinical assessment reveals the following:
- Alert, intermittently agitated, following commands.
- Airway variable (clear on sitting forward/semi-obstructed in left lateral position).
- Moderate facial bleeding.
- Lung fields clear.
- RR 18.
- P 112.
- BP 110/70 mmHg.
- SaO$_2$ 94% with oxygen held near.

Question 25.2
How would you secure the airway?

Discussion 25.1
The traumatised and difficult airway presents a challenging emergency clinical situation, especially in the relatively isolated and resource-depleted pre-hospital and retrieval environment. The critical decision required is whether the PHRM team should establish a definitive airway before departure, or support the airway and observe the patient en route to a definitive facility. When making this decision, there are a number of factors to consider. Some of these are outlined below and can be considered in terms of patient factors, team factors, transport platform factors, as well as assistance and advice.

Patient factors
Airway
Current
- Is there postural variability in airway patency? If so, such a precarious airway will be difficult to assess or support during the return journey.

Trend over time
- Has there been relative stability in airway patency for a prolonged period of time? A deteriorating airway will require early intervention.

Neck anatomy
- Are the landmarks for a surgical airway preserved?

Breathing
Respiratory pattern and work of breathing
- Aspiration of blood, tissue or foreign material, in addition to partial upper airway obstruction will significantly increase the patient's work of breathing.

Aspiration risk
- Is the patient struggling with ongoing bleeding or secretions?

Circulation
Haemorrhage control issues
- Facial trauma is often associated with brisk haemorrhage. General anaesthesia and a secure airway may allow for temporising haemorrhage control. Note that initial neuromuscular blockade may transiently worsen haemorrhage and the team should be prepared for this. Direct pressure will be easier with a secure airway.

Disability
Mental state and patient compliance
- Is the patient calm and compliant or agitated? It should be assumed that the patient has made a significant attempt to end his life and that his mental state is unstable. Pain, anxiety and hypoxia are likely to be compounding factors during transport. The risk to the air crew in this situation should be considered (see Case 40).

Team factors

Clinician experience
All PHRM team members should be trained and experienced in the management of the difficult airway and be proficient in the performance of a surgical airway.

Available equipment

Adequate suction will be vital. As the scene is some distance from the aircraft, oxygen supplies may be limited. Advanced airway equipment, including a range of laryngoscope blades, tracheal tubes, airway adjuncts and equipment for the performance of a surgical airway, are mandatory.

Transport platform factors

Access to airway during transport

Stretcher-loading configurations and restricted cabin areas that do not allow for clear access to the patient's neck and airway will profoundly limit any in-flight intervention.

Transport times and multiple transfers

The longer the transport time and the greater the number of transfers, the higher the chance of patient deterioration. This includes transfers from air medical to land-based platforms. It should be noted that the landing site is 1 km (0.6 miles) from the patient and that the mode of transport to and from the landing site will need to be considered. In such remote areas, civilian vehicles may be the only option. The tasking agency may be best placed to address such logistical issues while the team prepares for departure.

Noise/communications

The team must be able to communicate via a voice-activated or 'open microphone' communications system and should plan in advance for the possibility of dealing with an in-flight airway emergency.

Lighting

There must be adequate lighting if emergent, in-flight intervention is to be possible. Always communicate with the pilot before illuminating the cabin, especially in a medical emergency.

Assistance and advice

A physician experienced in emergency airway management

Advice and clinical direction from such a resource, accessed via the clinical coordination centre, may assist and support the team in both the decision-making process and the performance of any planned intervention. In the end, the best assessment of the situation and the most appropriate plan can only be made by the team faced with the immediate challenge. The PHRM team must therefore have the requisite experience, skills and knowledge. Telemedicine has enabled this level of clinical oversight.

Given the distance to a major trauma hospital, the patient's relatively precarious airway patency, early signs of increased work of breathing and ongoing haemorrhage and agitation, the securing of a definitive airway pre-departure is preferred. With shorter transport times, road transport options, nearby hospital facilities with specialist personnel and equipment (allowing for a staged retrieval) and more physiologically stable patients, a conservative 'support and observe during transport' plan may have been appropriate. In these latter circumstances, the cricothyroid membrane should be marked, equipment made immediately available and a clear plan verbalised to all team members (including the pilot).

Discussion 25.2

Techniques available to secure such an airway in the isolated out-of-hospital environment should not necessarily be compared with the relatively controlled and semi elective environment of a large tertiary hospital. While techniques such as awake fibre-optic intubation and gaseous induction have been used effectively in pre-hospital and retrieval situations, such techniques are highly equipment- and operator-dependent. Regardless, any technique that requires oropharyngeal manipulation is likely to be challenging and to significantly increase clot disruption and bleeding. Given the upper airway disruption and likely inability to ventilate the patient with a self-inflating bag valve mask should intubation prove difficult, a 'standard' rapid-sequence induction should be approached with caution. Despite the predicted difficulty and significant bleeding, an alternative option may be the 'awake look' with adequate topical anaesthesia. Operator experience will guide the final decision here.

A surgical cricothyroidotomy under local anaesthetic is the authors' preferred approach. The neck (and specifically the laryngeal structure) is preserved and accessible. With analgesia, reassurance (and potentially low doses of a sedative agent such as a benzodiazepine or ketamine), the patient could be suitably positioned. The cricothyroid membrane should be marked and anaesthetised using local anaesthetic with adrenaline. A small amount of local anaesthetic can be slowly injected into the upper trachea at this time to reduce coughing and discomfort that may occur with the ensuing manipulation. Adequate pre-oxygenation should occur and a clear plan should be verbalised to the team.

The technique of surgical cricothyroidotomy is described in Appendix 1.1.5.

Key points

- Carefully consider patient factors, team factors and transport options before every tasking.
- The surgical airway should be considered early and not left as a final option in peri-arrest scenarios.

SECTION B

Retrieval theme

Foreword to the Retrieval Section

Equity. In its simplest terms, Pre-Hospital and Retrieval Medicine is about ensuring our communities and patients have equity of access to high level clinical care, irrespective of where they live. Our ultimate goal, at both a system and professional practice level, is to provide the safest, highest quality patient care in transit, providing patients timely access to life changing and life saving treatment options.

It doesn't matter which service we work for, the vehicle platform we work on, the colour of of our uniforms or the country we live in, patients expect and deserve to be transported and cared for as safely as possible. They trust us to provide this in the challenging out of hospital environment. Fundamental to these principles, our standards of care require to be contemporary and our clinical and aviation personnel trained to the highest level.

I have had the privilege of working with the original authors over many years. Their combined experience and expertise bring together a spectrum of Pre-Hospital and Retrieval Medicine cases that provides important learnings and reflections for practitioners of all levels. I have no doubt that this compilation will have an enduring positive contribution to improving the standard of patient care in the Pre-Hospital and Retrieval environment.

Dr Mark Elcock PSM
MBChB FACEM FRCEM
Chair, ACEM Conjoint Committee Pre-Hospital & Retrieval Medicine
Executive Director, Aeromedical Retrieval & Disaster Management Branch, Queensland Department of Health, Australia
A/Prof (Adjunct) College of Public Health, Medicine and Veterinary Sciences, James Cook University, Australia

Incident

A 56-year-old woman has collapsed and presented by ambulance to a regional hospital without on-site neurosurgical support. On admission, she was deeply unconscious and required intubation and ventilation in the emergency department. Examination findings at that time revealed bilateral brisk reflexes, hypertension (BP 180/100 mmHg) and small, non-reactive pupils. A CT head scan has now been arranged, which will require the patient to be transported to the radiology department, which is located on another level of the hospital building.

Relevant information

- **Additional local resources:** 8-bed specialist staffed intensive care unit (ICU), anaesthetic support services.
- **Regional resources:** Dedicated pre-hospital and retrieval service with clinical coordination and tertiary neurosurgical centre 300 km (185 miles) away.

Question 26.1

Outline your plan for safe patient transfer to and from the radiology department.

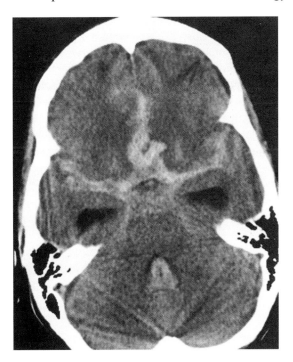

Question 26.2

What does the CT head scan reveal? What should now occur?

Question 26.3

Outline how the interhospital transfer of this patient to the neurosurgical receiving hospital 300 km (185 miles) away differs from the previously required intrahospital transfer for CT head scan.

Discussion 26.1

Intrahospital transport of critically ill patients occurs frequently. Transports are usually required to facilitate critical investigations and interventions, or to move the patient from one critical-care area (e.g. emergency department) to another (e.g. ICU). Critically ill patients with minimal or no physiologic reserve undergoing such transports are at risk of clinical deterioration, and adverse events are well reported (Haydar et al 2020).

To minimise potential adverse events, a structured approach for all intrahospital critical-care transports is required. Intrahospital transport guidelines and protocols may vary regionally. A broad outline is detailed below.

Risk–benefit assessment

Patients undergoing invasive ventilation and who require high levels of intensive care support should not be transported for non-urgent interventions or investigations. In this scenario, the need for urgent imaging, potential intervention and ongoing care outside the emergency department clearly supports the requirement for patient transport.

Patient stabilisation

- Although acute threats to life have been addressed, a definitive diagnosis is unclear. Further investigation is therefore required before any therapeutic options (if any) are considered. Thus, in this scenario, patient transport for definitive investigation can be considered part of the stabilisation process and should occur without delay. Prolonged periods of time in the emergency department performing invasive procedures and attempting complete physiologic normalisation are not appropriate.
- Clinical reassessment should occur swiftly, systematically, and, whenever possible, with the patient already supported by the equipment that will be used during transport.
- The airway should be checked and secured, ventilation and oxygenation optimised, adequate and patent vascular access secured, and drainage devices measured and emptied. Sedation and analgesic requirements should be addressed and any drugs required for transport (including additional infused agents) pre-drawn and labelled for immediate use.
- Neuroprotective care should be provided, despite the current undifferentiated nature of the presentation (see Case 10). Specifically, hypotension, progressive hypertension, hypoxia, hypercarbia or hypocarbia and hyperglycaemia should be actively managed.
- Ensure that the patient's clinical record remains with the team caring for the patient at all times.

Communication and coordination

Handover of care

This will be required if the intrahospital transport team are not the current treating team. Clinical handover should be between nominated team leaders and be clear, concise, structured and documented (see Case 18).

Team brief

- The assembled team (see below) should reassess the patient's clinical condition, the need for transport and predicted clinical requirements.

- Hospital-based protocols and pre-defined checklists (see Appendix 4) assist significantly and avoid the oversight of simple but critical requirements, such as adequate oxygen and available suction for the transport.

Receiving unit(s)

- The initial receiving unit will be the radiology department. Communication should confirm an agreed time for the investigation. This will allow the team to arrive with enough time to transfer the patient safely into the CT scanner.
- Following the investigation, consider again the destination of the patient, which may vary dependent on the CT findings. Possibilities include the emergency department, the ICU or an operating theatre. All relevant units should therefore be made aware of the pending transport and investigation, as well as the working diagnosis and current clinical plan.

Specialist clinicians

If not already involved, a senior neurosurgical doctor and radiologist should be contacted.

Transport route(s)

This should be decided prior to departure. Where possible, the route should avoid common public access areas, lifts and clinically isolated, poorly lit, exposed, narrow or cramped areas (limiting 360-degree patient access).

Contingency plan(s)

As a team, consider and verbalise the worst-case scenario. Plan how you will respond should this occur. This may include a plan to move to the nearest appropriate area for resuscitation, which may vary during the journey.

Communication devices

A fully charged, dedicated and serviceable phone should be carried during the transport. This will be required should there be a need to call for urgent assistance, or in order to facilitate ongoing clinical communication. Personal mobile phones may be considered back-up devices.

Staff

Clinical

A team consisting of at least two healthcare professionals should be free from other duties. Both team members should be thoroughly familiar with the transport process, equipment and environment. The team should possess the requisite skills and knowledge to independently manage critically ill patients in transit and to deal with anticipated emergencies.

Non-clinical

Assistance with safe patient, trolley and equipment movement will be required. Hospital orderlies or security staff are often part of the team and should be included in relevant briefs and contingency plans.

Equipment

Transport equipment should be:

- Regularly checked and serviceable
- Fully charged, with power cords accessible to facilitate use of mains power in the event of delay
- Lightweight, robust and ideally standardised throughout the hospital
- Securable in transit (not resting on the patient) but readily accessible

- Relevant to the clinical requirements of the patient and safe in the required area (e.g. magnetic resonance imaging)
- Dedicated for the transport (transport 'bridges' or gantries are commonly used).

In addition:

- Dedicated transport packs or boxes ensure safe carriage of consumable items, resuscitation equipment and drugs
- Equipment required for emergency airway management (e.g. bag valve mask, laryngoscope, airway devices and tracheal tubes) should be immediately available
- In this case, the available equipment in the radiology department should be clarified:
  - Does it meet the required standards, or will the patient need to remain on the transport equipment?
  - Are there compatible oxygen/air outlets or will ongoing portable oxygen be required?

Monitoring

- As a minimum, intubated and ventilated patients requiring intrahospital transport should have the following monitoring instituted:
  - Continuous waveform capnography
  - Continuous pulse oximetry
  - Continuous invasive or intermittent non-invasive BP
  - Continuous 3-lead ECG.
- Ideally, a cardiac-monitoring device should also be able to provide cardiac defibrillation and external cardiac-pacing capacity. If not, an additional device that does provide these functions should be secured and available in transit.
- Patients requiring transport with more advanced monitoring in situ should be considered on a case-by-case basis. For example, ongoing ICP monitoring is critical to ensure avoidance of profound unmonitored falls in cerebral perfusion pressure in an ICU patient with a severe head injury, whereas pulmonary artery pressure monitoring may be excluded from the transport requirements in the haemodynamically stable patient.

Documentation and review

- Contemporaneous and concise documentation of the transport process is mandatory.
- An audit of all transports should occur on a regular basis and incidents or events should be captured within the hospital or transport unit's quality and safety framework (see Case 52).
- The initial and ongoing educational requirements of all staff involved in intrahospital transports should be addressed.

Discussion 26.2

The CT head scan reveals blood within the subarachnoid space with evidence of acute hydrocephalus. This is a neurosurgical emergency, which requires immediate consultation with a specialist neurosurgeon regarding ventricular decompression. The CT images will need to be viewed by the neurosurgeon at a distant location. A concise description of the historical events and the patient's current clinical condition should be provided. In this setting, even fixed and dilated pupils should be interpreted with caution as complete reversibility has been described (Scotter et al 2015).

The key question at this point relates to how to ensure ventricular decompression occurs as rapidly and safely as possible. There may be a surgeon other than a neurosurgeon at the referral centre with the clinical skills to perform such a procedure. With increasing use of telemedicine a specialist neurosurgeon can guide the local surgical team on how to perform certain time-critical, life saving procedures if appropriate. Rarely, the rapid transport of a neurosurgeon with appropriate equipment to the referral facility may be an option, although this may add significant delays to time to definitive care. In most instances, such cases will require emergency interhospital retrieval. Involving the medical coordinator and tasking agency to set up the teleconferencing is important to keep all parties in the loop.

Discussion 26.3

Like intrahospital transports, a structured approach will ensure potential adverse events are minimised and much of what is outlined above is applicable here. However, when compared with intrahospital transports, interhospital critical care medical retrieval may differ in terms of both logistical and clinical complexity.

Risk–benefit assessment

This assessment now includes aviation and other logistical considerations. For example: What is the weather like? Are the roads busy and congested? Which transport platforms are available? Are there any patient issues that would preclude non-pressurised air transport? (See Case 27.)

Patient stabilisation

Now that the diagnosis is clear and the therapeutic requirements are known, the required transport can again be seen as part of the therapeutic process.

Prior to the arrival of the retrieval team, the referral hospital should ideally establish invasive arterial access for continuous pressure monitoring. An indwelling urinary catheter and nasogastric tube should also be placed. Central venous access will ultimately be required if vasoactive infused agents are required, although these may be administered peripherally in the short term (Cardenas-Garcia 2015). Neuroprotective strategies should be established and maintained.

Communication and coordination

- All communications should occur through the clinical coordination centre.
- Early advice to the referral facility is a key component of this process.
- The referral and receiving destinations, retrieval team(s) and transport agencies require clear communication, including the rapid notification of delays or variations to the transport plan.
- Given the required transport distance of 300 km (185 miles) and the clinical requirements of the patient, rapid-rotary wing transport is preferred. However, the final decision of the most appropriate transport platform will be influenced by a large number of variables (see Case 27).

Staff

Clinical

- There should be a dedicated PHRM team trained, audited and governed in the clinical, logistical and aviation aspects of retrieval medicine.

- The team should be adequately attired and have appropriate PPE for air medical operations.

Non-clinical

- The air crew or road ambulance personnel are key stakeholders in the retrieval process. PHRM services actively integrate with such personnel to develop high-functioning, multidisciplinary extended teams.

Equipment

In addition to the issues discussed in the first part of this case (Question 26.1), equipment for air medical transport (including packs and monitoring devices) must be approved for such use, able to be adequately secured during transport (while remaining accessible), robust enough to withstand the out-of-hospital and aviation environments, and ergonomically designed to ensure safe carriage and loading. The total weight of all the medical equipment should be kept to a minimum. A suggested equipment list can be found in Appendix 2.1.

Sufficient battery capacity should be ensured to comfortably last the entire trip. Oxygen requirements at altitude can be anticipated (see Case 27) and total oxygen required should be carefully calculated (see below). It is good practice to double the anticipated battery and oxygen requirements to cater for unexpected delays. Placement of the patient in a vacuum mattress should be considered if multiple stretcher moves are required during the retrieval in order to facilitate patient movement and minimise the risk of lines and tubes being dislodged.

Documentation and review

- Contemporaneous and concise documentation of the transport process is mandatory and should ideally be recorded electronically.
- Audit and quality assurance activities (including incident and event reporting) need to include the communication and coordination process, logistic and aviation considerations and patient outcomes, in addition to the clinical care delivered to the patient in transit (see Case 52). This may also be recorded electronically, ideally using the same platform used for contemporaneous medical notes.
- Regular multidisciplinary audit provides an effective whole-of-service tool with regard to meeting these audit and quality assurance requirements.
- Feedback both from and to the referral and receiving staff is an important additional consideration.

Oxygen requirements during transfer

$$2 \times \text{transport time in minutes} \times (MV \times FiO_2 + \text{ventilator driving gas})$$

MV = minute volume

FiO_2 = inspired oxygen fraction

Ventilator driving gas is dependent on ventilator make. Most modern ventilators do not use compressed oxygen for this purpose

(Note the transport time is doubled for safety)

Sample calculation for retrieval of 1-hour duration:

MV = 6 litres per minute

FiO_2 = 0.6

$$2 \times 60 \times (6 \times 0.6 + 0) =$$
$$120 \times 3.6 = 432 \text{ litres of oxygen}$$

Key points

- Critically ill patients are at risk of clinical deterioration while in transit between critical care areas, and a risk–benefit assessment is required when considering any patient transport.
- Risks can be minimised by applying a standardised approach to patient transfer.
- When considering inter-hospital transfer of critically ill or injured patients (retrieval), additional clinical and logistical consideration is required.

References

Cardenas-Garcia J, Schaub KF, Belchikov YG, et al. Safety of peripheral intravenous administration of vasoactive medication. J Hosp Med 2015; 10(9):581–585.

Haydar B, Baetzel A, Elliott A et al. Adverse events during intrahospital transport of critically ill children: a systematic review. Anesth Analg 2020; 131(4):1135–1145.

Scotter J, Hendrickson S, Marcus HJ, Wilson MH. Prognosis of patients with bilateral fixed dilated pupils secondary to traumatic extradural or subdural haematoma who undergo surgery: a systematic review and meta-analysis. Emerg Med J 2015; 32(8):654–659.

Additional reading

Appendix 4 – Transfer checklist.

Australasian College for Emergency Medicine, Australian and New Zealand College of Anaesthetists and College of Intensive Care Medicine of Australia and New Zealand. Guidelines for transport of critically ill patients. Author, 2015.

Evans C, Creaton A, Kennedy M. Oxford specialist handbook of retrieval medicine. Oxford University Press, 2016.

Intensive Care Society. Guidance on: the transfer of the critically ill adult. Author, 2019.

Lowe A, Hulme J. ABC of transfer and retrieval medicine. Wiley Blackwell, 2015.

Nathanson M H, Andrzejowski J, Dinsmore J, et al. Safer transfer of the brain-injured patient: trauma and stroke 2019: Guidelines from the Association of Anaesthetists and the Neuro Anaesthesia and Critical Care Society. Anaesthesia 2020; 75(2):234–246.

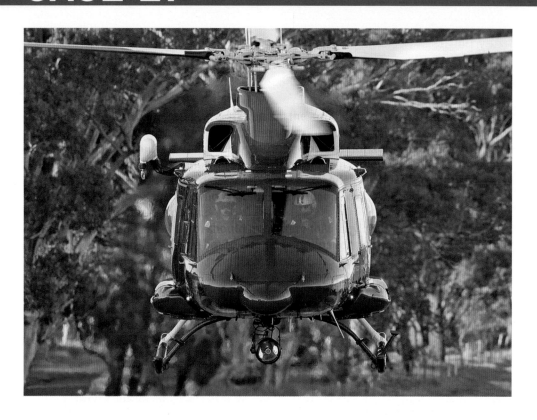

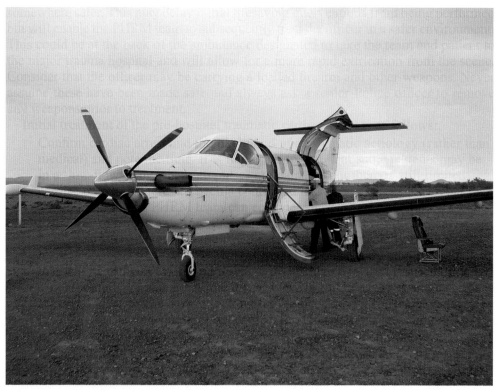

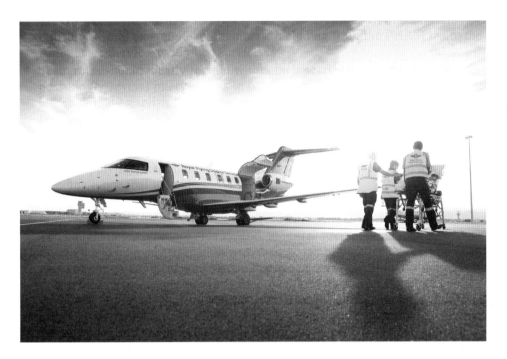

Incident

Following a fall from farm machinery, a 40-year-old female has an intracranial haemorrhage and spinal injuries and requires retrieval from a regional hospital. She is intubated and ventilated with the following ventilatory settings:

- Tidal volume 450 mL.
- RR 12 breaths per minute.
- Positive end expiratory pressure (PEEP) 5 cm H_2O.
- Inspired oxygen 28%.

Clinical information

- P 85.
- BP 140/80 mmHg.
- SaO_2 98%.

Relevant information

- **PHRM team transport options:** Fixed-wing turbo prop, fixed-wing jet and rotary-wing aircraft available.
- **Local resources:** One land ambulance.
- **Retrieval options:** Specialist quaternary neurosurgical and spinal hospital 370 km (230 miles) away.
- **Other:** Ambient conditions: Heavy rain 15°C (59°F).

Question 27.1

Discuss the key points of flight physiology.

Question 27.2

What are the key differences between the different types of fixed-wing and rotary-wing retrievals?

Question 27.3

Which transport platform would you choose in this scenario?

Discussion 27.1

Gas expansion

Boyle's Law, which relates to the expansion of gases, is the principal gas law to remember in the context of flight physiology. Essentially, gas will expand as altitude increases and atmospheric pressure decreases. As altitude decreases, the opposite occurs. Therefore, during an aeromedical evacuation, gas volume will vary. A change in altitude from sea level to 8000 feet (2500 metres) will expand an enclosed volume of gas by 35%. Relevant gas-filled structures that may be affected are listed in the box below. Slow changes in altitude can minimise the effects of gas expansion.

Gas-filled structures

Physiological body spaces
- Middle ears.
- Facial sinuses.
- Stomach and intestine.

Pathological body spaces
- Pneumothoraces.
- Intracranial air.
- Surgical wounds.
- Dental caries.
- Intravascular bubbles (see Case 46).

Equipment
- Tracheal tube cuffs.
- Pressure bags.
- Air in IV-fluid bags, giving sets or pressure-monitoring lines.
- Pneumatic or vacuum splints (the latter will lose rigidity at altitude).

Hypoxia

The relevant gas law in this instance is Dalton's Law. As altitude increases and atmospheric pressure decreases, the partial pressure of oxygen will fall at the alveolar interface unless supplemental oxygen is administered. A fall in alveolar oxygen partial pressure results in lower oxygen delivery to the tissues. Oxygen saturation for healthy adults will drop to around 94% at 6000–8000 feet (1800–2500 metres), which is the usual cabin pressure for commercial aircraft. This drop will be more significant in patients with underlying pulmonary or vascular disease, or conditions with reduced oxygen-carrying capacity (i.e. anaemia).

Oxygen requirements at altitude can be predicted (see box below). The administration of oxygen can usually be controlled by monitoring oxygen saturations or blood oxygen partial pressure via arterial blood gas assessment. Note that a patient requiring 70% inspired oxygen to avoid hypoxia at sea level would require 80% inspired oxygen at 4000 feet (1200 metres) to maintain a sea-level equivalent partial pressure of oxygen. Above 10,000 feet (3000 metres), the patient would become hypoxic even if the inspired oxygen concentration was 100%.

Relevant gas laws and oxygen requirements at altitude

Boyle's Law
- For a fixed amount of gas at a constant temperature, pressure and volume are inversely proportional (i.e. Pressure × Volume = constant).

Dalton's Law
- The total pressure exerted by a gaseous mixture is equal to the sum of the partial pressures of each individual component in a gas mixture.

Oxygen requirements at altitude
- (Current FiO_2 × barometric pressure 1) / (barometric pressure 2) = FiO_2 required.

FiO_2 = inspired oxygen fraction.
Barometric pressure 1 = current barometric pressure.
Barometric pressure 2 = barometric pressure at destination or altitude.

Management issues

In addition to administering supplemental oxygen, hypoxia can also be prevented by altering cabin pressure or flying below around 2000 feet (600 metres). On fixed-wing air ambulances, it is possible to fly with the cabin pressurised. This may be partial (e.g. to 8000 feet [2500 metres] equivalent even if the aircraft altitude is 35,000 feet [11,000 metres] or complete [sea-level cabin]). A sea-level cabin is usually possible if the anticipated cruising altitude is below 20,000 feet (6000 metres). Although cabin pressurisation will prevent gas expansion and hypoxia, overall aircraft performance is reduced (ground speed and range) and fuel use is increased. A brief discussion with the pilot will confirm cabin pressurisation feasibility. Cabin altitude should be documented on the medical notes. Remember, the patient's location may not be sea level, in which case, cabin pressure need only match that at the departure location (a 'ground-level cabin').

At altitudes below around 2000 feet (600 metres), it is unlikely that serious altitude-related problems will occur (including the often-feared complication of occult pneumothorax expansion). At higher altitudes (usually associated with longer transport times), close attention should be paid to the patient and the equipment affected by pressure changes. In the ventilated patient, any pneumothoraces must be checked for and may require drainage before departure dependent on peak altitude. A nasogastric tube should be passed to decompress the stomach. The tracheal tube cuff should be inflated to minimally occlusive volume at the altitude of departure, then checked with a manometer and adjusted accordingly, following ascent and descent (see Case 58). Although different techniques to minimise altitude-related variations in cuff pressure have been described, there is no evidence of effectiveness in reducing tracheal mucosal injury (Britton et al 2014).

Pneumatic splints can be affected by altitude, which may compromise limb perfusion. Conversely, vacuum splints or mattresses will lose stiffness at altitude. Air in intravenous fluid bags can expand at altitude and this may speed up flow, while the opposite applies on descent. Some older ventilators can be affected by altitude, with increases in certain parameters (e.g. tidal volume) occurring as barometric pressure falls; however, modern transport-specific ventilators will automatically compensate for altitude. Decompression illness is rare, only being an issue if an emergency loss of cabin pressure occurs at high altitudes (so-called explosive decompression). However, scuba diving 24 hours before a flight can lead to decompression sickness at commercial pressures of 6000–8000 feet (1875–2500 metres).

Other stresses of flight (that can affect patients and crew) include:

- Gravitational forces during turns, take-off and landing can cause transient haemodynamic compromise (e.g. by venous pooling). Patient position in the aircraft can help in this aspect (e.g. horizontal placement).
- Vibration forces, especially in rotary-wing aircraft, can affect the patient (e.g. clot disruption), passengers and equipment. Clinical examination is difficult, and monitors may be influenced by artifact.
- Turbulence can lead to motion sickness, fear and physical injury.
- Noise can be overt or covert (e.g. high-frequency jet turbines), both of which are debilitating in the short term (increased fatigue) and injurious in the long term (hearing loss). For this reason, hearing protection is mandatory for the PHRM team, and should be considered for the patient.
- Temperature in the cabin can usually be controlled but it is worth noting that external ambient temperature decreases by about 2°C (3.6°F) for each 1000 feet (300 metres) of altitude (the lapse rate).
- Humidity in the air decreases at altitude and can lead to dehydration.
- Confined space, poor lighting and limited mobility in the cabin make the delivery of clinical care challenging and should be mitigated where possible (e.g. pre-emptive access to equipment and drugs required in the event of clinical deterioration).

Discussion 27.2

Choosing how to transport a patient to hospital is heavily influenced by resource issues, patient condition, weather, geography and distance.

In general, road transport is preferred for distances less than 100 km (60 miles) as it is most resistant to the weather, and a road ambulance usually has a plentiful supply of medical equipment on board. Paradoxically, it can be quicker to do tasks within this 100 km radius by road, even when aeromedical resources are available, after factoring in the time taken to get the PHRM team airborne.

The differences between fixed-wing turboprop, jet and rotary-wing transfers are summarised below.

Differences between fixed-wing and rotary-wing transfers

Aircraft	Rotary-wing (Bell 412)	PC-12	PC-24 Jet
Speed	200–280 km/h (125–175 mph)	470 km/h (292 mph)	720 km/h (447 mph)
Useful range	240–320 km (150–200 miles) refuel stops likely	~1600 km (900 miles)* *range decreases with sea-level cabin, load >2 patients/1 team*	~2700 km (1500 miles)* *range decreases with sea-level cabin, load >1 patient/ 1 team*
Altitude	0–10,000 feet (0–3000 m) (unpressurised)	0–30,000 ft (can maintain sea level to 13,000 ft)	0–45,000 ft (can maintain sea level to 23,000 ft)
Fuel consumption	Uses 700lb fuel per hour	Uses 500lb fuel first hour, 400 lb/hr thereafter	Uses 1500 lb fuel first hour, 1000 lb/hr thereafter *(~double fuel for 1.5x speed)*
Response	2–10 minutes	20 mins if crew on base *(flight planning takes longer due to longer distance/weather considerations)*	20 mins if crew on base *(flight planning takes longer due to longer distance/ weather considerations)*
Flexible landing sites	Yes (can land at scene)	Airstrip required (1000 m length × 10–15 m wide)	Airstrip required (1200 m long × 18 m wide)
Useful for physical rescue	Yes	No	No
Secondary transfer required	Possibly but point-to-point transfers are possible	Yes	Yes
Weather affected	More frequently affected High temperature reduces range	Minimal (can fly above weather; fog can limit as requires 2000 m visibility)	Minimal (can fly higher above weather, fog less limiting – requires 800 m visibility as multiengine)
Vibration	Marked	Subtle	Subtle
Deck angle	N/A	6° takeoff/landing	15° takeoff/landing

Differences between fixed-wing and rotary-wing transfers—cont'd			
Aircraft	Rotary-wing (Bell 412)	PC-12	PC-24 Jet
Turbulence	Rare	Usually predictable	Usually predictable, less pronounced
Ability to work in cabin	Extremely limited	Constrained but possible	Less constrained with greater head clearance
Comms	GRN, satellite phone, 4G often accessible in-flight; Internal communication system (ICS) required in flight for effective communication	GRN, satellite phone Wifi capable, 4G often accessible in-flight; higher-speed internet possible with additional installed hardware and costly data	GRN, satellite phone Wifi capable, no 4G, higher-speed internet possible with additional installed hardware and costly data

Discussion 27.3

Based on the available information, the ideal platform in this scenario is fixed-wing. The distance to cover is quite long for a helicopter and refuel stops are likely. In addition, the fixed-wing aircraft will be able to fly above the poor weather. Finally, the working conditions in the fixed-wing cabin will be considerably better than in a helicopter cabin. The choice between jet and turbo prop in this instance will depend on availability, cost and, potentially, landing site. In this scenario, a turbo-prop aircraft would be adequate.

Key points
• Different retrieval platforms present variable benefits and limitations, both clinically and logistically.
• All available retrieval platforms should be considered by the PHRM team and the clinical coordination and tasking agency.
• Consider the impact of different transport platforms on both staff and patients.

Reference

Britton T, Blakeman T, Eggert J, et al. Managing endotracheal tube cuff pressure at altitude: a comparison of four methods. J Trauma Acute Care Surg 2014; 77(3):S240–S244.

Additional reading

Blumen IJ, Lemkin DL. Principles and direction of air medical transport. Air Medical Physicians Association, 2006.

Evans C, Creaton A, Kennedy M. Oxford specialist handbook of retrieval medicine. Oxford University Press, 2016.

King JC, Franklin RC, Robertson A, et al. Review article: primary aeromedical retrievals in Australia: an interrogation and search for context. Emerg. Med. Australas. 2019; 31(6):916–929.

Lowe A, Hulme J. ABC of transfer and retrieval medicine. Wiley Blackwell, 2015.

Teichman PG, Donchin Y, Kot RJ. International aeromedical evacuation. N. Engl. J. Med. 2007; 356(3):262–270.

Analyse images i–x and the incidents below.

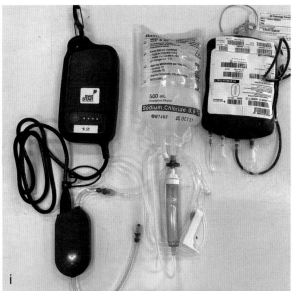

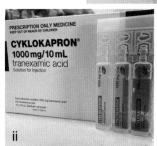

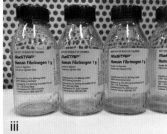

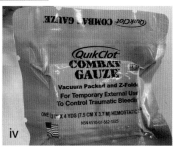

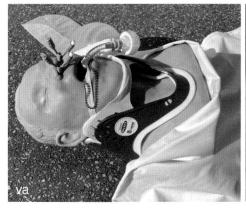

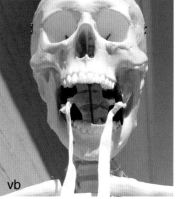

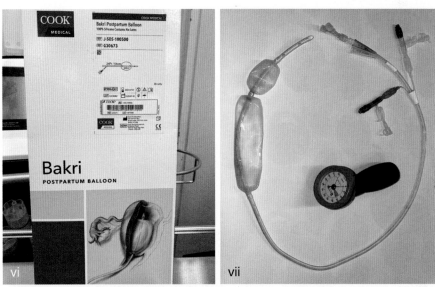

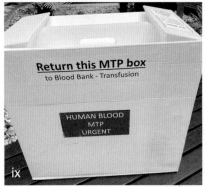

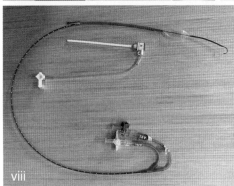

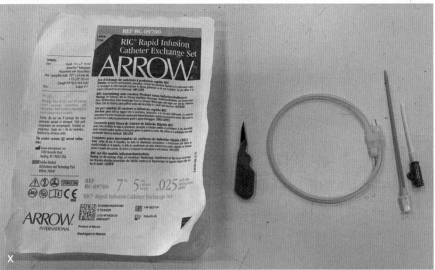

  i – Blood warmer
 ii – Ampoule of TXA
iii – Ampoule of Fib Conc (FC)
 iv – Haemostatic dressing
  v – Epistats and bite blocks
 vi – Bakri balloon
vii – Sengstaken tube
viii – Retrograde endovascular balloon occlusion of the aorta (REBOA) catheter
 ix – Massive transfusion pack (MTP) shipper
  x – Rapid infusion catheter RIC line

Relevant information

For each incident below, assume the patient is in a rural facility and the PHRM service has been tasked to assess, stabilise and transfer the case. All the above equipment is available on the PHRM base and can be safely transported to scene.

- **PHRM team transport options:** Rotary-wing aircraft.
- **Additional resources:** Rural facility nurses and single-handed rural doctor.
- **Retrieval options:** Quaternary centre with all sub-specialities: 35 minutes by air.
- **Other:** Weather clear 25°C (77°F).

  Discuss what items you would take to each incident and describe your initial management.

Incident A

A 30-year-old primiparous woman has just delivered a healthy child. Post delivery, she developed postpartum haemorrhage (PPH) and clinically deteriorated. Current observations are: P122, BP 82/45, GCS 15, ongoing significant bleeding PV.

Incident B

A 56-year-old man with known Child-Pugh C cirrhosis has presented with haematemesis. The rural facility reports at least 600 mL of fresh blood in the vomit. Current observations are: P95, BP 105/50, GCS 13 (E3V4M6). No further haematemesis in the past 2 hours.

Incident C

A 42-year-old man was working in construction when he was struck in the face by a heavy metal beam about 10 minutes ago. He is bleeding profusely from the nose, mouth and right ear. He has been laid on his left lateral side. Current observations are: P110, BP 120/60, GCS 6 (E1V1M4)

Incident D

A 24-year-old female cyclist has been involved in an MVA with a refuse truck. The on-scene reports were that the truck ran over both her legs. She was transported to the rural facility with a pelvic binder in situ. Current observations are: P125 Systolic BP between 80 and 90, GCS 14 (E3V5M6).

Question 28.1

For each scenario, select which items of equipment may be of benefit in managing the case. Each piece of kit can be used multiple times or not at all. Outline the pros and cons of each of the items selected in the given scenario. Are there any items of equipment that would be suitable in all the scenarios?

Discussion 28.1

All scenarios

i) In all circumstances where blood is administered, it should ideally be warmed immediately prior to use. Modern devices for warming have become smaller, lighter and more portable, mainly as battery technology improves. Devices such as the MEQU (pictured) can heat blood or other fluids from 5°C (41°F) to 37°C (98.6°F) at flow rates up to 150 mL/min. Weighing in at less than a kilogram, these devices are suitable to be carried all the time and on all transport platforms.

iii) Fibrinogen concentrate is available as a refrigerated blood product that can be reconstituted and administered on-scene if required. The benefits of administration of FC in the absence of any coagulation testing are unclear. Viscoelastic haemostatic assays (VHAs) such as rotational thromboelastography (ROTEM) are generally required to demonstrate a low fibrinogen level, although direct fibrinogen measurement is equally feasible. Such measurements are rarely possible in the PHRM environment. Equally, as above, the ability to take blood products is also limited. For patients with catastrophic bleeding it may be acceptable to 'blind' administer FC on the assumption that the patient will be coagulopathic. Such use must be carefully monitored and audited.

ix) The massive transfusion pack is widely used in the hospital setting. The complexity of managing blood products, such as fresh frozen plasma (FFP) or platelets has generally precluded their widespread use in the PHRM environment. However, effective processes, communication and clinical governance mean that arranging urgent pick-up of a suitable MTP can be feasible. This depends on:

- Location of patient
- Location of blood bank in relation to PHRM base
- Nature of tasking (e.g. time critical)
- Transport platform (space and weight).

Products carried in an MTP might include red cells, FFP, platelets, cryoprecipitate, factor concentrates and fibrinogen concentrate. PHRM services utilising an MTP process will likely already be carrying red cells and, possibly, other blood products, and this is likely to reduce the risk of errors related to blood-product carriage and documentation. The key to successful implementation of blood and blood-product carriage in PHRM revolves around robust clinical audit and governance, and good communication with the local blood bank.

x) In cases of significant haemodynamic compromise due to blood loss, large-bore intravenous (IV) access is an important step. Obtaining IV access in patients with haemodynamic compromise can be challenging, and, frequently, access will end up being narrow-bore. In such instances it may be useful to dilate the existing venepuncture to increase the calibre. The rapid infusion catheter (RIC) is an example of such a kit and it utilises a Seldinger approach to dilate a smaller-gauge IV catheter into a larger size that may be more suitable for fluid resuscitation. It is important to recognise that attempting an RIC can render the existing IV access unusable. Therefore, it is prudent to have a second functional IV access prior to attempting an RIC.

Scenario A

ii), vi), viii)

TXA is a standard of care following PPH (Shakur et al 2017). If not given at the referring hospital, at least 1g of TXA should be administered on arrival by the PHRM team, with a view to a second dose if bleeding continues. The use of intrauterine balloon occlusion (e.g. Bakri balloon) is a useful adjunct to haemorrhage control in PPH. In the PHRM environment there are rarely alternative options in the event of ongoing bleeding. Consider the '4 Ts':

- Tone – massage the uterus and administer syntocinon +/– ergometrine. Ongoing blood loss may require synthetic prostaglandins (e.g. misoprostol suppository)
- Tissue – ensure the placenta has been delivered and no remnants remain
- Trauma – examine for vaginal or perineal tears
- Thrombin – avoid hypothermia and consider blood product replacement (as above).

The use of REBOA is recognised in severe PPH (Ji et al 2020). REBOA is further discussed below in scenario D.

Scenario B

vii)

The most likely pathology in this case is bleeding from a peptic or duodenal ulcer; however, bleeding from gastro-oesophageal varices is also feasible. For ulcer disease, the administration of high-dose proton pump inhibitors is an initial step, although this has not been proven to be effective in managing acute haemorrhage. The most important step will be timely transfer to a centre capable of performing endoscopic treatments and this should be a priority. For variceal disease, balloon tamponade (e.g. Sengstaken tube +/- modifications) is an option, and services may have this equipment available on the PHRM base. Many services will not carry these devices routinely so timely instruction from the clinical coordination centre will be required to ensure the PHRM team picks up the equipment prior to departure.

Use of balloon occlusion: (See also Case 33)

- Familiarity with the available device (training, education and practical sessions)
- In the PHRM environment, the patient should be intubated and ventilated prior to insertion
- Confirmation of position prior to full inflation using local imaging or pressure monitoring of device balloons
- Securing device in position to allow traction to continue en route

Other drugs should be considered, some of which are unlikely to be carried routinely and may need collection from the PHRM base prior to departure. Drugs such as terlipressin or octreotide may have a modest effect in managing acute variceal bleeds.

Current evidence suggests TXA is not indicated in gastrointestinal bleeds (Roberts et al 2020).

Scenario C

ii), iv), v)

Severe maxillofacial haemorrhage following trauma poses particular challenges in the PHRM environment. The airway may be compromised, especially in the supine patient, and blood loss can be significant. Priority should be placed on securing the airway, especially in the patient with a reduced GCS. An Epistat is an inflatable device that uses 2 balloons to either directly control haemorrhage or offers splintage of facial fractures in conjunction with bite blocks and a hard cervical collar. Epistats will need careful positioning, especially as most patients are candidates for base-of-skull fractures, and incorrect positioning is possible as for nasopharyngeal airways and nasoenteric tubes.

TXA should be given to this patient (Shakur et al 2010).

Haemostatic agents should be considered as an adjunct in significant visible haemorrhage. In this patient, lacerations to the head, neck or face should be considered for use of haemostatic dressings. Impregnated bandages can be used to apply direct pressure, or the agent can be added directly to the wound. Care is needed to avoid the eyes and mucous membranes.

The short-term use of direct sutures is also an effective way of gaining haemorrhage control, especially for wounds to the head and neck.

Scenario D

ii), viii)

This patient has a significant mechanism and high suspicion for major abdomino-pelvic injury. In the trauma centre, this patient would receive prompt imaging followed by interventional radiology or surgery, if required. In the PHRM environment, the focus should be on minimising scene time, adequate splintage (e.g. pelvic binder), imaging if possible (e.g. FAST), adequate IV access and judicious replacement of fluid loss with blood and blood products. However, in this instance, the patient may remain haemodynamically unstable, or deteriorate further due to the nature of the injury and distance from definitive care. For PHRM services that carry REBOA, the siting of a suitable gauge sheath in the common femoral artery (CFA) should be considered in this case. At the very least a sheath can be used as an arterial line and, in the worst case, a REBOA catheter could be deployed (Zone 1) if the patient deteriorated en route. In the absence of a pre-hospital REBOA catheter, a standard arterial line in the CFA is acceptable, as it may later be dilated to an adequately sized sheath. Balloon inflation time is critical in REBOA and, if deployed, careful note must be made of balloon inflation time. Partial balloon inflation and intermittent balloon inflation are currently unproven methods in managing balloon inflation time.

A balanced approach to time spent on-scene to deliver critical life-saving interventions is key in this case.

TXA should be given to this patient as per CRASH-2 (Shakur et al 2010).

Key points

- Carriage of blood and blood products in the PHRM environment is rapidly becoming a standard of care.
- Temperature control of blood products and the ability to warm blood prior to administration is essential.
- Emerging agents and devices to help manage acute haemorrhage should be available to modern PHRM services.

References

Ji SM, Cho C, Choi G, et al. Successful management of uncontrolled postpartum hemorrhage due to morbidly adherent placenta with Resuscitative endovascular balloon occlusion of the aorta during emergency cesarean section – a case report. Anesth. Pain Med. 2020; 15(3):314–318.

Roberts I, Shakur-Still H, Afolabi A, et al. Effects of a high-dose 24-h infusion of tranexamic acid on death and thromboembolic events in patients with acute gastrointestinal bleeding (HALT-IT): an international randomised, double-blind, placebo-controlled trial. The Lancet 2020; 395(10241):1927–1936.

Shakur H, Roberts I, Bautista R, et al. (CRASH-2 trial collaborators). Effects of tranexamic acid on death, vascular occlusive events, and blood transfusion in trauma patients with significant haemorrhage (CRASH-2): a randomised, placebo-controlled trial. Lancet 2010; 376(9734):23–32.

Shakur H, Roberts I, Fawole B, et al. (WOMAN Trial Collaborators). Effect of early tranexamic acid administration on mortality, hysterectomy, and other morbidities in women with post-partum haemorrhage (WOMAN): an international, randomised, double-blind, placebo-controlled trial. Lancet 2017; 389(10084):2105–2116.

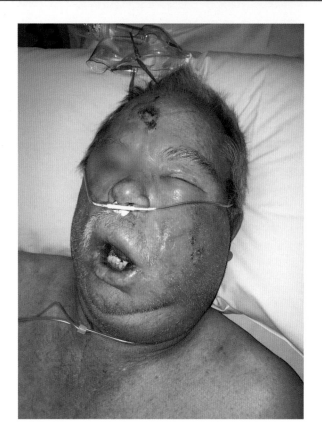

Incident

A 72-year-old male has presented to a rural hospital 220 km (137 miles) away with facial swelling and fever. He lives alone and rarely presents for medical assistance. His relevant medical history includes poorly controlled Type 1 diabetes, hypertension and obesity. Over the past hour, he has developed biphasic stridor, loss of voice and is now unable to move his jaw or swallow his own saliva. On request, the local medical officer has forwarded an image to the coordination centre (see image above).

Relevant information

- **PHRM team transport options:** Rotary-wing aircraft.
- **Additional resources:** Local medical officer and nursing staff. Difficult airway equipment available prior to departure.
- **Other:** Nil.

Question 29.1

Outline your approach to airway management both prior to departure and on arrival.

Discussion 29.1

The image forwarded from the local medical officer shows extensive erythema and facial oedema predominantly on the left side. This includes the periorbital, maxillary, buccal, sublingual and submandibular soft tissues. There are several small abrasions over the left cheek. Dentition is at least partially intact and appears carious. Given the known history of IDDM, presence of fever and progressive facial swelling, head and neck cellulitis or deep-space infection is suspected. His airway is very clearly threatened, and given the working diagnosis, is unlikely to improve in the short term. Definitive airway management during the retrieval is likely to be required and should be planned for.

Pre-departure

Equipment

Suggested airway equipment for a standard retrieval response is outlined in Appendix 2. As it is not practical to have extensive difficult airway equipment always available, an additional pack for known or predicted difficult airway management should therefore be immediately available prior to PHRM team departure.

An example of a difficult airway pack can be found in the box below.

Intubating fibreoptic scope (may be single use and of varying diameter) and screen (if applicable)

Aintree intubating catheter

100 mm Bermann Airway

Percutaneous cricothyroidotomy kit

Catheter mount with scope access port

Non-invasive ventilation mask with scope access port and securing strap

Lignocaine 2% and adrenaline 1:200,000 (20 mL).

High-flow airway atomising device

Personnel

The PHRM team should be trained in the management of predicted difficult airways and should have a thorough knowledge and working understanding of the contents of any additional difficult airway pack. However, even the most senior PHRM doctors may not have had extensive experience in the management of such challenging airways. Where possible, the most senior and experienced clinician should be included in the responding PHRM team, either in addition to or as a replacement for less experienced doctors.

On arrival

Following patient assessment on arrival, a decision regarding the most appropriate approach to definitive airway management can occur. In this case, significant soft tissue distortion, tongue swelling, limited mouth opening and prominent dentition, in addition to limited physiological reserves, should lead the team to strongly consider an awake fibre-optic intubation (AFOI). An in-depth review of AFOI is beyond the scope of this discussion but is provided via further reading below.

A brief overview of an approach to AFOI is as follows:
- Planning
  - Assess nasal patency and decide if the nasal or oral route will be attempted.
  - Assess anterior neck and plan for potential surgical airway as a rescue procedure in the event of airway loss.

145

- Assess patient compliance and sedation requirements.
- Explain what is planned to the patient.
- Assign team roles and share the plan/mental model.
- All equipment checked and drugs drawn.
- Patient location and positioning
  - Optimise 360-degree access.
  - Ensure back-up oxygen, adequate suction and lighting.
  - Consider hospital theatre space if available.
  - Have the patient semi-recumbent and bed height appropriate for the fibre-optic operator.
- Oxygenation
  - Apply supplemental oxygen either orally or nasally depending on the planned route of airway access (this oxygen source should remain in place throughout the procedure).
- Sedation
  - Establish secure IV access.
  - Consider sedative choices available and doses. Ideally, the lowest doses required to facilitate a calm and compliant patient without apnoea or significant physiological side effects is the goal.
  - Common agents include:
    - Fentanyl (or other opiate analogues if available)
    - Midazolam
    - Ketamine
    - Propofol
    - Dexmedetomidine infusion.
- Antisialogogue for secretion reduction
  - Atropine or glycopyrrolate.
  - May not provide significant benefit for 30–45 minutes.
- Vasoconstrictor to reduce airway oedema and bleeding risk
  - Co-phenylcaine (lignocaine plus phenylephrine containing 5 mg of lignocaine per spray).
- Airway topicalisation
  - Required for analgesia and to suppress cough and gag reflexes.
  - Utilises a combination of lignocaine strengths and routes of administration (e.g. nebulisation, topical spray or atomising device).
  - In this case, 5 mL 4% nebulised lignocaine in addition to nasopharyngeal co-phenylcaine and 'spray as you go' 4% lignocaine (total of 11 mL) would be effective.
  - Ensure maximum local anaesthetic dose is calculated and not exceeded (8–9 mg/kg total topical lignocaine).
- Equipment selection
  - Tracheal tube selection should consider the diameter of the nasal passage chosen and the length required to ensure adequate depth of tube placement.
  - Pre-warming a tracheal tube (with warm water) can improve malleability and ease of placement.
  - Adequate tube lubrication is critical.

- When utilising the oral route, an introducing airway (such as the Bermann airway) is preferred. This is similar to a Guedel airway but is cut away at the side. However, given the oral soft tissue distortion, the nasal route would be preferred in this case.
- Fibre-optic tube placement via the nasal route
  - Ensure an adequate image through the fibrescope is achieved.
  - Preload the selected tracheal tube onto the fiberscope.
  - By standing behind the patient, relative orientation is preserved (e.g. your left is the patient's left).
  - Under direct vision, navigate the nasal passage to the posterior nasopharynx.
  - Further topicalisation can be administered via the fibrescope port.
  - Consider the '3 step rule' of 'Stop. Centre. Move.' to acquire and maintain orientation and successful passage of the fibrescope.
    - Stop – regularly as you navigate the airway.
    - Centre – your next target in the fibrescope's field of view.
    - Move – to the target only once centred.
    - (Repeat)
  - Under direct vision, topicalise and intubate the vocal cords.
  - Confirm direct vision of the tracheal rings.
  - Advance the tracheal tube over the fibrescope, inflate cuff and confirm end tidal CO_2.
  - Administer general anaesthesia and muscle relaxants.

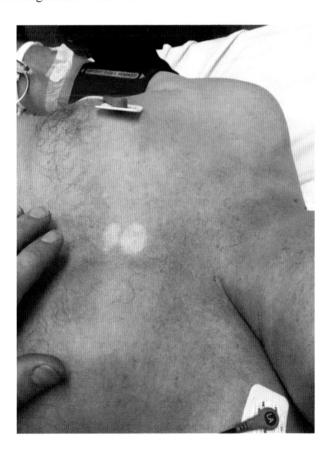

Following FOI and establishment of invasive ventilation, the patient becomes progressively hypotensive with BP of 70/35 mmHg. His heart rate is 115 bpm sinus. His central capillary refill is delayed beyond 10 seconds (see image above).

Question 29.2

How will you assess and manage his shocked state?

Halfway through the return flight, his rhythm changes to atrial fibrillation with a rapid ventricular response (156 bpm).

Question 29.3

Is it safe to attempt cardioversion mid-flight? If so, is it likely to be effective?

Discussion 29.2

A rapid clinical reassessment should occur including confirmation of tracheal tube position. If high doses of sedative anaesthetic agents are infused, these should be temporarily paused. The likely cause is sepsis with septic shock. As with polytrauma, acute myocardial infarction, and stroke, early identification and appropriate immediate management in the initial hours after development of sepsis improves outcomes.

Blood should be drawn for blood gas and lactate analysis if available. Point-of-care pathology devices should be available as additional items for PHRM teams responding to critically unwell patients. A fluid challenge should be rapidly infused and repeated as required looking for an improvement in both systolic BP and capillary refill. If there is a volume-resistant shocked state, peripheral inotropic support should be commenced. Noradrenaline can safely and effectively be infused through an adequate peripheral cannula (Cardenas-Garcia 2015) (see Case 26). If diluted as 3 mg noradrenaline in 50 mL or equivalent, each mL per hour equates to 1 microgram per minute. Commence the infusion at 10 mL per hour (10 micrograms per minute) and titrate to SBP.

Blood cultures should be taken and packed for transport with the patient, and broad-spectrum antibiotics administered. The choice of antimicrobial agents for PHRM teams will be regionally variable. However, it is worth noting that many retrieval tasks will be to medical facilities where basic, broad antimicrobial agents are already available. Furthermore, many critically ill patients requiring retrieval will have failed to respond to available antimicrobials, may be immunocompromised (as in this case), and will have been potentially exposed to multi-resistant organisms (MRO). For these reasons, it is advisable to carry broad-spectrum agents with potential activity against MROs (such as piperacillin/tazobactam, meropenem and vancomycin). In this case, cover inclusive of anaerobic organisms (given the potential dental origins of head and neck infection) should be given. As an example, piperacillin/tazobactam in combination with vancomycin should be administered. This should occur without delay.

Ongoing targeted resuscitation will require placement of invasive arterial and central venous lines. The same attention to aseptic technique (ANZICS 2021) and use of ultrasound guidance as would occur in the receiving facility ICU should be applied. A urinary catheter should also be placed to monitor hourly urine outputs.

Discussion 29.3

Cardioversion can occur mid-flight, but communication to and approval from the pilot and aircrew is mandatory as defibrillation may interfere with aircraft electronics.

In this case, atrial fibrillation with rapid ventricular response is likely secondary to sepsis with septic shock. Cardioversion is unlikely to provide sustained sinus rhythm. Electrolyte imbalance should be sought and corrected. Cautious antiarrhythmic therapy can be considered such as amiodarone (150 to 300 mg loading with or without a subsequent infusion).

Key points

- PHRM services should have the capacity to manage difficult airways including the use of fibre-optic techniques
- Adequate topical anaesthesia is critical to safe and effective AFOI.
- Early and aggressive resuscitation and appropriate broad spectrum anti-microbial agents improve outcomes in severe sepsis.

References

ANZICS. Central Line Associated Blood Stream Infection (CLABSI) Prevention. Online. Available: https://www.anzics.com.au/clabsi/. 26 July 2021.

Cardenas-Garcia J, Schaub KF, Belchikov YG, et al. Safety of peripheral intravenous administration of vasoactive medication. J. Hosp. Med. 2015; 10(9):581–585.

Additional reading

Bradley P, Chapman G, Greenland K et al. Topicalisation and sedation for awake fibreoptic intubation. 2019. Online. Available: https://www.anzca.edu.au/resources/sig-resources/2019-airway-management-sig-afoi-topicalisation-sed.aspx. 26 July 2021.

Society of Critical Care Medicine. Surviving Sepsis Campaign. Online. Available: https://www.sccm.org/SurvivingSepsisCampaign/Home. 26 July 2021.

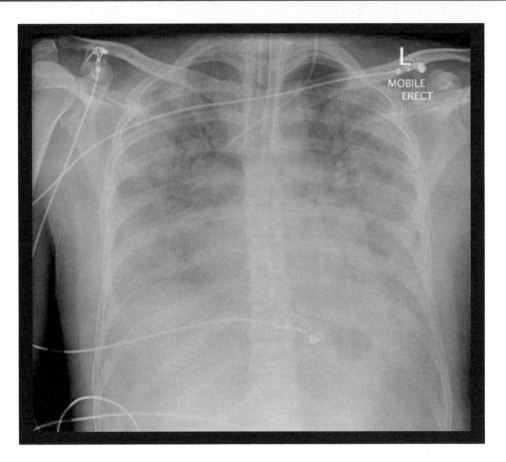

Incident

A 38-year-old male has presented to a rural hospital emergency department 450 km (280 miles) away with 3 days of increasing breathlessness, cough and fever. On arrival he was hypoxic, agitated and in severe respiratory distress. He has been intubated and ventilated by a local anaesthetist who has also placed invasive arterial and central venous lines. A mobile chest X-ray has been taken post intubation and is available to the coordination centre.

The local team has now called for clinical assistance and requested a retrieval.

Relevant information

- **PHRM team transport options:** Fixed-wing turbo-prop aircraft.
- **Local resources:** One land ambulance.
- **Other:** Ambient conditions: Heavy fog, 3°C (37°F), 21:00 hours.

Clinical information

On arrival of the PHRM team:

- Intubated size 8.0 TT 20 cm at the lip. Audible cuff leak.
- Positive pressure ventilation.
  - Synchronised intermittent mandatory ventilation (SIMV).

- Tidal volume (TV) 700 mL.
- Respiratory rate (RR) set at 12 bpm.
- PEEP 5 cm H_2O.
- Pressure support (PS) 15 cm H_2O.
- Actual respiratory rate 35 bpm.
- Pulse 137 sinus rhythm. BP 95/55. Urinary catheter in place draining 40–50 mL/hr.
- Sedated with propofol at 15mL/h (150 mg/hr). Grimacing.
- Temperature 39.8°C (103.6°F).

Question 30.1

What will be your initial management plan?

Question 30.2

Outline your ventilation strategy for the retrieval.

Question 30.3

Calculate the P:F ratio. What additional therapeutic options could be utilised to manage the increasing hypoxia? What other issues should be considered?

Discussion 30.1

The audible leak suggests the airway is at risk and requires immediate attention. This should be made clear to the local team and occur without waiting for a detailed handover. The team should rapidly prepare for re-intubation, utilising a checklist to ensure all equipment is available and the plan is clearly understood. If the initial intubating clinician is available, ask them about the grade of view at initial laryngoscopy. Consider utilising an airway exchange catheter to safely guide tube re-placement.

Tracheal tube migration in the setting of poor lung compliance and high airways resistance is common if the tube has not been adequately secured and once the tracheal tube is re-placed attention should focus on this important detail. One technique utilising a cloth tie is detailed in Appendix 1.1.7.

The patient is inadequately sedated and not muscle relaxed. Both will be critical for ongoing management – particularly relating to controlled ventilation. The blood pressure should be confirmed and supported with small volumes of fluid and vasopressors if required, to allow for adequate sedation. An opiate infusion should be added for sedation and benzodiazapines should be considered. Large volume fluid resuscitation should be avoided to minimise extravascular lung water (see below).

A 'top to toe' assessment should occur noting key findings, ensuring correct placement of devices, and planning for any required interventions. Lung ultrasound will assist in differentiating lung pathology (see Case 39). If available, a bedside point-of-care cardiac ultrasound may also assist in excluding acute heart failure as a contributing pathology (see Case 44).

Discussion 30.2

This patient has presented with acute, severe hypoxaemia and bilateral interstitial lung infiltrates. In the absence of isolated, acute heart failure, he has acute respiratory distress syndrome (ARDS).

It should be noted that this patient requires a long-distance, fixed-wing retrieval. Additional road ambulance transfers are also required. As a result, total ventilated patient transport time is likely to be in excess of 2 hours. Therapeutic interventions during this phase of care will have positive downstream clinical effects. However, omissions in care or harmful therapies may impact negatively on clinical outcomes. This is certainly applicable to invasive ventilation of the patient with ARDS where further injury can occur with poor ventilatory strategy (ventilator associated lung injury – VALI) (Frank & Matthay 2003).

A 'lung protective' ventilation strategy is required where the aim is to avoid or minimise known secondary insults to the injured or at-risk lung. These are detailed, together with key management principles, in the following table:

Injury mechanism	Management
• Volutrauma ○ The overdistension of alveolar lung units where trans-pulmonary pressures exceed 30 cm H_2O. ○ Results in disruption of alveolar basement membrane and intracellular junctions in addition to lung-connective and vascular-tissue injury. ○ Resultant cellular injury leads to inflammatory response (biotrauma).	• Limit TV to 6 mL per kg of body weight. • Limit measured plateau pressures to no more than 30 cm H_2O. • Reduce TV to 4–5 mL/kg if required. • Tolerate hypercapnia if pH > 7.2 ('permissive hypercapnia').

• Barotrauma
○ The overdistension of lung where trans-pulmonary pressures exceed 50 cm H_2O.
○ Mechanical disruption of lung results in classic barotrauma:
  ○ Pneumothorax
  ○ Pneumomediastinum
  ○ Subcutaneous emphysema
  ○ Arterial gas embolism.
	• As above.

• Atelectatrauma ○ The cyclic collapse and re-expansion of alveolar lung units at end expiration. ○ Results in alveolar cellular injury and inflammation (adding to biotrauma).	• Avoid end expiratory alveolar collapse with titrated PEEP. • Limit 'driving pressure' (plateau pressure – PEEP) to 12–15cm H_2O. • Limit excessive IV fluid use to minimise extravascular lung water.
• Biotrauma ○ Mechanical injury leads to cellular inflammatory mediator release and resultant local, regional and systemic inflammatory response and multi-organ dysfunction.	• Lung-protective ventilation strategy • Consider early use of neuromuscular blocking agents (NMBA).

Continued

Injury mechanism	Management

• Oxygen toxicity
   ○ Cellular oxygen-free radical injury.
   ○ Potential for adsorption atelectasis with higher fractional inspired oxygen concentrations.
	• Limit FiO_2 via recruitment of additional lung units using PEEP (consulting a PEEP: FiO_2 table).
	• Tolerate relative hypoxia (SaO_2 > 88%).

As you are preparing to depart for the airport, the pilot calls to inform you that the fog has worsened, and that no aircraft are able to take off or land until the morning. The fog has affected all potential alternative airfields in the region and at the retrieval destination. Only one land ambulance is available in the region which is unable to be used for such a long-distance road transfer. The time is now 23:30 hours.

Following discussion with the tasking agency, it is decided that the PHRM team will be required to remain at the local hospital until the following morning and manage the patient there with assistance from the local medical team.

A repeat arterial blood gas has just been taken with ventilatory settings of SIMV 400, RR 24, PEEP 15 cm H_2O and FiO_2 0.8 and reveals the following:

- pH 7.27.
- $PaCO_2$ 57 mmHg (7.6 kPa).
- PaO_2 68 mmHg (9.1 kPa).

Discussion 30.3

- P:F ratio is 85 (68/0.8). ARDS severity can be divided into:
  - Mild – P:F ratio 200–300
  - Moderate – P:F ratio 100–200
  - Severe – P:F ratio <100
- Neuromuscular blockade
  - Adequate deep sedation and neuromuscular blocking agents (NMBA) will allow for a controlled, lung-protective ventilation strategy and avoid patient/ventilatory dysynchrony
  - NMBAs may have a survival benefit for hypoxic patients (P:F < 150) with ARDS if used in the first 48 hours of invasive ventilation (Papazian et al 2010)
  - Adequate muscle relaxation and sedation reduces oxygen consumption (as will reduction of fever).
- Prone position ventilation
  - Improves oxygenation via enhanced ventilation: perfusion matching, secretion drainage and alveolar recruitment
  - Not without significant risk during patient movement (e.g. extubation, device displacement, patient or staff injury) and while in the prone position (e.g. orbital, peripheral nerve and skin-pressure injury, haemodynamic instability and enteral feeding intolerance)
  - There are significant challenges with retrieving patients in the prone position; however, it has been described successfully in the PHRM environment (DellaVolpe et al 2016).

- Inverse ratio ventilation
  - Increased inspiratory times until the inspiratory time is longer than the expiratory time (I:E > 1)
  - However, this may worsen gas trapping and increase the risk of barotrauma.
- Minimise extravascular lung water
  - Minimise fluid inputs
  - Consider diuretics.
- Maintain haemoglobin > 70 g/L to optimise oxygen-carrying capacity.
- Optimise cardiac output and lung perfusion using inotropic support.

Other therapies that may not be immediately available include pulmonary vasodilators such as inhaled nitric oxide (iNO) and nebulised prostacyclin. (See Cases 61 and 66).

Additional considerations include the following:

- General critical care patient management
  - Placement of nasogastric tube (NGT)
  - Adequate analgesic and sedation requirements
  - Glycaemic control
  - Thromboprophylaxis.
- Fatigue management
  - Communicate with the coordination centre, the PHRM team and local teams regarding patient monitoring and management requirements overnight
  - Plan for PHRM team meal and rest breaks
  - Possibilities for team rotation in the event of further delays.
- Extracorporeal membrane oxygenation (ECMO) should be considered early and the case discussed with the most appropriate ECMO centre.

Key points

- The retrieval phase of care presents an opportunity for positive therapeutic interventions. However, harm can occur in this phase if beneficial therapies are not provided or provided in a suboptimal fashion. Ventilatory strategy to avoid lung injury is a good example of this.
- PHRM teams should be prepared, mentally and physically, for variations in the pre-arranged retrieval plan.
- The vast majority of non-ventilatory strategies (such as inhaled pulmonary vasodilators, prone positioning, etc.) to manage ARDS are feasible in the PHRM environment.

References

DellaVolpe JD, Lovett J, Martin-Gill C, Guyette FX. Transport of mechanically ventilated patients in the prone position. Prehosp. Emerg. Care 2016; 20(5):643–647.

Frank JA, Matthay MA. Science review: mechanisms of ventilator-induced injury. Crit Care. 2003; 7(3):233–241.

Papazian L, Forel J-M, Gacouin A et al. Neuromuscular blockers in early acute respiratory distress syndrome. N Engl. J. Med. 2010; 363:1107–1116.

Additional reading

Bein T, Grasso S, Moerer O et al. The standard of care of patients with ARDS: ventilatory settings and rescue therapies for refractory hypoxemia. Intensive Care Med. 2016; 42(5):699–711.

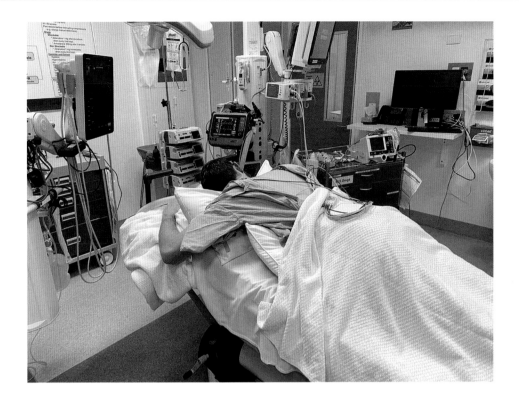

Incident

The following morning, the 38-year-old male detailed in the previous case has deteriorated further. Although he remains haemodynamically stable, the PHRM team has struggled overnight to maintain oxygenation and adequate ventilation despite neuromuscular blockade, inverse ratio ventilation, cautious diuresis and up-titration of PEEP. They have positioned the patient prone with the assistance of the local hospital team (see picture above).

Clinical information

His current ventilation settings are as follows:
- Synchronised intermittent mandatory ventilation (SIMV) volume control.
- Tidal volume (TV) 380 mL.
- Respiratory rate (RR) 28 bpm.
- PEEP 18 cm H_2O.
- Plateau pressure (Ppl) 35 cm H_2O.
- FiO_2 1.0.

The most recent arterial blood gas some hours after prone positioning is as follows:
- pH 7.18.
- $PaCO_2$ 64 mmHg (8.5 kPa).
- PaO_2 61 mmHg (8.1 kPa).
- HCO_3 22 mmol/L.
- Lactate 1.8 mmol/L.

Relevant information

- **PHRM team transport options:** Fixed-wing turbo prop aircraft.
- **Local resources:** One land ambulance.
- **Other:** Ambient conditions: Fog has cleared and local airfield is now open. Nearest ECMO centre with specialist retrieval team is 400 km away.

Question 31.1

What are the indications for ECMO in the setting of acute respiratory failure?

Question 31.2

What are the options for establishing ECMO in this case? Can this occur at the local hospital?

Question 31.3

What potential ECMO retrieval emergencies should be planned for?

Question 31.4

Unrelated to this case, what other extracorporeal support therapies could be applied in the PHRM setting?

Discussion 31.1

Venovenous (VV) ECMO involves venous blood from the patient being accessed from the large central veins, pumped through an oxygenator and then returned to the venous system near the right atrium. It provides support for severe respiratory failure and requires an intact circulation and adequate cardiac function for blood circulation. VV ECMO improves the patient's oxygenation by adding oxygen to blood that then passes through the lung to the systemic circulation. Oxygen is provided and carbon dioxide (CO_2) is removed via the oxygenator's gas/blood interface membrane. Removal of CO_2 allows the level of ventilatory support to be reduced, which may reduce ventilator-induced lung injury. Mechanical ventilation is continued, but with 'lung rest settings' (low TV, PEEP to maintain alveolar opening, low Ppl and low respiratory rates).

VV ECMO should be considered in cases of severe ARDS with $PaO_2/FiO_2 < 80$ and/or when mechanical ventilation becomes dangerous (because of the increased tidal volumes and plateau pressures) and despite optimisation of ARDS management, including high PEEP, neuromuscular blocking agents, and prone positioning.

VV ECMO indications

- Refractory hypoxia ($PaO_2:FiO_2 < 80$) and/or worsening respiratory acidosis ($pH < 7.2$) despite optimal ventilation strategies (high PEEP, neuromuscular blocking agents, and prone positioning).
- Unsafe nonprotective ventilation settings are consistently required to support gas exchange (with or without barotrauma).
- Air leaks or bronchopleural fistulae.

Contraindications

ECMO is unlikely to be successful for patients with:
- Nonrecoverable respiratory failure, who are not candidates for transplantation
- Preexisting conditions incompatible with recovery (severe neurologic injury, end-stage malignancy)
- Relative contraindications to therapeutic anticoagulation (such as active bleeding)
- Preexisting severe multi-organ failure
- Allogeneic stem cell transplantation
- Advanced age
- Prolonged pre-ECMO mechanical ventilation.

Ultimately, the decision to initiate ECMO is made on a case-by-case basis following discussion with the tertiary ECMO specialist clinical team. These discussions should be facilitated by the PHRM coordination centre.

Discussion 31.2

Team and location

If expert ECMO support cannot be provided locally, eligible patients will require retrieval to an ECMO specialist centre. Three types of ECMO retrieval are described:
- Patient retrieval to an ECMO specialist centre prior to ECMO cannulation and initiation
- ECMO cannulation and initiation at the referring site and retrieval to ECMO specialist centre on ECMO (known as primary transport)
- Patient on ECMO (established locally) and transferring to another ECMO site (secondary transport).

In this case, the two options are to either transport the patient utilising standard ventilatory supports to an ECMO specialist centre or utilise a specialist ECMO retrieval team to respond to the regional centre for cannulation and ECMO establishment (primary ECMO transport). As this patient is already profoundly hypoxic and hypercarbic despite maximal support therapies, a long-distance retrieval requiring road and fixed-wing transport is likely to be hazardous, and cannulation and establishment of ECMO are ideally provided by a responding team from the specialist ECMO centre.

While very few PHRM services currently have the capacity or expertise to provide primary ECMO transports, secondary ECMO transports are increasingly performed by generic PHRM service teams.

Circuit options

For VV ECMO, venous cannulae are most commonly placed in the right or left femoral vein for drainage and right internal jugular vein for infusion. The femoral cannula tip lies at the junction of the inferior vena cava and right atrium, and the internal jugular cannula tip lies at the junction of the superior vena cava and right atrium (see image below). A double lumen cannula such as the Avalon® (placed in the right internal jugular vein) may be used as an alternative, which is large enough to accommodate 4–5 L/min of blood flow.

Discussion 31.3

There are a number of commonly encountered ECMO emergencies that all ECMO specialists and PHRM team members involved in ECMO retrieval need to be aware of and prepared for.

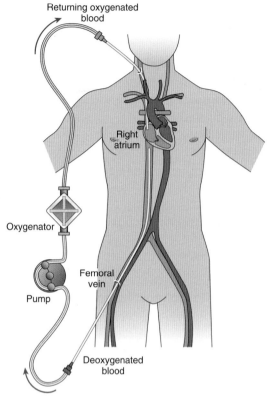

Figure 31.1 VV ECMO circuit. Source: Jessica Spellman, Lauren Sutherland, 2022, edited by Edmand Cohen, Cohen's Comprehensive thorasic Anesthesia, first edition.

Pump failure

Most transport ECMO circuit pumps are centrifugal in nature. Pump rate (one determinant of blood flow) is therefore measured in revolutions per minute (RPM). Absolute pump failure is therefore defined as a pump RPM of zero.

Potential causes of pump failure include:

- Pump head disengagement
- Electrical motor failure
- Battery failure (no electrical power supply).

Pump failure in VV ECMO will have immediate patient impact, leading to hypoxia, hypercarbia and potentially sudden haemodynamic collapse.

Pump failure can potentially be avoided by maintaining the pump head in a safe position during the retrieval (see image A below) and minimising ECMO console time on battery.

In the event of pump failure, immediate return to conventional full ventilation should be established. A rapid examination of the circuit should then look to identify easily reversible problems (such as battery failure where there is electrical power supply immediately available).

Manual pump support utilising a hand-crank to re-established oxygenated blood flow will be required if pump restoration is not immediately achievable (see image B below). To do this, the pump head (rotaflow) or the integrated pump head and oxygenator (Cardiohelp) will need to be moved to the crank handle housing. For

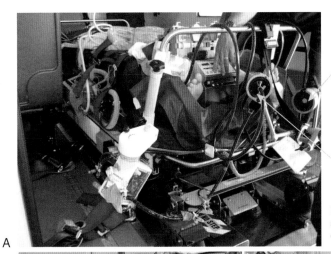

Hand crank handle housing
(rotaflow system)

Pump head only (rotaflow
system – with separate
oxygenator and pump head)

A

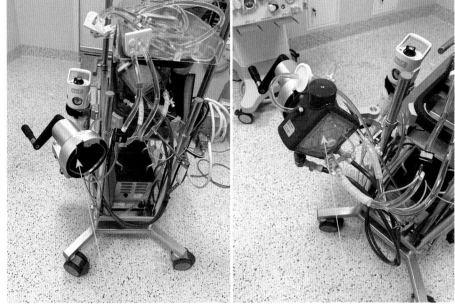

B

Hand crank handle housing
(cardiohelp system)

Integrated oxygenator and pump head
(cardiohelp system)

Figure 31.2 Images of commonly used ECMO transport circuits.

this reason, the hand-crank arm should be identified within easy reach of the team throughout the retrieval, a plan for who will access and use it should be made, and a run-through of the required process conducted prior to departure from the referral hospital.

Circuit air embolism

Circuit air embolism is an introduction of air into any part of the extracorporeal circuit. This can occur with poor de-airing procedure during cannulation or due to a breach of the ECMO circuit on the access (pre-pump) side. The effects of air entry into the circuit include air build-up in the pump head, which may eventually lead to pump failure (see above). Return of large volumes of air to the patient will lead to pulmonary air embolism and potentially cardiovascular arrest.

Prevention of air embolism includes meticulous attention to de-airing the circuit during cannulation and circuit connection. In addition, circuit connector fracture or circuit disintegration is recognised following repeated exposure to alcohol-based solutions which should therefore be avoided.

If large volumes of air are seen within the circuit, the circuit return line should be clamped and the pump switched off to prevent introduction of air into the patient. Management should then proceed as per pump failure. In the event of clinical air embolism, the patient should be positioned head down. The existing CVC line can potentially allow for aspiration of air from the right heart. Finally, circuit de-airing and correction of the source of the problem will be required.

Accidental de-cannulation and circuit rupture

Inadvertent de-cannulation (removal of either the access or return cannula) can be partial or complete. Complete de-cannulation leads to hypoxaemia, rapid blood loss from the cannula site and potential haemodynamic collapse. In this event, a rapid assignment of team roles is required to simultaneously address the following:

- Re-establish conventional ventilation
- Clamp the remaining line and switch off the pump
- Volume resuscitation for hypovolaemia +/– vasopressors
- Direct pressure application to the bleeding cannula insertion site.

If the cannula is partially removed and there is inadequate residual lung function, the cannula can be pushed back in its original location until the side holes are covered (if confident to do so). Note, this is a temporising procedure only and, due to potential infection risk, formal replacement of the cannula may be required at the receiving ECMO centre.

In the transport environment, the greatest risk of de-cannulation relates to tension on circuit lines or fouling of the circuit on other objects during transport and transfers. This can be prevented by ensuring one of the PHRM team is assigned the role of 'spotting' the circuit during transfers, to ensure lines are free. In addition, adequate securing and anchoring of the cannula during cannulation is critical. There are various techniques described for this. The use of insertion-site sutures is avoided given the requirement for anticoagulation and the higher risk of line-related infection.

Circuit rupture can be caused by accidental circuit line cutting or a break in any of the circuit components. As mentioned above, prolonged exposure to alcohol-based solutions increases the risk of circuit disintegration. Like de-cannulation, circuit rupture leads to rapid blood loss, hypoxia with haemodynamic collapse, in addition to potential air embolus. While early circuit disintegration is unlikely, damage to the circuit from sharp instruments (such as scalpels or scissors) remains a risk in the PHRM environment. The management of circuit rupture is similar to that of de-cannulation. However, clamping of the circuit on either side of the circuit breach can allow for sterile circuit repair using a sterile connector. Given the requirement for rapid circuit clamping in response to many of the above emergencies, specific line clamps should be immediately available throughout the transfer and retrieval.

Oxygenator failure

Oxygenator failure is usually seen after a prolonged period of ECMO and is usually related to a build-up of thrombus in the oxygenator membrane, leading to decrease in the gas-exchange function. Impending oxygenator failure, therefore, results in worsening gas exchange in addition to increasing trans-membrane pressure (TMP). If left untreated, full membrane failure can result.

Preventive measures include early circuit anticoagulation – usually with patient heparinisation to a target activated clotting time (ACT).

Discussion 31.4
Veno-Arterial (VA) ECMO

VA ECMO involves venous blood being accessed from the large central veins, pumped through an oxygenator and then returned to a major artery (usually the proximal aorta). It provides support for acute, severe cardiac pump failure (sometimes with associated respiratory failure). A venous cannula is usually placed in the inferior vena cava or right atrium for drainage while an arterial cannula is placed in the right femoral artery for re-infusion (see Fig. 31.3 below). Femoral access is preferred and, as a result, there is a risk of distal limb ischaemia of the ipsilateral lower extremity. This can be avoided by inserting an additional (smaller-calibre) arterial cannula distal to the femoral artery cannula, which redirects a portion of the oxygenated return blood to the distal limb.

Following cardiac surgery with an inability to separate from cardiopulmonary bypass (CPB), central cannulation of the right atrium and aorta may be maintained to allow for ongoing CPB via the transport ECMO circuit.

Flow rates on VA ECMO reflect native cardiac output (up to 4–5 L/min). As a result, flow from the return, arterial cannula can significantly increase cardiac afterload on an already failing left ventricle (LV). Off-loading of the LV is therefore occasionally required, with the use of an intra-aortic balloon pump (IABP) being one option described. Aeromedical transport of patients requiring both VA ECMO support and

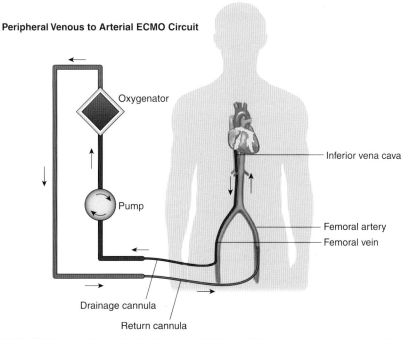

Peripheral Venous to Arterial ECMO Circuit

Oxygenator

Inferior vena cava

Pump

Femoral artery

Femoral vein

Drainage cannula

Return cannula

Figure 31.3 VA ECMO circuit. Source. Joni L. Dirks, Julie M. Waters, 2022, Cardiovascular Therapeutic Management.

IABP presents additional logistic and clinical challenges but has been successfully conducted (see images below).

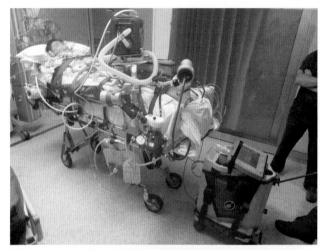

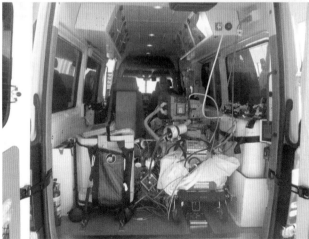

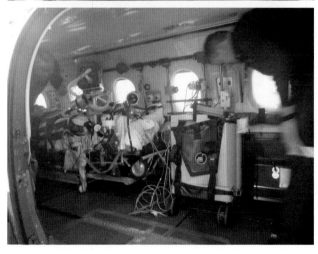

Extracorporeal Cardiopulmonary Resuscitation (ECPR)

ECPR is the use of VA ECMO to augment resuscitation following cardiac arrest where ROSC is unable to be achieved with standard cardiopulmonary resuscitation (CPR).

Patient selection for ECPR is critical to enhancing clinical outcomes, and positive prognostic determinants include:

- Age 18–65 years
- Witnessed arrest with bystander CPR
- VF/VT rhythm or signs of life during resuscitation
- No-flow time < 5 minutes (Fagnoul et al 2014).

In addition, the ideal therapeutic window for ECPR is within 60 minutes following cardiac arrest. Pre-hospital care systems offering access to ECPR therefore need to consider the time required for the initial ambulance response, the time for standard resuscitation on scene, the time required for patient extrication and transport, the logistics of maintaining quality chest compressions en route to the hospital and the time required to perform cannulation and establish VA ECMO on hospital arrival. To achieve the 60-minute window, many pre-hospital systems deploy mechanical CPR devices with early identification and transport of potential ECPR candidates to an ECPR-capable hospital. However, some advanced PHRM service models can deliver ECPR in the pre-hospital arena, thus eliminating the difficulties of providing quality CPR in transit and significantly reducing 'low-flow' time and thus systemic and cerebral ischaemia (Lamhaut et al 2017).

Key points

- Access to ECMO technology in the PHRM setting has revolutionised the management of previously unsurvivable, acute cardiorespiratory failure.
- The establishment of specialist ECMO retrieval teams has seen this area further evolve to allow safe ECMO transport (primary and secondary) to specialist ECMO centres.
- The role of PHRM services in the establishment of extracorporeal support has also expanded, specifically for out-of-hospital ECPR.

References

Fagnoul D, Combes A, De Backer D. Extracorporeal cardiopulmonary resuscitation. Curr. Opin. Crit. Care 2014; 20(3):259–265.

Lamhaut L, Hutin A, Puymirat E, et al. A pre-hospital extracorporeal cardio pulmonary resuscitation (ECPR) strategy for treatment of refractory out hospital cardiac arrest: an observational study and propensity analysis. Resuscitation. 2017; 117:109–117.

Pillai AK, Bhatti Z, Bosserman AJ, et al. Management of vascular complications of extra corporeal membrane oxygenation. Cardiovasc. Diagn. Ther. 2018; 8(3):372–377. doi: 10.21037/cdt.2018.01.11.20.

Additional reading

Agency for Clinical Innovation. ECMO (extracorporeal membrane oxygenation) services in NSW. ACI, 2020. Online. Available: https://www.aci.health.nsw.gov.au/__data/assets/pdf_file/0003/624279/ACI-ECMO-Adult-Clinical-Practice-Guide.pdf.

Singer B, Reynolds JC, Lockey DJ, O'Brien B. Pre-hospital extra-corporeal cardiopulmonary resuscitation. Scand. J. Trauma, Resusc. Emerg. Med. 2018; 26:21.

Incident

A 48-year-old woman known to mental health services with a background of depression has re-presented to a rural general hospital. She had been assessed in the hospital's emergency department 24 hours earlier with an exacerbation of chronic lower back pain and discharged home with a supply of simple analgesics (paracetamol and codeine phosphate). She informed the ambulance team that she had taken an overdose of 'tablets' around 2 hours prior to calling them, and empty packets of both amitriptyline and paracetamol/codeine were found on-scene, along with some other unidentified tablets. She subsequently became significantly drowsier during transport to hospital.

Clinical information

Observations on arrival to rural hospital:

- GCS 12 (E3, M5, V4).
- P 134.
- BP 90/40 mmHg.
- RR 9.
- SaO_2 99% on mask oxygen.

The attending doctor has faxed through an ECG to the PHRM team. This poor-quality fax is pictured below.

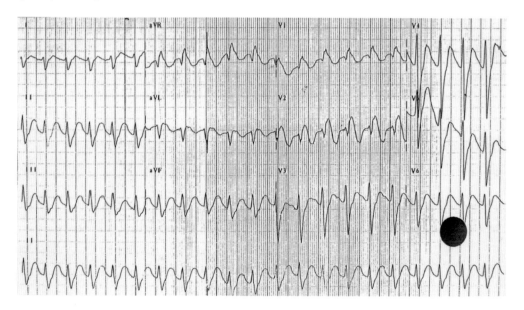

Relevant information

- **PHRM team transport options:** Fixed-wing aircraft.
- **Additional resources:** Regional hospital. Airway competent staff on-site. No on-site laboratory service. No ICU facilities. Land ambulance and crew.
- **Retrieval options**: Tertiary referral hospital.
- **Other**: Flight time 50 minutes.

Question 32.1

What additional information is relevant and how might the retrieval coordinator obtain this?

Question 32.2

What pre-retrieval advice should be given to the referral hospital medical staff?

Question 32.3

What are the priorities of the retrieval team when they arrive on site?

Discussion 32.1

Relevant information when coordinating a retrieval response can be considered as either critical ('need to know') or important ('nice to know'). Critical information will usually have an impact on the immediate actions required to both support this patient in her current location and mobilise a PHRM team to retrieve her.

Critical information

- Which medications she has ingested (both type and quantity).
- Her access to any other medications.
- Likely time(s) of ingestion.
- Availability of laboratory capacity to investigate ingestion.
- Availability of medical staff with anaesthetic skills at the referring hospital.
- Availability of potential therapeutic agents at the referring hospital:
  - *N*-acetylcysteine (NAC).
  - Sodium bicarbonate and/or hypertonic saline.
  - Naloxone.
- Availability of the PHRM team and aircraft.
- Bed availability at receiving ICU.

Important information
Past medical history

- Factors that might increase her risk of liver injury following paracetamol overdose:
  - Chronic alcohol abuse.
  - Hepatic microsomal-inducing drugs (e.g. carbamazepine).
  - Potential glutathione depletion (e.g. malnutrition).
  - Pathological causes of liver injury such as viral hepatitis.
- Sustained-release, chronic or repeated supratherapeutic paracetamol ingestion will alter the ongoing toxicology management.

Other relevant comorbidities

- Heart disease.
  - May increase risk of developing TCA-related cardiac complications and limit tolerance to large fluid volumes and sodium loads.

- Past mental health history.
  - Stability of mental state and recent alterations to medications.
  - Previous hospital admissions.
  - Social supports and family.

Resources available to obtain relevant information

The patient
- Accuracy and completeness of history may be limited.
- Progressive obtundation is probable. Ask the local medical staff to obtain as much information as possible from direct questioning before this occurs.

Local medical staff
- The patient may be well known at the hospital, general practice or in the community.
- Staff may be aware of next of kin or contact person (see below).
- Past medical records on file.

Local pharmacy
- Current medications including doses and available quantities.

Family and friends
- May have access to her house to look for potential ingested medications.

Mental health services
- Likely to have access to current medication regimen.
- Will be involved in ongoing care and will be able to notify her usual community mental healthcare team or psychiatrist.

Poisons information
- Varies regionally.
- Many countries have dedicated around-the-clock poisons information services available by phone or via the web to medical staff and, in less detail, to the general public.
- A clinical toxicologist is usually available to give high-level advice to the coordinator and PHRM team.

Discussion 32.2

While tasking the PHRM team to respond, the coordinator should provide clinical support and critical care advice to the referring hospital. It is important that the rationale for the advice given be relatively explicit as the regional hospital medical staff may not have extensive experience in the management of critically ill patients, let alone those with complex poisonings.

This patient has taken a life-threatening polypharmacy overdose and is likely to deteriorate significantly prior to the arrival of the retrieval team. The local medical team will need to provide a series of critical interventions in a short time span and may need to be provided with advice regarding the delivery of these. The retrieval coordinator will be required to ensure that the local team is aware of the expected time course of evolution of her poisoning, and the interventions required to provide stability, and will be required to ensure that these occur as efficiently as possible.

The codeine component of her analgesics may explain the depressed conscious state, but not her haemodynamic compromise or ECG. Sinus tachycardia and hypotension with a low diastolic pressure suggest peripheral alpha blockade, while the ECG findings of a sinus tachycardia, prolongation of the QRS, rightward axis with a terminal R wave in aVR suggest sodium channel blockade. These findings, in combination with her requirement for mental health support, should immediately raise the suspicion of tricyclic antidepressant (TCA) toxicity. Note that the degree of QRS widening following TCA ingestion reflects the risk of seizures, wide complex arrhythmia and cardiac arrest.

Tricyclic antidepressant toxicity typically escalates rapidly in the first few hours after ingestion and peaks at around 6 hours post ingestion. This patient will require immediate serum alkalinisation through a combination of sodium bicarbonate administration, intubation and gentle hyperventilation, in addition to haemodynamic support and seizure control.

Additionally, it is likely that a significant amount of paracetamol (and codeine phosphate) has also been ingested. The risk of paracetamol-induced hepatic injury increases significantly if antidotal therapy with acetyl cysteine is initiated more than 8 hours after ingestion, and treatment should be initiated on-site or with the retrieval team if a paracetamol level cannot be performed within this timeframe.

Airway

- Rapid clinical deterioration is highly likely given the collateral history and ECG abnormalities.
- Despite the relatively high-scoring current GCS, this patient should undergo early anaesthesia, tracheal intubation and controlled ventilation.
- Assuming there are staff available with the requisite skills to do so, this should occur as soon as possible and before the PHRM team arrive.
- Avoidance of acidaemia following TCA poisoning is critical (see below). Hypoventilation and hypercarbia during the induction of anaesthesia must be avoided.
- A modified RSI technique with assisted mask ventilation prior to induction should be used. Doing so will ensure that any fall in pH associated with apnoea following induction is minimised. This will be of particular benefit if any difficulty is encountered during intubation.
- Pre-induction plasma alkalinisation with sodium bicarbonate should also occur (see below).

Breathing

- Acidaemia will decrease TCA plasma protein binding, increase plasma levels of free drug, and increase the ionised fraction of free drug trapped in the vascular compartment. This combination of kinetic effects increases toxicity and, conversely, creating an alkaline serum reduces it.
- Once intubated and ventilated, $ETCO_2$ should be monitored and low–normal (30 mmHg [4 kPa]) levels targeted. The serum pH should be maintained at 7.45–7.55.

Circulation

- Both the borderline hypotension, ECG changes and acidaemia should be treated with sodium bicarbonate (initially 1–2 mmol/kg over 3 to 5 minutes, titrated to narrowing of the QRS and aiming for a serum pH of 7.45–7.55. Maximum cumulative total of bolus doses should not exceed 6 mmol/kg, and the serum pH should not be allowed to exceed 7.55.

- Once intubated, the target serum pH can generally be achieved with hyperventilation alone. Occasionally a bicarbonate infusion may be required but will not be effective unless the patient is mandatorily hyperventilated.
- Hypotension should also be corrected with intravenous fluid resuscitation.
- Infused vasoactive agents are advised for volume-resistant hypotension.
- Hypertonic saline solutions are effective in improving sodium channel blockade. However, sodium bicarbonate, with the combined benefits of high-dose sodium and an alkalinising agent, is preferred.

Gut decontamination

- The routine use of gastric lavage is not recommended.
- Activated charcoal (1 g/kg) may reduce plasma paracetamol and TCA concentration if given early.
- If given, charcoal should be administered by nasogastric tube following tracheal intubation for airway protection.

Other

Regularly check the pH and electrolytes

- The PHRM team should plan to take a portable point of care testing unit with them.

N-acetylcysteine

- Death from paracetamol poisoning should not occur in patients treated with N-acetylcysteine (NAC) within 8 hours of acute ingestion.
- In view of the uncertain history, NAC (if available) should be commenced immediately by the referring hospital staff until further assessment in the receiving ICU.
- NAC is infused in a two-stage intravenous infusion giving a total dose of 300 mg/kg over 20 hours.
  - Infusion 1: 200 mg/kg in 500 mL of 5% glucose over 4 hours.
  - Infusion 2: 100 mg/kg diluted in 1000 mL of 5% glucose over 16 hours.
  - If not available locally, the coordinator should advise the PHRM team to take NAC with them. This is unlikely to be a standard agent in the PHRM team's drug pack but should be available on base.

In addition

- A urinary catheter should be placed.
- Invasive arterial access should be sited for blood pressure monitoring and repeated blood sampling.
- Central venous access may be needed if vasoactive-infused agents are required.
- A blood sample should be drawn and held for later comparative assessment of paracetamol level, liver function and coagulation studies.
- Avoid long-acting muscle relaxants if possible as they may mask seizure activity.

Discussion 32.3

On arrival the retrieval team's priorities are the following.

- Obtain and confirm a history of the presenting events, in hospital progress and interventions.

- Perform a screening examination of the patient.
- View all relevant investigations.
- Ensure
  1. The patient is intubated and has correctly positioned and secured tracheal and gastric tubes
  2. That the target pH range has been achieved, and adopt or continue a ventilation strategy to maintain this
  3. That the patient is volume replete and haemodynamically supported with adequate blood pressure and end-organ perfusion
  4. That acetylcysteine has been commenced and is running at an appropriate rate and dose
  5. That appropriate resuscitative medications are drawn up or immediately available
     - Bicarbonate (for the management of broad complex arrhythmia)
     - Long-acting benzodiazepine (for seizure management)
  6. That appropriate vascular access and invasive monitoring have been obtained and are secured
  7. That the retrieval coordinator and receiving facility are aware of any significant developments.

Key points

- Good information facilitates good decision making, particularly when coordinating a PHRM team response to a critically ill patient at a distant location.
- Early intervention following TCA overdose reduces the risk of potentially fatal cardiovascular and neurological sequelae. The threshold for such intervention should be low, particularly when air medical transport is required.

Additional reading

Murray L, et al. Toxicology handbook, 3rd ed. Elsevier, 2015.
National Poisons Information Service: www.toxbase.org.
Therapeutic Guidelines Limited. Toxicology and toxinology guidelines. Author, 2021.
Toxicology and Toxinology, Therapeutic Guidelines Limited, Australia 2021.

Incident

A 59-year-old male alcoholic has been taken to a small rural emergency department by the local ambulance with an episode of haematemesis. He has known alcoholic liver disease and 1 week earlier was discharged from the regional referral centre also following an episode of haematemesis. During that admission he had a gastric endoscopy and had a number of oesophageal varices injected and banded.

Relevant information

- **PHRM team transport options:** Fixed-wing aircraft available.
- **Additional resources:** GP-led 10-bed hospital with nursing staff. Nil local surgical or anaesthetic capabilities, basic x-ray capabilities.
- **Retrieval options:** Hospital is 10 minutes' drive from local airfield. The fixed-wing flight time is 45 minutes from airfield to airfield with the major receiving centre 30 minutes' drive from the airport.
- **Other:** Nil.

Clinical information

The local GP has managed to obtain a 20G IV cannula in the left ante-cubital fossa and given 500 mL of lactated ringers/Hartmans and reported the following findings:
- HR 126 Regular.
- BP 110/76.
- RR 18.
- Sats 98% on 2L via nasal specs.

Question 33.1

Discuss any specific equipment, pharmacological and fluid considerations for retrieving this patient.

On arrival at the local hospital the GP reports that the patient has had two further vomits of bright red haematemesis, and you note the suction cannister (see picture below).

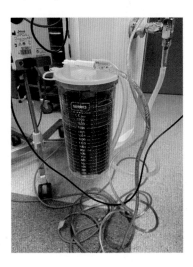

On your examination the patient is sweaty, grey and agitated.
- HR 141.
- BP 85/66.
- RR 24.
- Sats difficult to record due to poor perfusion.

Question 33.2

Discuss your management plan.

The patient is successfully intubated and put onto a transport ventilator. At this point, the patient has another haematemesis and the decision is made to place a Sengstaken-Blakemore tube.

Question 33.3

Describe the use of a Sengstaken-Blakemore Tube in the retrieval environment.

Question 33.4

Describe the following x-rays, your process for securing the tube in place and any particular considerations required for the flight back to the receiving facility.

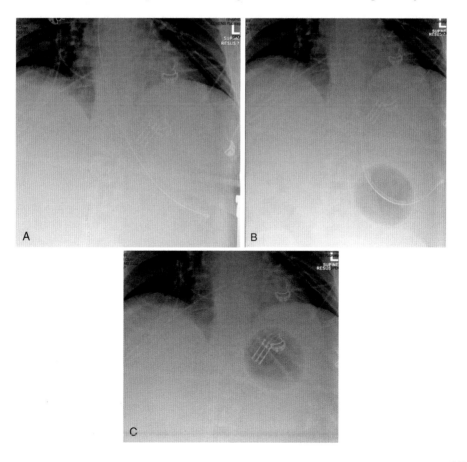

Discussion 33.1

This patient has known varices and liver disease and is likely to be coagulopathic and at risk of further bleeding. Modern PHRM service models will have a separate dedicated pack set for the management of patients with life-threatening GI haemorrhage. This should contain medication useful in the management of oesophageal varices such as terlipressin or octreotide, both of which can be given intravenously. Although evidence of benefit in acute GI bleed remains equivocal, proton pump inhibitors are routinely administered in these patients and would also be reasonable to have available. The addition of a gastric tamponade device such as a Sengstaken-Blakemore or Minnesota tube may be life-saving.

The team should take red blood cells and, if available, further blood products or fibrinogen concentrate in the form of a massive transfusion pack (MTP) (see Case 28).

Discussion 33.2

There are 1.5 litres of blood in the suction cannister. Clinically, the patient appears to have hypovolaemic shock with signs of cerebral hypoperfusion. They have ongoing GI bleeding and this will be difficult to manage in the back of an aircraft with the additional risk of aspiration should their mental state continue to deteriorate. Given their ongoing bleeding they are likely to require placement of a Sengstaken-Blakemore tube to facilitate management during retrieval. This will necessitate protection of the airway with intubation and ventilation prior to insertion.

In the first instance, better additional IV access should be obtained to allow some degree of volume replacement prior to induction. Options for this would be to use a rapid infusion catheter (see Case 28) to upgrade the current access or establish additional peripheral vascular access. If this is proving difficult then central access should be considered. Given the likely coagulopathy this should be in a site that is easily compressible and performed under ultrasound guidance. The femoral vein is ideal in this situation.

Pre-induction fluid loading should be with packed red cells via a portable blood warmer (see Case 28) and other blood products if available.

Terlipressin or octreotide should also be commenced at this point.

Discussion 33.3

A Sengstaken-Blakemore tube (SBT) (below) is used to control ongoing upper GI haemorrhage due to oesophageal varices, despite pharmacological intervention and coagulopathy correction. The device has two balloons – oesophageal and gastric. The gastric balloon alone controls bleeding in most cases by applying direct pressure to the gastric cardia (oesophageal blood supply) under traction. Generally, this is sufficient to arrest bleeding, but in some circumstances the oesophageal balloon may be required, which applies tamponade to the oesophageal variceal vessels directly.

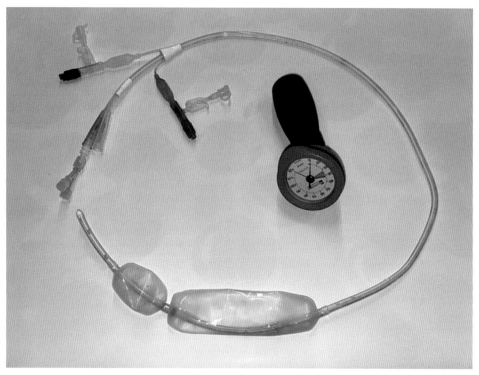

SBT and cuff manometer

There are different varieties of balloon tamponade device available, and teams should be familiar with the equipment available to them. Regardless of the device used, both balloons should be tested prior to insertion. If radiology is unavailable, then the pressure in the inflated gastric balloon should be measured (at a specified volume) using a cuff manometer prior to insertion to allow for pressure comparison post insertion. Once the balloons have been tested the stylet within the SBT should be lubricated by injecting some normal saline down the stylet port. This will help facilitate stylet removal once the tube is in place.

Measure the distance in an arc traced from the xiphisternum to the bridge of the nose via the earlobe using the tube against the patient to establish insertion depth (as a general rule, an insertion depth of 50 cm will be safe in the majority of patients). Lubricate the external tube with some lubricant gel and then insert the tube into the patient's oesophagus. This can be done either orally or nasally and may require the use of a laryngoscope and Magill forceps to assist with placement. Care needs to be taken not to damage the balloons with either instrument. The nasal route is much easier to secure for the transport process but needs to be weighed up against the risk of epistaxis, especially in the coagulopathic patient.

Discussion 33.4

Reviewing the x-rays (images A and B), the stylet can be seen safely within the confines of the stomach and remains so with the balloon inflated with 250 mL of air.

With traction on the tube, the x-ray shows it well positioned against the gastric cardia (image C). If x-rays are unavailable, measure the balloon pressure with the manometer to ensure it is at a similar pressure to that measured prior to insertion and definitely no more than 15 cm H_2O greater than the initial test pressure.

Generally, a hanging saline bag with a cloth tube tie is used to apply constant traction to the SBT. However, this is impractical in the retrieval environment. An alternative technique is the use of a dressing pad bolster taped to the tube at the nose (ideally) or mouth (see image below). The tube depth at the nose or mouth should be noted and regularly checked to ensure SBT migration has not occurred.

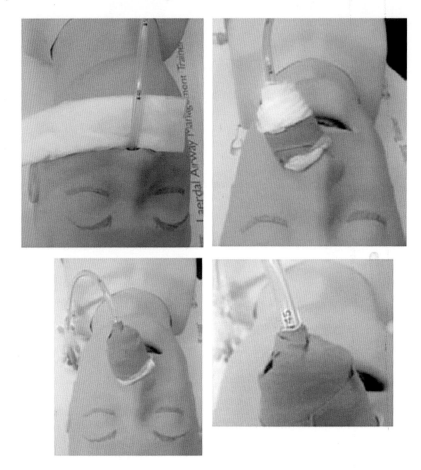

In the unlikely event of ongoing haemorrhage, despite an adequately inflated gastric balloon, the oesophageal balloon may require inflation. The oesophageal balloon should have a pressure of 25–35 cm H_2O and definitely not more than 40 cm H_2O.

A pressurised cabin, ideally at sea or ground level, will minimise volume changes in the balloons. Balloon-pressure monitoring using the manometer should occur throughout the retrieval, in particular when ambient pressure changes during flight, especially at take-off, maximum altitude and landing. This is particularly important for the oesophageal balloon where the risk of mucosal injury is greater.

Key points

- Balloon tamponade devices may be life-saving in cases of acute GI haemorrhage and should be available to PHRM teams.
- Such devices when combined with appropriate pharmacological agents may form an additional specialty equipment pack available prior to departure.
- As with all low-frequency high-consequence procedures, PHRM teams should undergo regular training to ensure safe and effective use of such equipment.

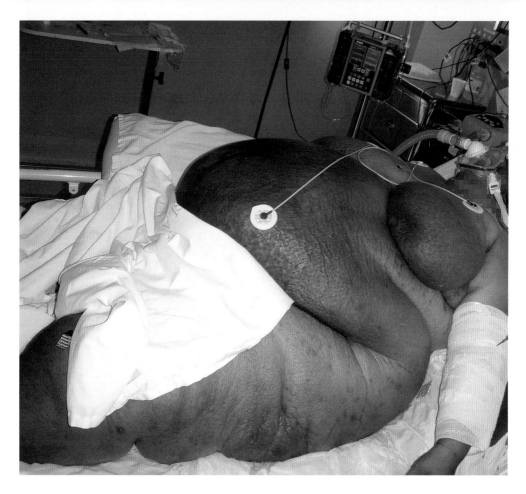

Incident

A 39-year-old woman with a history of hypertension, Type 2 diabetes and chronic renal impairment has presented to an isolated regional hospital 1100 km (690 miles) away. The local medical officer reports that she has significant respiratory distress requiring non-invasive ventilatory support and a high percentage of inspired oxygen. She responds to pain only. A urinary catheter was placed 3 hours ago but she has been anuric since. She is in atrial fibrillation with a ventricular rate of 138 beats per minute. Her blood pressure is not able to be measured. Her last recorded weight was 217 kg (480 lb).

Relevant information

- **PHRM team transport options:** Range of civilian and military fixed- and rotary-wing aircraft.
- **Local resources:** Hospital with local GP and nursing staff. Road ambulance single-stretcher capacity.
- **Retrieval destination:** Large tertiary referral hospital ICU.
- **Other:** Nil.

Question 34.1

What further information could be obtained by the clinical coordination team to help formulate a retrieval plan?

Question 34.2

What difficulties can be expected in the clinical assessment and management of this patient?

Question 34.3

Assuming it is appropriate to do so, how should she be transported to the retrieval destination?

Discussion 34.1

Clinical

This patient has overwhelmed the level of clinical care available at her current location and therefore critical care retrieval is required. The early clinical advice given, and clinical plans for the responding PHRM team, may well be influenced by further information. Further questions may include:

What is the usual level of physical functioning?
- Is she house or even bed bound?
- Does she function at the limit of her physiologic reserve even when 'well'?
- Is there any exercise capacity?

What is the time course of the current illness?
- Is this the clinical picture of sudden heart failure or progressive pneumonia or a combination?
- Is non-invasive ventilation likely to be adequate for the duration of the retrieval or would early invasive ventilation be indicated?

What current physiological support is required?
- She has high oxygen requirements at the moment, which may impact on transport platform selection.

What clinical investigations are available to aid diagnosis?
- Chest radiograph?
- Point-of-care blood analysis?
- Ultrasound?

Skill and knowledge at referral hospital
- If early intervention is advised, do the staff have the clinical capability to manage such a complex patient?

Logistics

Regional variation will guide the clinical coordinator in this regard. An in-depth knowledge of local transport assets (including their availability and patient weight limitations) and regional geography is required. Knowledge of available specialist bariatric patient transport equipment, platforms or even teams may also have an impact on the plan. In broad terms (and on top of the usual logistic considerations when coordinating a retrieval response), additional considerations include:

PHRM team response options
- Outbound and return legs may be achieved using differing transport platforms.

Referral facility layout and support
- Current location of patient.
- Lifts or ramps requiring negotiation.
- Personnel at the referring centre to assist in patient movement.

Patient transport options
- Hospital to aircraft at referral centre.
  - Regional ambulance capacity (including stretchers, vehicles and staff).
- Air asset capability and availability.
  - Range, speed, cabin pressurisation, loading mechanisms and capacity, stretcher bridge systems and equipment/patient restraint.
- Aircraft to hospital at receiving centre.
  - Local ambulance capacity.

PHRM team requirements
- Familiarity with potential use of novel transport platforms.
- Additional personnel for predicted logistical or clinical challenges.
- Additional/specialised equipment.

Discussion 34.2

Assessment

Most aspects of the clinical assessment are more difficult in the morbidly obese patient. In particular, non-invasive blood pressure may be inaccurate. A ratio between arm circumference and cuff breadth of 3:1 is required. The 'long large adult' cuff should be used with patients who weigh in excess of 130 kg (285 lb). Such a cuff may need to be included in a 'special response' pack for morbidly obese patients. In critically ill, obese patients, in whom blood pressure is labile and infused vasoactive agents may be required, invasive arterial pressure monitoring is preferred. However, arterial access may be problematic (see below).

Examination of the respiratory and gastrointestinal system is impaired because of large amounts of subcutaneous fatty tissue. In addition, most bony surface anatomy landmarks are obscured. Investigations (even simple venesection) may prove difficult and radiological examinations are complex to perform and image quality is often poor. The ability of using telemedicine in this case will allow the clinical coordination team to accurately assess the patient's clinical status in conjunction with the local medical team. The local team will also need to measure the patient's width and girth to determine which stretcher and, hence, transport platform may be used.

Management

Airway

Airway management in the morbidly obese patient is challenging, even for the most experienced airway clinician. Anatomical and pathophysiological abnormalities in the obese predispose to difficulty maintaining the airway when conscious level is impaired. In addition, functional residual capacity (FRC) is reduced and, even with effective pre-oxygenation, such patients rapidly desaturate after relatively short periods of apnoea. Acute critical illness only compounds this reduction in physiologic capacity.

To make matters worse, with inadequate preparation, the incidence of a difficult airway during rapid-sequence induction and intubation may be significantly higher in this group. In addition to the common predictors of a difficult airway (see Case 6), a large neck circumference may also predict difficulty, as would a known history of obstructive sleep apnoea. For these reasons, the PHRM team should ideally have access to difficult airway equipment (see Case 29).

Patient positioning is critical when managing the airway of the morbidly obese patient. Specifically, the patient's thorax and head should be elevated such that the external auditory meatus is level with the patient's sternum (the 'ear to sternal alignment') (Levitan & Kinkle 2007).

Ventilation

Non-invasive ventilatory techniques are challenging in the morbidly obese patient and given this patient's current location, physiological compromise and predicted clinical course intubation and ventilation will be required. Notwithstanding acute pulmonary pathology, the airway pressures of ventilated morbidly obese patients are high as a result of reduced thoracic and upper abdominal compliance. Diaphragmatic excursion is also limited. Positive end expiratory pressure (PEEP) is routinely required and high levels may need to be considered. Should pleural decompression or drainage be required, navigating the extensive subcutaneous tissues may provide added complexity.

Circulation

Peripheral and central venous access is difficult. Portable ultrasound guidance will be very useful in this regard. Similarly, arterial access for invasive pressure monitoring may prove problematic. In both cases, longer cannulae may need to be used to account for the depth of subcutaneous tissue. In emergency settings or when obtaining central access proves impossible, there should be a low threshold for utilising an intraosseous access device. Again, a longer device will need to be selected.

Discussion 34.3

There are, in fact, multiple components to the transport. Regional variation will have an impact on the final decision of transport platform(s) and process. In general, multiple movements of the patient from one stretcher to another should be avoided to minimise harm to both the patient and all personnel. Any transport platform considered should therefore accommodate the same stretcher if possible. The patient, the PHRM team and equipment restraint must also be considered when non-standard transport vehicles are utilised.

The first consideration is how to transport the patient from the bed to an appropriate stretcher (specific bariatric stretchers are commonly used). There are a number of devices available (including hover mattresses – see figures 34.1 and 34.2)) which may be present at the referring facility. If not, such equipment will need to be taken by the PHRM team who may have access to a dedicated bariatric retrieval pack specifically for this purpose. The second consideration is how to secure monitoring and supportive equipment with the patient. An equipment bridge is ideal but standard bridges may not be fit for purpose.

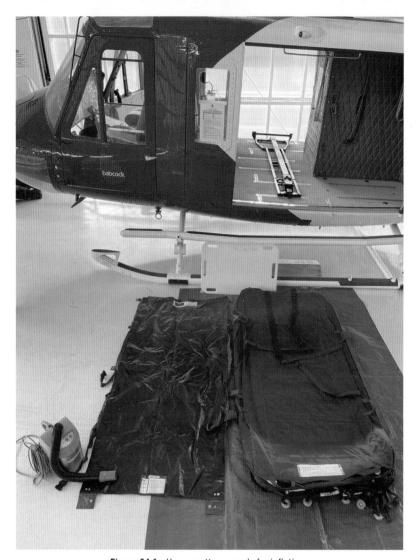

Figure 34.1. Hover mattress ready for inflation.

The next consideration is the movement to an air transport platform. Many rotary-wing aircraft are capable of bariatric patient transport. Aircraft range, speed, the need for refuelling, and the absence of a pressurised cabin, will all need consideration. If a fixed-wing aircraft is selected, a road ambulance trip is unavoidable, and negotiation of any lifts or ramps out of the hospital complex may require a number of non-clinical assistants. Although a road trip for the whole retrieval is possible, the distance is significant, will require several legs, and the region may then be without any ambulance capacity for several hours.

At 217 kg (480 lb), this patient is at the weight limit for many commonly used civilian air medical transport platforms. Increasing frequency of bariatric patient transport and retrieval has necessitated the development of enhanced aircraft and stretcher load capacity (e.g. up to 300 kg) and different methods of patient loading to improve staff health and safety. Although a rare requirement, military assistance in such circumstances (e.g. utilising the ambulance drive on load capacity of platforms such as the C130 or C17 aircraft – see Case 54) has been successfully reported.

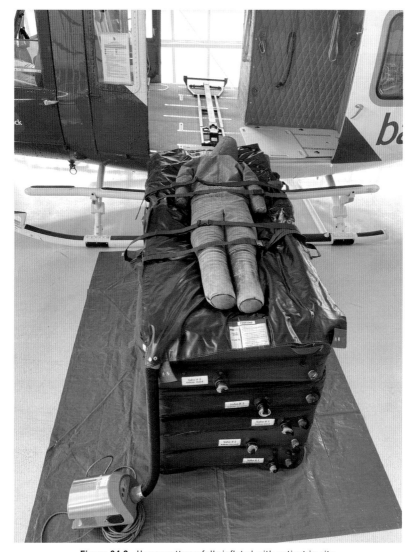

Figure 34.2. Hover mattress fully inflated with patient in situ.

Key points

- The growing need to retrieve and transfer morbidly obese patients presents numerous clinical and logistic challenges.
- Specialised vehicles, stretchers, air frames and medical equipment are increasingly utilised.
- Extensive pre-retrieval preparation and planning will assist in a safe transfer for both patient and attending team members.

Reference

Levitan RM, Kinkle WC. Pocket guide to intubation, 2nd edn. Airway Cam Technologies, 2007.

Additional reading

Burtenshaw A, Benger J, Nolan J. Emergency airway management, 2nd edn. Cambridge University Press, 2015.
Jones C. Retrieval and transfer of bariatric patients in NSW. Curr Anaesth Crit Care 2010; 21(5):287–291.

Incident

A 34-year-old male has presented to his local GP-run rural hospital in Australia, 25 minutes after a witnessed snakebite to his right foot. He was not wearing socks or footwear at the time, and drove himself to hospital. The attending doctor describes the patient as nauseous but otherwise asymptomatic, and has rung for management advice at 35 minutes post bite.

Clinical information

Observations on arrival to hospital:
- GCS 15.
- PR 105.
- BP 155/60.
- Saturations 98% on air.
- The doctor describes minor bleeding from a scratch at the reported bite site, but has not yet examined the patient.

Relevant information

- **Aircraft:** Fixed-wing (flight time: 30 minutes) or rotary wing (flight time: 50 minutes).
- **Local resources:** No on-site laboratory or blood products. No staff with advanced airway capabilities. No ICU facilities. Polyvalent antivenom available. No monovalent antivenom available.
- **Other:** Helipad on hospital grounds. Road transport via ambulance without medical support possible (drive time 80 minutes).

Question 35.1

What are the principles of snakebite management?

Question 35.2

What information do you need from the attending doctor's examination findings?

Question 35.3

Is it preferable to use polyvalent or monovalent antivenom? How is appropriate antivenom selected?

The attending doctor's physical examination findings are:
- Minor bite site bleeding on the right foot
- No lymphadenopathy
- No mucosal bleeding
- Partial ophthalmoplegia and subtle ptosis
- No weakness of the remaining motor cranial nerves or muscles of respiration

Question 35.4

What immediate management is required?

Question 35.5

Does the patient require retrieval, and if so what platform should be used?

Question 35.6

What key issues need to be re-assessed at the point of team arrival?

Discussion 35.1

The principles of snakebite management are as follows:
- Deliver resuscitative care in line with standard ALS guidelines.
- Slow venom distribution with a pressure bandage AND immobilisation.
- Evaluate for evidence of envenoming.
- Determine the appropriate antivenom for use if envenoming is suspected.
- Administer antivenom early if envenoming is suspected.
- Deliver medical support for venom-induced complications:
  - Haemorrhage
  - Paralysis
  - Rhabdomyolysis
  - Thrombotic microangiopathy
  - Acute kidney injury.

Discussion 35.2

The attending doctor's examination should target findings of envenoming, as presence indicates the need for antivenom. The clinical features of envenoming are:
- Coagulopathy (examine for evidence of spontaneous bleeding)
  - Australian snakes may cause either consumptive coagulopathy (brown, tiger, taipan, rough-scaled snake and hoplocephalus species) or an anticoagulant effect (mulga, Collet's snake, red-bellied black snake).
  - Spontaneous haemorrhage is considerably more likely with consumptive coagulopathy.
  - Coagulation parameters and bleeding risk due to consumptive coagulopathy DO NOT normalise following antivenom administration, but will normalise more rapidly in response to clotting factor replacement IF a neutralising dose of antivenom has been administered.
  - Coagulation parameters due to anticoagulant coagulopathy WILL normalise following antivenom administration, but bleeding risk is low.
  - With the exception of brown snake, the presence of consumptive coagulopathy is associated with a risk of neurotoxicity.
  - Anticoagulant coagulopathy is not associated with a risk of neurotoxicity.
  - Point of care INR analysers are unreliable in the assessment of venom-induced coagulopathy and should not be used. False positives and false negatives are both possible.
  - Whole blood that remains non-clotted beyond 20 minutes after being put in a glass container suggests coagulopathy and therefore envenoming. The type of container used is critical to the validity of this test.
- Neurotoxicity (examine for evidence of descending paresis and/or ventilatory failure)
  - Tiger, taipan and rough-scaled snake cause a mixture of pre- and post-synaptic neurotoxicity, generally accompanied by consumptive coagulopathy.

- Death adder causes primarily post-synaptic neurotoxicity, without coagulopathy.
- The typical pattern of evolution involves a descending paresis, involving the cranial motor nerves before the neck muscles, then the muscles of the chest wall and ventilation, and finally limb muscles.
- Antivenom will reverse post-synaptic toxicity, and will halt the progression of (but NOT reverse) pre-synaptic neurotoxicity. Therefore, antivenom should be administered as soon as neurotoxicity is detected.
- Myotoxicity (examine for muscle belly tenderness to palpation)
  - May be caused by tiger, taipan, rough-scaled snake, mulga, Collet's snake, or red-bellied black snake.
  - Creatine Kinase (CK) levels will not begin to rise until myotoxicity is established, and the progression of myotoxicity may be halted (but NOT reversed) by the administration of antivenom.
- Thrombotic microangiopathy and/or acute kidney injury
  - Clinically silent pathologies that are demonstrated by laboratory evaluation.
  - The incidence and severity of acute kidney injury may be reduced by early use of antivenom for other primary indications (typically the finding of consumptive coagulopathy).

Discussion 35.3

Monovalent antivenom contains an antibody load sufficient to neutralise the maximal anticipated venom load for its defined species of snake. Polyvalent antivenom contains this neutralising capacity for each of the medically relevant snake species, and consequently is a significantly larger volume and protein load. Polyvalent antivenom carries a greater risk of an adverse reaction than do monovalent antivenoms.

Appropriate antivenom may be selected by:

- Coupling the observed envenoming syndrome with knowledge of the local snake fauna. Most clinical toxicologists use this approach, and their advice is available through hospital-based toxicology services in most states, or the national Poisons Information Centre network. In regions where two species with similar envenoming syndromes co-exist, two monovalent antivenoms may be used together (and remain a lower risk than polyvalent).
- Use of a Venom Detection Kit and a sample of venom swabbed from the bite site. The VDK cannot be used on blood and has a high false positive rate when used on urine samples. A positive VDK indicates the type of antivenom to be used IF the patient is envenomed, but DOES NOT diagnose envenoming.
- Use polyvalent antivenom if neither of the previous approaches is possible.

Discussion 35.4

The attending doctor's assessment suggests neurotoxicity and therefore envenoming. Immediate management required is:

- Application of pressure bandage (see image over page)
- Immobilisation of the affected limb
- Secure intravenous access
- Administer 1 vial of polyvalent antivenom (dilute in 500 mL saline and administer over 20 minutes)

- Monitor for complications of antivenom administration (pyrogenic and/or anaphylactic reactions)
- Monitor for progression of neurotoxicity, and provided airway and ventilatory support if required.

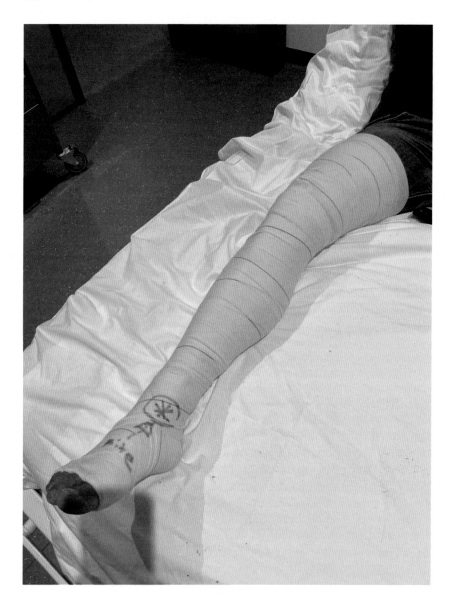

Discussion 35.5

The patient is developing neurotoxicity in a hospital that lacks the ability to manage airway and ventilatory issues and must be retrieved using a team and transport platform that can deliver this high-level support. Road transfer without a retrieval team is not appropriate, but either air platform would be reasonable. The ability to land a helicopter on hospital grounds makes this an attractive option.

Discussion 35.6

Once on-site, the team will need to re-evaluate:
- For the clinical signs of envenoming and their rate of progression
- The adequacy of pressure immobilisation
- Time, type and dose of antivenom used
- The response to, and potential complications of, antivenom administration.

The team arrives at the patient 2.5 hours post bite. The patient is lying in bed with an adequate pressure bandage in place and an immobilising splint on the affected leg. One vial of polyvalent antivenom was administered 90 minutes post bite. A re-assessment of the patient demonstrates:
- GCS 15.
- He appears short of breath with a weak and ineffectual cough. Blood-stained saliva is pooling in his mouth.
- An emesis bag at the bedside contains several hundred mL frank blood.
- No oropharyngeal oedema.
- No wheeze or stridor, no urticaria.
- Respiratory rate: 20 with small tidal volumes.
- Saturations 95% on air.
- PR 120.
- BP 90/50.
- Established ophthalmoplegia and ptosis.
- He is unable to lift his head from his pillow and is evidencing diaphragmatic breathing.

Question 35.7

What additional management is required?

Question 35.8

Is more antivenom required? How might an expert opinion be obtained to support this decision?

Discussion 35.7

The assessment suggests progressing neurotoxicity with an imperilled airway and ventilatory failure, together with venom-induced coagulopathy (likely consumptive) and haemorrhagic shock. There does not appear to be evidence of antivenom-associated anaphylactic shock. The immediate management interventions are:
- Rapid sequence induction of anaesthesia, intubation and subsequent provision of adequate sedation
- Mechanical ventilation with provision of adequate minute ventilation and oxygenation
- Volume resuscitation (preferably with packed cells)
- Provision of clotting factors (if available) after confirming that a neutralising dose of antivenom has been given.

Discussion 35.8

The antivenom dose required to ensure venom neutralisation is a topic of some controversy, although most would consider 1 vial of polyvalent antivenom to be adequate. Factors that might prompt consideration of further antivenom (without obligating it) would include multiple bites or a prolonged attachment time during bite. An expert opinion may be obtained to support this decision from a tertiary hospital-based toxicology service, or from the national Poisons Information Centre network.

Key points
• All potentially venomous snake bites should initially be managed with a pressure bandage and immobilisation.
• Clinical features of envenomation will vary with snake species and degree of envenoming.
• Relevant antivenoms may be available at local hospitals or carried by the PHRM team.

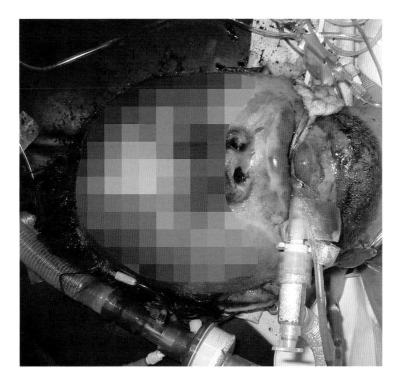

Incident

A 40-year-old mining worker has been involved in a gas explosion and subsequent fire. He has sustained burns to the face and circumferentially to both lower limbs (totalling 25% burn surface area [BSA]). He was intubated and ventilated on arrival at a regional hospital emergency department approximately 3 hours ago and now requires retrieval to a specialist burns centre.

Relevant information

- **PHRM team transport options:** Rotary-wing.
- **Additional resources:** Regional hospital staff.
- **Retrieval options:** Major trauma hospital with specialist burns facility 90 minutes by air.
- **Other:** Patient weight estimated to be 80 kg (175 lb).

Question 36.1

Describe the findings illustrated in the picture above.

Question 36.2

Outline the specific issues relevant to the management and safe retrieval of this patient.

Question 36.3

What would be the indication for lower limb escharotomy in this retrieval environment? If indicated, how should the procedure be performed?

Discussion 36.1

There is a significant facial burn injury, which appears to include areas of both deep partial thickness (wet, erythematous) and full thickness (dry and pale or charred) burn injury involving the entire face but not the neck. There is extensive associated tissue oedema. Both nares are heavily coated with soot, blood or charred tissue. There is a dressing over the left anterior shoulder. An oral tracheal tube is visible at the lips and has been pre-cut. A gastric tube is also visible adjacent to the tracheal tube. A tracheal tube tie is in situ but partially obscured by the tissue oedema. Ventilation circuitry is visible, including sidestream $ETCO_2$ chamber and sampling tubing.

Discussion 36.2

Pre-departure

Assessment

Although overt, the burn injury may be only one of a number of serious injuries. The mechanism of an explosion should flag the need to consider blunt, penetrating and blast trauma pathophysiology. Seek collateral history if available (e.g. from coworkers) and clarify the patient's past medical history, tetanus status, known allergies and current medications. Also clarify the nature of the pre-hospital scene including enclosed-space fire exposure (raising the risk of carbon monoxide, cyanide and prolonged super-heated gas inhalation) and additional trauma mechanisms such as a secondary fall from height. The clinical findings and therapeutic interventions, both pre-hospital and in the emergency department, should also be reviewed. Questions to ask would include:

- Apart from airway protection, were there other indications for intubation, such as respiratory failure, unconsciousness, evidence of a head injury?
- What radiological investigations have been done?

A thorough head-to-toe clinical review should then occur with specific focus on airway security, vascular access and evidence of additional injuries. At this time, a formal assessment can be made of the percentage of BSA, noting that simple erythema is not included in this calculation. A suggested assessment and management proforma for this purpose can be found in Appendix 1.5.

Interventions

The initial concern here is airway security as a pre-cut tracheal tube has been placed and facial tissue oedema is likely to progress. The tracheal tube will need to be replaced as extubation in transit is a real possibility if the current tracheal tube remains secured to the swelling facial tissues. This is a high-risk procedure.

Involvement of on-site senior anaesthetic personnel is advised. If available, additional 'difficult airway' equipment (e.g. airway exchange catheter, fibre-optic scope as part of a difficult airway pack) (see Case 29) should be taken by the PHRM team. A contingency plan, including emergency surgical airway (note the neck is relatively spared) should be made and clearly articulated to all team members (see Cases 6, 25 and Appendix 1.1). If a fibre-optic scope is available (either locally or via the PHRM team), inhalational burn injury can also be ascertained.

The correct placement of the orogastric tube should be confirmed as gastric stasis is common.

At least two points of vascular access should be secured (preferably away from any burnt skin) and resuscitative fluid requirements calculated. There is significant regional variation regarding fluid resuscitation guidelines following burn injury. The receiving burns unit protocol should be utilised where possible. The modified Parkland formula is commonly used and described below.

In this case:

$$\text{Total fluid (first 24 hours)} = 2 \text{ to } 4 \text{ mL} \times \% \text{ BSA} \times \text{patient weight (kg)}$$
$$= 4000 \text{ to } 8000 \text{ mL}$$

Half of this fluid should be given over the first 8 hours (from time of injury, not time of assessment) and the remainder over the ensuing 16 hours. Use a crystalloid solution.

It is suggested that fluid therapy be started if BSA is greater than 15–20% and fluids should be titrated to a urine output of at least 0.5 mL/kg/hour (greater if myoglobinuria is present), so a urinary catheter should be placed if not already in situ.

Other blood results should be checked before departure as correction may be required. If inhalational injury is strongly suspected or confirmed, or there is evidence of progressive rhabdomyolysis with myoglobinuria, fluid requirements are likely to exceed predicted fluid calculations.

Cooling of burns is most effective within the first three hours but should occur for no more than 20 minutes as hypothermia is a greater risk beyond this time. Cool running water is the preferred method. After 20 minutes of cooling the burn area, the patient should be actively warmed to prevent hypothermia.

Antibiotics have no proven role at this stage of treatment.

Patient packaging

Packaging should ensure easy access to intravascular devices. The burn area should be dressed to reduce heat loss and improve analgesia. Cling film is ideal and can be applied longitudinally on limb areas (not wrapped circumferentially). Facial burns may be covered with paraffin gauze. In general, topical creams should be avoided on the face. Be sure to address good eye care (removal of macroscopic particulate matter and use of artificial lubrication).

The legs should be elevated and, if indicated, escharotomy considered (see below). Non-burn-related trauma should be addressed including immobilisation of long bone fractures and full spinal precautions.

In-flight

Monitoring

With extensive burn injury, monitoring may be problematic. For example, ECG electrodes may not adhere to the chest wall and SaO_2 traces may be absent or poor (or inaccurately high in the setting of carbon monoxide toxicity). In addition, there may be limited non-burnt areas for central venous or invasive arterial access. In the absence of non-burnt skin, vascular access may be achieved through the burn.

Common problems in the retrieval and transport setting are the assessment of depth of anaesthesia and the adequacy of analgesia in ventilated patients without closed head injury. Pupil reaction may not be measurable with severe facial and periorbital oedema. The endogenous sympathetic release associated with extensive tissue insult may make interpreting physiologic signs of awareness or pain difficult.

Avoidance of repeated muscle relaxation and consideration of the use of a dissociative anaesthetic agent with significant analgesic potency such as ketamine is recommended.

Measure core temperature constantly and continue to actively warm the patient. Check the blood sugar levels intermittently.

Ongoing care

The patient's destination should be made clear prior to departure. Discussion with the specialist burn team awaiting the patient should be facilitated through the coordination centre.

Psychological support or other social supports for family may be required.

Discussion 36.3

Escharotomy in the pre-hospital or retrieval environment occurs uncommonly. In this setting, limb escharotomy should only be considered after consultation with the receiving burns unit team. In general, limb escharotomy would be reserved for situations involving critical limb ischaemia with very prolonged times to definitive care (e.g. > 3 to 4 hours).

If limb escharotomy is deemed necessary, the procedure should be conducted in the referral hospital operating theatres and the expertise of local surgical staff called upon. In emergency or out-of-hospital settings, the basic principles for performing lower-limb escharotomy are as follows:

- Ensure adequate analgesia.
- Ensure strict asepsis.
- Place the lower limb in a neutral position.
- Commence the incisions longitudinally in healthy unburnt skin (see Appendix 1.5).
- Stay lateral (mid axial) and avoid the common peroneal nerve laterally and long saphenous vein medially.
- Continue the incision into subcutaneous fat on both sides of the limb.
- Run a finger along the incision to ensure complete deep fascia division.
- Apply a sterile dressing and reassess for improved distal perfusion.
- Document the procedure, any complications and outcome, and be sure to hand over what you have done at the receiving hospital.

In addition, severe thoracic burns (not present here) resulting in a thickened truncal eschar may profoundly impact on chest wall elasticity and compromise patient ventilation. Emergency thoracic escharotomy in the pre-hospital environment is required in such circumstances. The technique for thoracic escharotomy is described in Appendix 1.5.

Key points

- The core components of good, acute, severe, burn injury management include:
  - Accurate assessment
  - Management of life-threatening events (actual and potential)
  - Fluid resuscitation
  - Pain control
  - Wound management and infection control
  - Early specialist burns unit referral and transfer.
- Exact burn management guidelines will vary regionally. Communicate early with the receiving burns unit.
- A small number of patients will require life- or vital-tissue-saving escharotomy in the pre-hospital or retrieval environment. When required, this must be timely and adequate.

Additional reading

Australian and New Zealand Burn Association (ANZBA) website. Online. Available: www.anzba.org.au. 26 July 2021.

British Burn Association (BBA) website. Online. Available: www.britishburnassociation.co.uk. 26 July 2021.

CASE 37

The following questions relate to the tasking and coordination of physician-led PHRM teams (see also Cases 22 and 42). Tasking and clinical coordination are key aspects of pre-hospital and retrieval medicine. Triage, resource allocation and high-level clinical oversight are core elements to this process.

The following incidents should be considered to be independent of each other for the purposes of this case. In each case, the decision to task, coordinate and support the PHRM team rests solely with you as the clinical coordinator. You have information technology, maps and communications equipment available to you.

Incident A

A rural facility has called to request a retrieval. On the phone is a single-handed rural practitioner with limited anaesthesia experience who tells you about a 22-year-old obese female who has taken a polypharmacy overdose. The location is in a small town 35 minutes away by fixed-wing aircraft. The patient was GCS 3 with an obstructing airway, so the practitioner has intubated the patient who is now reported as 'self-ventilating via the tube attached to a bag and valve'. Despite reporting no complications with the procedure, you can hear noisy breathing in the background. The doctor used suxamethonium for intubation and is now keen to administer longer-acting neuromuscular paralysis. The doctor has attached an $ETCO_2$ monitor which is reading '0' and on further questioning the doctor believes the monitor is broken.

Question 37.1

Discuss possible clinical issues and options while still on the phone to the rural practitioner, and consider suggestions for follow-up of the case.

Discussion 37.1

This incident involves acute clinical issues, but also communication. Noisy breathing following intubation suggests tracheal tube misplacement or leak, and the situation could rapidly deteriorate if longer-acting neuromuscular paralysis is administered. The complexity of the incident is compounded by distance – even if the PHRM team leaves immediately, it will not arrive in time to help with the airway issue. In addition, communication solely via telephone increases the chances of miscommunication. As coordinator, your first steps should be to prevent administration of neuromuscular paralysis and dispatch a PHRM team. Telemedicine would be beneficial in this case and, if available, this should be initiated as early as possible. Attempts should be made to ascertain whether the non-functional $ETCO_2$ monitor is in fact broken or simply is not recording CO_2 because the tracheal tube is misplaced (oesophageal) or leaking. Blowing into the monitor (using a fresh sampling circuit) can often demonstrate that it is functional. In the absence of further evidence to support correct placement of the tracheal tube, it should be removed, and the patient managed with simple airway techniques until arrival of the PHRM team.

While an error may have occurred, the doctor has been trying to manage a critically unwell patient, possibly at the limits of his abilities. Such clinicians are valuable assets in remote communities and it is important that they feel supported and offered educational opportunities for skills improvement. If an error has occurred, the appropriate process will need to be followed. This might include:
- Entry into the local incident-reporting system
- Feedback to the supervisor of the referring doctor

- Open multidisciplinary audit
- Root cause analysis (see Case 52).

Incident B

A motorcyclist has been involved in a collision with a four-wheel drive vehicle in the sub-urbs. Messages from the scene are staccato and unclear. It appears the patient is in extre-mis. A PHRM team has been dispatched but is still 20 minutes away by road. A message is received that the ambulance crew on-scene wish to depart to the nearest hospital, which is 5 minutes away and has several services including emergency medicine and anaesthesia, but is not a trauma centre. The quaternary trauma centre is 20 minutes away by road.

Question 37.2

Discuss the options in the case with particular reference to trauma systems.

Discussion 37.2

Two options are available regarding coordination decision making. Transport to the nearest as requested or a suggested diversion to the trauma centre with a PHRM team rendezvous en route.

The benefit of going to the nearest hospital is short lived as the infrastructure in that hospital is less able to deal with the predicted pathophysiological derangements of com-plex polytrauma. It is inevitable that the patient will need moving, but the consequence of subsequent secondary retrieval can lead to much longer times to definitive care. If the primary pathology requires specialist trauma surgery, then it is likely that the delay to definitive care will have an impact on patient outcome. However, the nearest hospital should have enough staff to generate a functional trauma team to receive the patient. In addition, some of the trauma pathology identified in the primary survey can be managed locally, allowing the patient to be stabilised prior to transfer. Certain trauma pathology (e.g. ruptured spleen) can be definitively managed locally but it is not possible to have knowledge of the trauma pathology at this early stage. Increasing the transport time will also have an impact on the ambulance crew who will now need to manage the critical trauma patient for far longer, with a subsequent impact on team psychology.

Such incidents are predictable and relatively common in ambulance practice, lead-ing to the concept of 'trauma bypass'. Systems for trauma bypass should be set up by the Ambulance Service and should link into trauma systems, PHRM and local hospital trauma practice. This will allow ambulance crews to assess trauma patients, make a clini-cal risk–benefit analysis, and decide whether to bypass or not with the support and back-ing of the ambulance service. This will also allow for clinical 'rendezvous' between the ambulance crew and the PHRM team if unstable trauma pathology is critically compro-mising the patient (e.g. chest decompression or airway intervention). Trauma bypass deci-sions must be subject to rigorous clinical governance and undergo clinical audit regularly.

In this instance, with the clinical information provided and assuming a system of trauma bypass exists locally, attempts should be made to take this patient to the quater-nary trauma centre with PHRM team rendezvous.

Incident C

A workplace incident has occurred at a factory 95 km from both the trauma centre and the PHRM base. A worker has suffered an amputation of the right hand in a guillotine-type device used for cutting paper. The patient has a makeshift tourniquet in situ, is already in the back of an ambulance and has almost arrived at the trauma centre (45 minutes by road). The factory foreman has been put through to you and informs you that he has retrieved the severed hand from the machine, and it looks 'otherwise undamaged'.

Question 37.3
Discuss your options and rationale.

Discussion 37.3
Considering the timelines in the question, the hand is still viable and reimplantation is a potential option. There is no need to call the inpatient teams at the trauma centre to confirm potential reimplantation as this could add significant delays to the process. Efforts should be made to retrieve the severed hand as safely and rapidly as possible. Dispatching the helicopter is an option but the clinical risk–benefit of using an aviation asset will need careful consideration and this includes other taskings, team availability, weather and landing sites. Of note, no clinical support is needed for the severed limb, but care of the hand during transport will be important. A road ambulance could be dispatched to collect the limb, but this may also be dependent on resource availability. The local Police force may be able to help and are arguably best placed to drive the limb under 'lights and sirens' to the trauma centre. The most rapid resource available should be tasked as this is a potential 'limb-saving' manoeuvre. Clear instructions on how to carry the limb will need to be passed to the Police service in a challenge-and-response format to ensure comprehension. The hand should be wrapped in a damp dressing or towel and placed in a sealed plastic bag, which should then be placed in a container filled with iced water. It is important that the hand is not packed in ice as this will cause tissue thermal injury.

Incident D
A 35-year-old primipara on her third cycle of IVF is pregnant with twins at 22/40. She lives with her partner in a rural property 175 km away. Her partner has called to report that the patient's waters broke a few minutes ago, both hind legs of a single twin have been partly delivered and the patient is in labour. There is a rural GP and an ambulance on the way to the property. Other staff in the ambulance coordination centre know the parents and appear distressed with the detail of this case and have requested an 'immediate helicopter dispatch' to assist at the scene.

Question 37.4
Discuss management and retrieval options in this case.

Discussion 37.4
Gestational age and the viability of the fetus is a significant issue in this case. The remote nature of the incident adds to the complexity of the required decision making. In addition, the fact that the patient is known to staff adds significant emotion to an already challenging scenario. While dispatching an aeromedical asset is plausible, the coordinator should reflect on team composition to best facilitate the case. A neonatal

team seems the initial team of choice, but considering that neither twin is yet fully delivered, it may be prudent to send a team that can manage the pregnant mother (see Case 42). It is unlikely that both teams can travel on the one asset, so rather than send one or other it may be better to take a few more minutes to gather information before dispatch.

A multiparty teleconference should be immediately set up with a neonatologist and an obstetrician to further analyse the case details. The neonatologist would be able to clarify the severity of the situation, especially regarding the partially delivered twin. In reality, the chance of survival for a 22/40 child partially delivered in the breach position over 4 hours from definitive care is extremely low and the focus should shift to the mother and keeping the second twin in utero for as long as possible. The obstetrician can also advise on management of the partial delivery plus the administration of tocolytics and steroids.

With the additional information from the teleconference, dispatch of a rotary-wing asset is now appropriate. Team composition should reflect management of the pregnant patient. A neonatal team could be kept on standby in this case. Despite the viability issues, it may be prudent to keep all options available.

Such a task carries significant emotional and psychological weight for all members of the team including team members in the coordination centre and the wider health service. As well as comprehensive case review and other clinical governance tools, such cases should trigger peer support intervention and subsequent wellness and wellbeing input.

Key points

- Clinical coordination teams should have access to advanced technologies to facilitate multiparty video and telephone calls to assist in case management.
- Clinical coordination models require flexibility to allow both medical and non-medical specialists to augment patient care.
- The skills and knowledge required for effective clinical coordination are unique to the PHRM environment.

CASE 38

Incident

A 49-year-old man with anuric chronic renal failure requires transfer to a tertiary centre for renal dialysis. He has missed his last two community dialysis appointments and now presents as breathless and mildly confused. He has a past history of anaemia, chronic obstructive pulmonary disease, previous myocardial infarction and heavy alcohol consumption.

Clinical information

- P 100.
- BP 105/60 mmHg.
- RR 25.
- GCS 14 (E4V4M6).
- SaO$_2$ 92% on air.

Blood analysis:

- PH 7.21.
- Potassium 6.1 mmol/L.
- Urea 39 mmol/L.
- Creatinine 845 μmol/L.
- Hb 90 g/dL.
- INR 2.2

Relevant information

- **PHRM team transport options:** Fixed-wing.
- **Local resources:** Local general practitioner. One land ambulance.
- **Retrieval options:** Tertiary centre 2 hours by fixed-wing.
- **Other:** Time 22:00 hours, Friday evening.

Question 38.1

Does the patient require retrieval or are they suitable for lower-acuity single-clinician transfer? What could be clinically optimised in this patient prior to departure?

Midway through the retrieval (in-flight), the patient vomits approximately 700 mL of fresh red blood into his oxygen mask.

Current clinical information

- P 130.
- BP 85/45 mmHg.
- RR 26.
- GCS 9 (E2V3M4).

Question 38.2

Discuss your management of this in-flight emergency?

The patient is now intubated and ventilated. Ten minutes post intubation, the patient suddenly becomes hypotensive (SBP 60 mmHg). The ventilator is alarming (see image over the page).

Question 38.3

How will you manage this development?

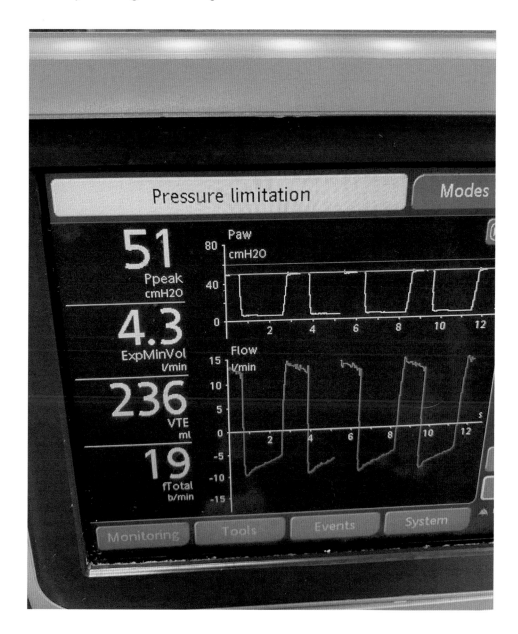

Discussion 38.1

The patient needs prompt dialysis, which will not be deliverable in the community given his acute presentation and the time of day.

The ultimate decision on retrieval versus low-acuity transfer will be dependent on the clinical condition of the patient, staff availability and transport logistics. Assuming there are no logistic limitations to aviation transfer, this patient demonstrates several clinical features of concern.

- New confusion
- Hyperkalaemia
- Acidaemia
- Anaemia in the setting of coagulopathy
- Elevated urea/creatinine ratio raising the possibility of upper gastrointestinal haemorrhage
- Respiratory compromise and potential intravascular volume overload.

Given the above, retrieval (as defined in Case 26) is required.

Prior to departure, there are several interventions that should be considered. Advanced systems with dedicated clinical coordination would be able to provide advice to the referring centre prior to the team's arrival. Telemedicine is increasingly utilised in this way (see Case 55).

- Adequate IV access
- Initial management of hyperkalaemia
- Reversal of coagulopathy
- Septic screen and consideration of antimicrobial therapy
- Some regional centres will have the ability to perform advanced vascular access (e.g. arterial lines) or respiratory support (e.g. continuous positive airways pressure [CPAP]) or blood transfusions, and this should be explored.

Discussion 38.2

A structured approach will be required to ensure that the chance of successful management is maximised. The following structure would be applicable to both the rotary- and fixed-wing environment.

Control

Prior to responding to the medical needs of the patient, alert the pilot via the communications system that there is a medical emergency in the cabin and seek approval to move out of your seat if required. It is important to clearly distinguish between medical emergencies and other (e.g. aviation) emergencies. Such communication through the aircraft's communication system should ensure all members of the PHRM team are aware of the clinical deterioration.

Airway

From the information given, the airway may be compromised with a reduced GCS and haematemesis. A parallel approach that encompasses airway assessment and basic manoeuvres (e.g. sitting up, positioning, suction) should occur in addition to preparation for potential advanced airway management in flight. A dynamic ongoing risk/benefit analysis should occur as prompt recovery or deterioration may require a new plan. Conditions for performing RSI in flight are high risk, and rescue airway options are limited. However, diverting to the nearest airfield may not be feasible at night, may only marginally improve operating conditions, but will add significant logistical problems and considerable time delay.

Bleeding

Confirm the origin of the bleeding (haematemesis or haemoptysis). This can be difficult, as blood coughed up gradually can be swallowed and subsequently vomited. Assuming haematemesis, the diagnosis is likely to be a peptic ulcer, although a variceal bleed cannot be ruled out. Reassess vital signs and see if the GCS is improving. Signs of encephalopathy are ominous in this situation and should lean the team towards securing the airway.

Treatment

Drug therapy for peptic ulcer disease has a role but is unlikely to prevent a re-bleed in the next few hours. Despite this, vitamin K and intravenous proton pump inhibitors should be considered. If a variceal bleed is thought likely, antibiotics should also be given. Other agents (e.g. somatostatin and vasopressin analogues) may be carried routinely but the team may find themselves without any appropriate agents. Likewise, most services will not routinely carry a device to provide oesophageal tamponade (e.g. Sengstakken-Blakemore tube – see Case 33). Fluid therapy will be challenging for this patient. Firstly, the patient initially appeared fluid overloaded and has no facility to excrete excess fluid. Secondly, extra fluid may elevate the blood pressure more than anticipated and may contribute to a gastrointestinal re-bleed.

Communications

When safe to do so, notify the tasking agency of this event so that the receiving hospital can be alerted to the patient's deterioration and the potential for higher-level care on arrival. Theoretically, this new information could generate resource issues at the receiving hospital (e.g. no intensive care beds, or a need for specialist gastrointestinal services), and the tasking agency may need to alter the final destination. The tasking agency can also arrange for blood and blood products to be brought to the airport.

Discussion 38.3

The diagnostic dilemma is whether this development represents a re-bleed or another pathology. A swift survey of the patient, monitors and equipment is indicated. The picture of the ventilator reveals a high airway pressure alarm. Tension pneumothorax is the prime concern, although dynamic hyperinflation is also possible (see Case 59). The history of chronic obstructive pulmonary disease increases the risk of bullous lung disease, which may lead to pneumothorax in the setting of positive pressure ventilation. Remove the patient from the ventilator and attempt slow hand-bagging for a few moments. Ensure the tracheal tube is patent and replace if required. Suctioning down the tracheal tube (TT) may demonstrate obstruction and, where there are secretions, these may be removed. Carefully assess and auscultate the chest, looking for signs of pneumothorax. Depending on findings and patient response, prompt needle decompression or simple thoracostomy would be indicated, followed by a formal chest tube if time allowed. Again, the pilot and the tasking agency must be notified of this occurrence. Document the cabin pressure at this time, and consider requesting adjustments in cabin pressure to facilitate further management of any pneumothorax.

Key points

- Unexpected occurrences during transport are not uncommon in the pre-hospital and retrieval environment.
- Always communicate acute changes in the condition of the patient to the entire aeromedical crew as well as the tasking agency.
- Predicting potential deterioration is a core skill in PHRM services and requires high-level clinician assessment and decision making.

Incident

The PHRM team has been tasked to retrieve a patient from a remote community clinic to a regional hospital for further investigation. The patient is a 70-year-old man with epigastric pain. He has a pulse of 120 beats per minute and a BP of 95/55 mmHg. The differential diagnosis includes acute myocardial infarction (MI), acute abdominal aortic aneurysm, acute pancreatitis, gastric ulcer disease.

Relevant information

- **PHRM team transport options:** Fixed-wing aircraft. Maximum two stretcher cases.
- **Additional resources:** Single-doctor clinic. One land ambulance.
- **Retrieval options:** Regional hospital 1.5 hours by air.
- **Other:** Equipment available – standard PHRM kit, which includes portable ultrasound.

En route, the tasking agency asks if you can review, and possibly bring back, a second patient from the same location. New clinical information:

- 15-year-old boy with abdominal pain following a fall from a bicycle with handlebars to the abdomen.
- Currently stable.

The tasking agency also informs you that the elderly patient's pain has worsened, although no further details are available.

Question 39.1

What are your options for possible retrieval of two patients? Illustrate your retrieval plan.

Clinical information

On arrival at the clinic, the elderly man's observations are:

- P 125.
- BP 90/50 mmHg.
- Severe abdominal pain.

The 15-year-old boy has normal observations but marked abdominal and left chest wall tenderness with shallow breathing.

Question 39.2

Discuss your assessment of each patient using the equipment available. Review Figure 39.1, Figure 39.2 and Figure 39.3 overleaf.

The following images are obtained using portable ultrasound.

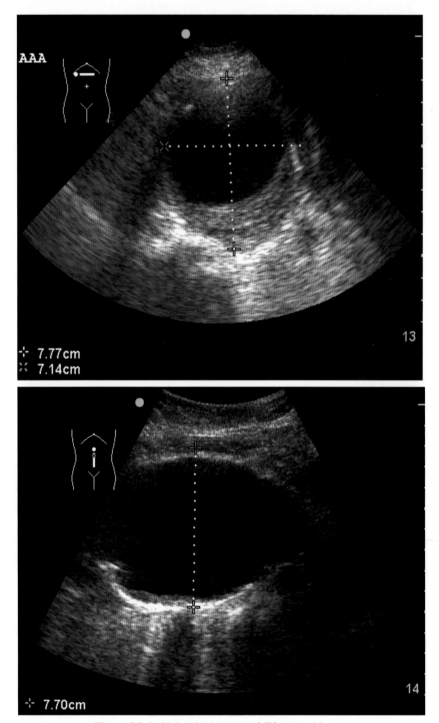

Figure 39.1 Abdominal scans of 70-year-old man

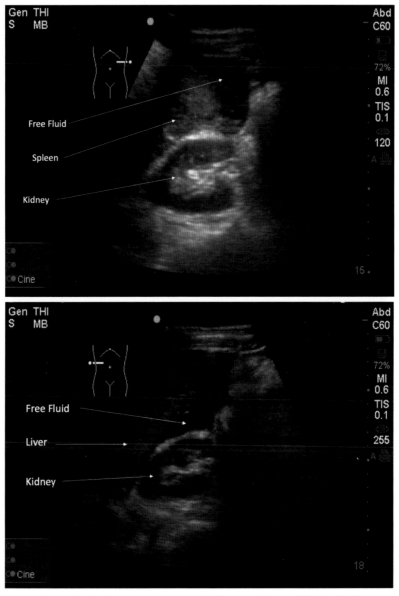

Figure 39.2 Abdominal scans of 15-year-old boy (LUQ & RUQ)

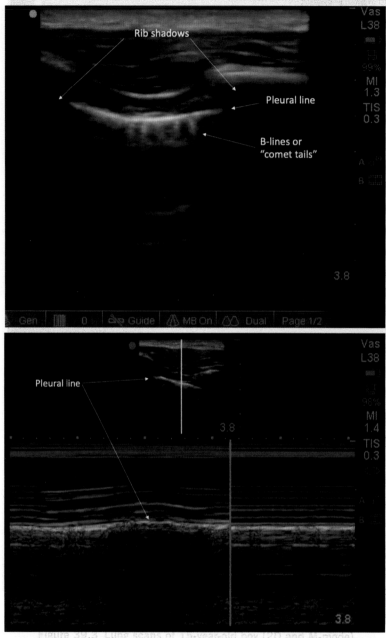

Figure 39.3 Lung scans of 15-year-old boy (2D and M-mode)

Question 39.3

Discuss your management plan. Highlight any concerns about taking both patients simultaneously.

Question 39.4

The clinic has two units of O-negative blood. Discuss.

Discussion 39.1

Optimisation of resources will often lead to the tasking agency trying to 'fill' an empty space on the aircraft, especially in remote areas. The PHRM team heading to scene needs to consider the practicalities of managing two patients on the return journey and make arrangements accordingly. The PHRM team should reserve the right to make a final decision on the transfer after assessing both patients but, at this stage, should agree in principle to do so. This is good for the patients (getting to their destination quicker) and the system (decreased cost per retrieval, and optimising scarce air medical assets). The entire team should be made aware of the new plan in order to prepare the second stretcher and think about any extra equipment required. The pilot may need to alter the flight plan to cater for extra weight and fuel issues and may potentially decline a second case if these factors are an issue. The potential for a parent or guardian with the second patient is an additional consideration.

Discussion 39.2

The availability of ultrasound provides the PHRM team with greater assessment capability in this scenario. If the service does not routinely carry ultrasound but crew members are competent point-of-care ultrasound users, it is worth asking in the referring hospital or clinic if they have ultrasound available. It is not uncommon for there to be an ultrasound machine somewhere in the clinic that is used for outpatients (e.g. obstetrics) by visiting specialists.

Point-of-care ultrasound (POCUS) is a core skill in emergency medicine and critical care and, increasingly, clinicians in the pre-hospital and retrieval field have crossover skills in this area.

In this scenario, ultrasound of the abdominal aorta (looking for an aneurysm) and basic cardiac echo (cardiac valve incompetence, ventricular volume, and possible early wall motion abnormality), in conjunction with the ECG, would be useful for the elderly patient. An extended focused assessment by sonography in trauma scan (E-FAST), looking for abdominal free fluid, pericardial fluid, pleural fluid and lung sliding, will be useful in the child.

These ultrasound exams themselves will take just a few minutes and should not be considered as adding excessive time to the retrieval. Depending on the final working diagnosis, the ultrasound may also be utilised to assist with arterial line and central venous catheter placement if required, or even difficult peripheral access.

Discussion 39.3

Figure 39.1 shows a large abdominal aorta. In the presence of the described symptoms and clinical exam, this patient has a leaking abdominal aortic aneurysm until proven otherwise. The key management strategy is expedient transfer to an appropriate surgical centre. With this information, the PHRM team can now notify the tasking agency and ensure the appropriate surgical and anaesthetic team is ready on arrival. Depending on the patient's condition and the systems in place, it may even be appropriate for the team to bypass the emergency department of the receiving hospital and proceed directly to the operating theatre.

It is also appropriate to discuss the likely diagnosis with the patient and his family. The mortality of this condition is high and the patient, depending on his circumstance, may elect not to have surgery. He may even have previously rejected or been assessed as unsuitable for surgery. It is important that the team act according to the patient's wishes in this scenario.

Medical management and stabilisation during transfer mirrors emergency department management of this condition. Large-bore intravenous access (an additional potential role for the ultrasound if IV access is difficult) should be obtained but fluid resuscitation kept to a minimum. Aim for a blood pressure at which the patient cerebrates normally (i.e. is able to maintain lucid conversation). Analgesia should be generous. During the flight, if safe to do so, the team can optimise the patient's preparation for theatre by placing an arterial line, urinary catheter and securing additional intravenous access. A central venous line will be difficult to site in the aircraft cabin using aseptic techniques and should only be sited prior to transport if intravenous access is poor. Under no circumstance should inserting a central venous line delay the team's departure. The same argument can be made for arterial line placement. A precipitous deterioration in the patient's condition mid-flight is likely to signal rupture of the aneurysm into the peritoneal cavity and, under these circumstances, is likely to be a pre-terminal event. The team (and the patient and their family) should be aware that this might occur and should have considered and discussed possible treatment options prior to departure. Intubation, ventilation and CPR may be attempted while the PHRM team reassesses the patient, but is unlikely to change the outcome. Limited laparotomy or lateral thoracotomy (e.g. to occlude the descending aorta) is not generally feasible or useful in this situation. The team should be prepared to withdraw active care and keep the patient comfortable if necessary.

Figure 39.2 shows fluid in Morrison's pouch (RUQ) and splenorenal space (LUQ). This constitutes a positive FAST scan and implies that the child is bleeding into his peritoneal space. The absence of hypotension or even a tachycardia is not uncommon in this age group and should not generate a false sense of security. Reassuringly, Figure 39.3 demonstrates good pleural sliding, B lines, a normal M-mode lung scan and absence of pleural fluid, helping to exclude concurrent pneumothorax and haemothorax. The child may need prompt surgery, although some paediatric surgeons may opt for a CT scan first, but either way they cannot stay in their current location where there are no appropriate surgical services. Once again, the tasking agency must be informed so as to facilitate an appropriate receiving team at the hospital. Intravenous access should be obtained, and good analgesia provided. Intravenous fluid should be kept to maintenance levels only, unless there is deterioration in the child's condition.

The advantages of taking both patients include:

- Prompt transfer to a hospital able to deal with both conditions
- Eliminates the need for a second trip to the clinic and its associated aeromedical risks and costs
- Satisfaction of both the patients' needs and those of the referring clinic.

In this situation, the team is left with little choice. Both patients need urgent transfer and leaving either patient, even for a few hours, could result in an adverse outcome. It is acceptable to ask the tasking agency if there is another resource available nearby to assist, but unless another aircraft can be on-site within the hour, this plan should be reconsidered. The PHRM team needs to accept the situation and should be prepared for any deterioration en route.

Discussion 39.4

Ideally, the team would have taken blood with them, either from the receiving regional hospital or from the PHRM service blood store if a blood carriage system is in place, but the diagnoses were unclear at that time. Taking the two units from the clinic for the flight home is an option, but there are issues that should be considered.

First, the blood is likely to be the only supply for that clinic and the surrounding regional area. If the blood is taken, it is likely that replacement blood will need to be urgently transported to the hospital. This may require a dedicated flight with associated risks and costs.

Second, at this moment, neither patient needs a blood transfusion, so the blood is actually being taken as a precaution. Should another patient need it at the referring clinic, it will no longer be immediately available.

Third, if the elderly patient deteriorates catastrophically to the point of needing a blood transfusion, will two units make any difference? The likelihood would be that the patient has ruptured his aneurysm, and, in the absence of immediate surgery, he would die with or without two units of blood.

If the team was required to choose one patient over the other for blood transfusion, the child would be the priority. Precipitous decline in his condition may well respond to a two-unit transfusion (a larger volume relative to circulating blood volume), potentially 'buying some time' during the transfer. In any case, the PHRM team should inform the tasking agency that the blood has been taken so a replacement can be arranged. If required, the PHRM team can also arrange for more blood to be taken out to the destination airport ready for the team's arrival (see Case 38).

Key points

- The PHRM team should utilise all available diagnostic equipment.
- The team may be required to deal with extra patients, especially at remote facilities.
- Consider the availability of blood and blood products before, during and after a tasking.

Additional reading

Harris T, Bystrzycki A, Mazur SM. Prehospital ultrasound. In Nutbeam T, Boylan M (Eds), ABC of pre-hospital emergency medicine, pp 57–62. Wiley Blackwell, 2013.

Harris T, Bystrzycki A, Mazur SM. The role of ultrasound in pre-hospital care. In Connolly JA, Dean AJ, Hoffmann B, Jarman RD (Eds), Emergency point-of-care ultrasound, 2nd ed., pp 425–439. Wiley Blackwell, 2017.

Incident

A 37-year-old patient known to local mental health services, and suffering from schizo-affective disorder and substance abuse, requires retrieval from a rural hospital to a secure psychiatric unit. The patient has been violent and has required sedation overnight. Currently, she is stable and sedated.

Relevant information

- **PHRM team transport options:** Rotary wing aircraft, maximum 2 stretcher cases.
- **Additional resources:** Rural GP and nursing staff. One land ambulance.
- **Retrieval options:** Regional psychiatric unit 30 minutes by air (rotary wing).
- **Other:** Nil.

On arrival, the patient appears calm and content. As the PHRM team introduces themselves, the patient physically attacks one of the team. With local colleagues, you are able to physically restrain the patient, who is now shouting abuse.

Question 40.1

Discuss your retrieval options and make an appropriate plan.

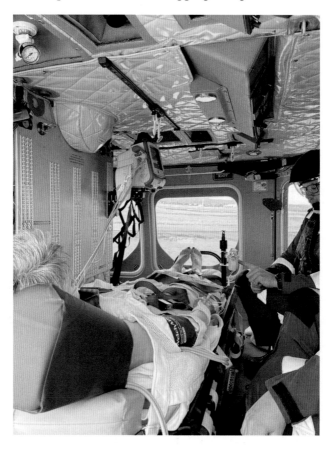

Study the picture above, taken inside the aircraft cabin.

Question 40.2

Referring to the picture, which retrieval option has occurred and what precautions have been taken?

Discussion 40.1

Retrieval of the acute psychiatric patient generates a unique set of problems for both the tasking agency and the PHRM team. Certain aspects relevant to tasking will be discussed in Case 42.

Risk assessment

The PHRM team will initially rely on the information and assessment provided by the tasking agency. On arrival, a clearer history and assessment can be expected. The recent psychiatric history is of great importance, and the team should ask about suicide attempts or ideation as well as observed violent or aggressive behaviour, especially towards healthcare workers (as in this case). Clinical assessment can be difficult, especially if the patient has been heavily sedated. The PHRM team may be tempted not to disturb the sedated patient to avoid waking her and causing further agitation. In fact, the opposite applies. The team must assess the patient, gain intravenous access as required and inform the patient about the plan. It is better that the patient becomes combative and uncooperative prior to departure rather than during the transfer. Ideally, patient assessment should be carried out with the entire PHRM team present (including the pilot). It is this entire team that the patient will be with for the next few hours and each member's opinion and advice should be acknowledged.

Risk assessment tools have been developed to risk-stratify mental health patients regarding suitability for transfer, including appropriate transport platforms. An example of such a tool can be found in Appendix 5.

Team discussion

After the assessment, the PHRM team should discuss the case. On the basis of this discussion, a decision can be made on the appropriateness of aeromedical transfer, the precautions needed, and a back-up plan for a mid-flight emergency. The entire team must be involved as everyone could be put at risk in the event of a problem. Remember, the pilot has ultimate authority over the aircraft and so must be involved in the decision-making process. Following this discussion, call the tasking agency to provide a sit rep.

Precautions

Mental health escorts

Once a decision has been made to proceed with aeromedical transport, an appropriate escort should be considered. Regional practice may dictate the requirement for additional dedicated staff to escort the patient in such scenarios. Escort selection may depend on the composition of your PHRM team and available resources. Depending on the physical stature of the PHRM team, the decision may be that no extra escort is required. If required, escorts are often mental health workers, specially trained ambulance officers or Police officers. It is also important to consider, in consultation with local psychiatric services, regional mental health legislation with regards to care and control orders, consent to treatment and inpatient treatment orders.

Sedation (see Case 20)

The patient may have received sedation already, which will wear off with time and the team should anticipate this. Minimum standards of 'safe sedation' must always apply with adequate monitoring, and intravenous access, oxygen saturations and continuous end-tidal carbon dioxide monitoring will be required. If safe sedation cannot be guaranteed, then consideration should be given to general anaesthesia with airway protection. This should occur prior to leaving the referring facility to avoid unexpected, urgent intervention in-flight. General anaesthesia should be considered a last resort as it complicates the transfer and care at the receiving facility, and may negatively impact on the patient's mental health and wellbeing.

Although advice on anti-psychotics and psychiatric risk assessment can be taken from a psychiatric specialist, the type of sedative(s) and level of sedation are best addressed by the PHRM team with the patient. Choice of sedative agents includes benzodiazepines, antipsychotics and dissociative anaesthestics (ketamine). Increasing use of ketamine for high-risk mental-health transfers has dramatically changed the landscape, specifically reducing the incidence of mental-health transfers requiring general anaesthesia.

Use of ketamine

- Consider low-dose benzodiazepine initially.
- Initial ketamine dose: 0.25–0.5 mg/kg slow intravenous push.
- Ketamine infusion: 200 mg in 50 mL = 4 mg per mL. Commence at 1–2 mg/kg/hour. For example, 20–40 mL an hour for the average adult, titrated to effect.

Physical restraint

Physically restraining patients is controversial (and may not be accepted practice in some jurisdictions) but should be considered for certain patients in the aeromedical environment to ensure staff and patient safety during transfer. If applied, custom-made restraints should be used and the patient informed of their use in advance. Also note that the standard safety harness on the stretcher will also need to be used, which may augment formal restraints.

Data on the use of physical and chemical restraint by the PHRM service should be collected and analysed to ensure that patient safety and quality has not been compromised by the ongoing use of these techniques.

Emergency plan

An unrestrained, violent patient in an aircraft cabin constitutes a serious risk to the aircraft and any negative consequences must be anticipated and prevented.

The team should have a plan in case the patient wakes abruptly and becomes violent. Further physical restraint by the team may be possible temporarily but a rapid take-down of the patient using pharmacologic agents will need to be considered. If the patient is on a ketamine infusion, additional bolus doses may suffice. In certain situations, further agents may be required (e.g. propofol). PHRM teams undertaking high-risk mental-health transfers will need to possess the necessary airway skills to deal with all eventualities, including the need to secure the airway in-flight.

Arrival

In the unlikely event that the patient required intubation and ventilation, alert the tasking agency, as an intensive care bed may now be required.

Discussion 40.2

The picture shows a psychiatric patient undergoing an aeromedical retrieval. Key points from the picture include:

- Patient/doctor position: the PHRM team is positioned close to the patient, making potential intervention easier.
- Monitoring: the patient is fully monitored including awake capnography.
- Access and pharmacology: the patient has two intravenous access points and is on a ketamine infusion. Further drugs should be readily available.
- Restraint: The patient has been secured using a customised transfer net.
- Equipment: airway equipment should be easily to hand including a bag valve mask.

Key points

- Team and patient safety are paramount during retrieval and transfer of acutely psychotic patients.
- Meticulous preparation and planning will allow a safe and uneventful retrieval.
- The pilot has the final decision for aeromedical retrievals that may put the aircraft or its crew at risk.

Additional reading

Le Cong M, Finn E, Parsch CS. Management of the acutely agitated patient in a remote location. Med. J. Aust. 2015; 202(4):182–183.

Parsch C S, Boonstra A, Teubner D, et al. Ketamine reduces the need for intubation in patients with acute severe mental illness and agitation requiring transport to definitive care: an observational study. Emerg. Med. Australas. 2017; 29(3):291–296.

CASE 41

Incident

A 60-year-old man has presented to a general hospital emergency department following sudden-onset headache and collapse. A CT scan reveals intracranial haemorrhage. He was intubated and ventilated on arrival with a pre-intubation GCS of 5 (E1, V1, M3). The tasking agency has sent the PHRM team 'early' to expedite the anticipated neurosurgical transfer.

Clinical information

Clinical information prior to arrival:
- P 58.
- BP 190/105 mmHg.
- SaO_2 100%.

Relevant information

- **PHRM team transport options:** Rotary-wing.
- **Additional resources:** Regional hospital, no neurosurgery or ICU on-site.
- **Retrieval options:** Regional neurosurgical centre 45 minutes by rotary-wing.
- **Other:** Nil.

Question 41.1

Outline your plan for initial clinical management.

A quick bedside review of the patient soon after your arrival reveals the following:
- P 60.
- BP 85/55 mmHg.
- SaO_2 93% on 50% inspired oxygen.
- Bilateral fixed and dilated pupils.

The neurosurgical team at the receiving hospital has now reviewed the CT scans and telephones as you arrive to say that 'the intracranial haemorrhage is inoperable and unsurvivable'. They are concerned that the patient may have 'already coned'.

Question 41.2

What are the options in this scenario? Are you able to diagnose brain death in this case?

Question 41.3

What are the key points of discussion with the family?

Discussion 41.1

The initial clinical management plan should focus on good neurointensive care. The patient should be managed 30 degrees head-up, making sure the tracheal tube tie is not applied too tightly (potentially impeding cerebral venous drainage). Although currently hypertensive, cerebral perfusion should be protected. A mean arterial blood pressure (MAP) of at least 80 mmHg should be targeted in the absence of invasive intracranial pressure monitoring. Vasoactive agents should be used if necessary. Hypoxia should also be aggressively avoided and ventilation must be controlled to achieve normocapnoea ($PaCO_2$ 30–35 mmHg [4.0–4.5 kPa]) correlated with an equivalent $ETCO_2$. If there is evidence of localising neurological signs, early consideration should be given to hypertonic solutions such as mannitol or hypertonic saline. In addition, large intraparenchymal cerebral haemorrhages are highly eleptogenic and seizure prophylaxis is often advisable (intravenous levitarectam 1.5 mg/kg). Euglycaemia and normothermia should be targeted. Induced hypothermia is not recommended in this scenario.

Discussion 41.2

There is no worldwide consensus on the definition or criteria for determining death. At the very least, a period of observation (4 hours) and specific bedside testing or investigations are required. This patient may be brain dead but the PHRM team are in no position to formally confirm that. The PHRM team could make the decision that any ongoing care is likely to be futile and, thus, leave the patient at the referring facility. However, there is no ICU, the local medical team is likely to feel overwhelmed by the management of such a case (even if palliative), and the wishes of both the patient and any family are, as yet, unknown. Another option is for the PHRM team to remain with the patient either to observe further clinical progress (to clinical brain death) or to assist the local medical staff in the palliative care process. However, if the former occurs and organ donation is possible, the referral facility may not have the capacity to support the preparation and harvesting process demanded of organ retrieval teams. The final decision will depend upon a number of factors, particularly the wishes of the patient's family. Notwithstanding this and, given the relatively short flight time, the best option is probably to commence resuscitation and, thus, meet some of the defined preconditions, and then prepare to transport the patient to the receiving ICU.

Patients who are progressing or who have progressed to brain death are often physiologically unstable. Without the ability to diagnose brain death, such instability will require management on the return journey. Ethically, the focus of such management remains on the patient's care. However, if brain death is later confirmed and the patient becomes an organ donor, there is added benefit for any potential organ recipient as tissue injury to potentially donated organs will be minimised.

Various physiologic challenges may be encountered as outlined below.

Autonomic (catecholamine) storm

- Usually transient.
- If antihypertensive agents are used, they should be short-acting.

Arrhythmias

- May be minimised by maintaining normal serum electrolyte concentrations, blood pressure, volume state and temperature.
- Standard therapy may be administered for atrial and ventricular arrhythmias (e.g. amiodarone or cardioversion).

Hypotension

- Often associated with low cardiac output states.
- An adequate perfusion pressure should be targeted (e.g. MAP >80 mmHg) by optimising volume status and use of vasoactive agents.

Diabetes insipidus (DI)

- DDAVP (desmopressin, 1-desamino-8-D-arginine vasopressin) or vasopressin (arginine vasopressin [AVP]) should be administered early in diabetes insipidus; however, these agents are rarely carried by PHRM teams.

Hypothermia
- Easier to prevent than reverse.
- Intravenous fluid should be warmed.

Respiratory
- Neurogenic pulmonary oedema is well described.
- Adequate oxygen and PEEP should be considered.

Discussion 41.3

This will not be easy. The family has probably been told that the PHRM team is coming to rapidly retrieve their loved one for potentially life-saving neurosurgery. Expectations and emotions will be running high. Now is not the time to discuss potential brain death and organ donation. However, the PHRM team should ensure time is spent with the family outlining the gravity of the situation. This should occur in a quiet, private room and involve the local medical team. This offers both immediate and latent support and shows the family that the PHRM team is a supportive extension of the local team and not a fly-in replacement. In discussing the deterioration since the team was tasked, it is important for the PHRM team leader to be clear that death is a very real possibility and that surgery is not thought by the specialist surgeons to offer any benefit. This may lead to further questioning and potentially a request from the family that nothing further be done, that the 'life support' be removed and the patient be allowed to die at the referring centre, likely to be closer to family and supports. Setting the scene concerning the potential outcome (death) and assuring them that you will do everything possible to ensure their loved one remains comfortable may be all that you can do at this time. If the patient is transferred, transport should be arranged for the family to the receiving facility.

If the family spontaneously asks about brain death and/or organ donation, then be open and honest. This is certainly a possibility, but neither brain death nor the option for organ donation can be confirmed now.

Key points

- Be prepared for a patient's condition to change dramatically while en route to a referral facility.
- The PHRM team may bring more than life-saving capability to a regional facility. Remember that you are there to also support local medical staff who may feel overwhelmed.
- Where appropriate, the PHRM team can provide expert support regarding acute end-of-life care.

Additional reading

Academy of Medical Royal Colleges. A code of practice for the diagnosis and confirmation of death. AORMC, 2010. Online. Available: https://www.aomrc.org.uk/reports-guidance/ukdec-reports-and-guidance/code-practice-diagnosis-confirmation-death/.

Australian and New Zealand Intensive Care Society (ANZICS). The ANZICS statement on death and organ donation, 4th ed. ANZICS, 2019.

Tasking and retrieval coordination are key aspects of pre-hospital and retrieval medicine (see also Case 22). The role demands high-level decision making, often in the presence of incomplete or confusing clinical information. Triage, resource allocation, effective interpersonal communication and clinical acumen are necessary requisite skills.

The following incidents should be considered to be independent of each other. In each case, the decision to mobilise, coordinate and support the PHRM team rests solely with you.

Incident A

A 24-year-old patient with schizophrenia has stopped taking medication and is now behaving bizarrely and threatening violence. He has been accepted for admission under the psychiatry team in a secure psychiatric unit. He is currently at a single-doctor clinic one hour flight by rotary-wing aircraft from the psychiatric unit, and has required moderate doses of sedative hypnotics to calm him down.

Question 42.1

Discuss the issues that should be considered when coordinating this retrieval.

Incident B

A 74-year-old man with severe chronic obstructive pulmonary disease (COPD) has presented to a nurse-only clinic 45 minutes' fixed-wing flight from the nearest appropriate hospital. He was reported to have a GCS 6 (E1, V1, M4) on arrival but has responded well to non-invasive ventilation (NIV) and is now GCS 13 (E3, V4, M6). He has been accepted for continuing NIV and optimisation by the regional hospital. The patient has been previously assessed as a 'poor' candidate for invasive ventilation by the local intensive care unit.

Shortly after arrival, the PHRM team phones through reporting that a second patient is also in the clinic. A 32 year old man has sustained a penetrating injury to the epigastrium with a screwdriver following an altercation 45 minutes ago. On examination his observations are normal but he has marked abdominal tenderness. Bedside ultrasound done by the PHRM team shows fluid in the right upper quadrant.

Question 42.2

How will you manage this scenario? Explain your decisions.

Incident C

A 25-year-old primigravid patient has spontaneously ruptured membranes at 29 weeks' gestation. She is having periodic abdominal pains and needs retrieval to a regional hospital with obstetric and neonatal facilities. The patient is located in a single-doctor-and-nurse clinic on a small offshore island, 15 minutes' helicopter flight from the hospital. The nurse has midwifery skills.

Question 42.3

What are the concerns with retrieving this obstetric patient? How would you go about coordinating it?

Discussion 42.1

Incident A

Retrieval of the acute psychiatric patient generates a unique set of problems for the coordinating and PHRM teams (see Case 40). The over-riding issue is team safety followed by patient safety. The coordinating staff (working with the local medical staff) are directly responsible for the initial assessment and risk management. Managing a mentally ill and unstable patient in the pre-hospital and retrieval environment is a significant challenge, especially if there is an aeromedical aspect to the retrieval plan.

Method of retrieval

A risk–benefit analysis should be conducted regarding the need for aeromedical transfer versus road transfer. Considerations include distance, weather, time of day and availability. Under normal circumstances, aeromedical retrieval could be considered for retrievals that would take over one or two hours by road. There are also occasions when the distance or the terrain precludes land transfer, in which case aeromedical retrieval will need to be considered. In such cases, the relative calm of the fixed-wing aircraft cabin is preferred to the rotary-wing equivalent. The tasking agency should also be aware that local resource issues may lead to reluctance among ambulance personnel to release a land ambulance and its crew for what could be several hours.

Urgency of transfer

Most aeromedical accidents happen at night and in bad weather (Aherne et al 2019, Holland & Cooksley 2005) (see Case 22). For this reason, psychiatric aeromedical retrievals should not take place at night or in bad weather. While psychiatric patients may have a life-threatening illness (particularly with regard to suicide risk), waiting until the following morning may be appropriate. If so, the local clinic will need to be supported in order to keep the patient under observation with sedation. Advice from an appropriate psychiatric specialist should be an integrated component of such support. The expanding role of telehealth systems has enabled improved remote assessment of mental health patients by psychiatric specialists. On occasion, patients can remain at the referring location, being managed remotely by the psychiatrist and obviating the need for a retrieval.

The coordinator should suggest the patient be kept nil by mouth for 6 hours prior to the PHRM team's arrival to allow safe sedation, intubation and ventilation if required.

Discussion 42.2

Incident B

While initially in extremis, the elderly patient has stabilised and will now require transport on NIV. The information suggesting that supportive care should be limited (i.e. 'not for intubation') needs to be confirmed. In addition, the wishes of the patient with regard to escalation of care may have been made clear in an 'advanced directive' or similar.

Despite normal physiology, the presence of free fluid on ultrasound is concerning for significant injury requiring prompt surgical intervention. Intravenous access should be obtained and good analgesia provided. Intravenous fluid should be kept to maintenance levels only, unless there is deterioration in the patient's condition.

Both patients need urgent transfer, and leaving either patient, even for a few hours, could result in an adverse outcome. Arrangements should be made with the pilots to take both patients, if feasible, with regard to aviation logistics. If another team and aircraft are immediately available, it may be an option to take the penetrating trauma case first.

The advantages of taking both patients include:

- Prompt transfer to a hospital able to deal with both conditions
- Eliminating the need for a second trip to the clinic and its associated aeromedical risks and costs
- Satisfaction of both the patients' needs and those of the referring clinic.

Discussion 42.3

Incident C

The obstetric patient offers another layer of complexity to the clinical coordination team who must also factor neonatal considerations into the retrieval equation (see Case 37). The key aspect to these scenarios is anticipation of delivery, and the nearest healthcare professional should attempt to assess this. Key tools for assessment are degree of cervical dilation, cervical effacement, and nature and frequency of contractions. In this scenario, the local clinic doctor should be able to assess the patient adequately. Based on this assessment, the patient will fall into one of two categories.

Anticipated delivery imminent

In this setting, it is generally accepted practice to avoid ante-partum retrieval. The coordinator should instead focus on providing clinical support for the island doctor. There are two components to this support: obstetric and neonatal. If available, an obstetrician should be involved in providing advice alongside the coordinator. Sending an obstetrician to the scene is rarely required, and the benefit of adding any non-standard retrieval staff should be weighed with the risks of sending staff into an unfamiliar environment. Many services will have a dedicated neonatal coordinator and retrieval team available (see the Paediatrics and Neonates section) and this team should be notified as soon as possible to allow prompt mobilisation.

Anticipated delivery unlikely within the next few hours

Under these circumstances, it is acceptable to retrieve the mother and infant in utero. Telephone advice from the obstetric service, including the administration of steroids and tocolytics should be forthcoming. The coordinator should alert the neonatal service and receiving obstetrician. In turn, the obstetrician should alert the operating theatre and other appropriate staff as required.

In this unpredictable scenario, it is quite possible that the assessment of timing of delivery is inaccurate and plans need to be kept flexible. Whenever possible, emergency delivery in the aircraft cabin should be avoided, and the PHRM team should be prepared to deliver the baby in the clinic and await the neonatal retrieval team's arrival, if necessary. Focused training programs that provide PHRM teams with the necessary knowledge and skills are available (see Advanced Life Support in Obstetrics [ALSO]: www.aafp.org/cme/programs/also.html).

Key points
• Tasking and coordinating of PHRM teams is not straightforward. It requires sound medical knowledge, astute clinical acumen, an understanding of local resources and an appreciation of regional geography.
• Ideally, tasking and coordination should be carried out by staff with active or recent PHRM team experience. This brings invaluable 'field knowledge' to this critical but sometimes complex process.

References

Aherne B, Zhang C, Chen W, Newman D. Systems safety risk analysis of fatal night helicopter emergency medical service accidents. Aerosp. Med. Hum. Perform. 2019; 90:396–404. doi:10.3357/AMHP.5180.2019.

Holland J, Cooksley DG. Safety of helicopter aeromedical transport in Australia: a retrospective study. Med. J. Aust. 2005; 182(1):17–19.

Incident

A bus has rolled over in the late evening some 450 km (280 miles) from your base location near a remote mining community. Initial reports suggest multiple casualties and numerous fatalities.

Patients are being extricated by passers-by and voluntary emergency services personnel and moved to a nurse-led clinic nearby. You are being sent to the clinic.

Relevant information

- **PHRM team transport options:** Fixed-wing. Two stretcher and one seated capacity.
- **Additional resources:** One land ambulance: Police and voluntary Fire & Rescue Services including experienced remote-clinic nurse.
- **Retrieval options:** Major trauma hospital 1.5 hours by air (additional short road transfer from the airport) or 6 hours by road.
- **Other:** Nil.

Question 43.1

What are the considerations prior to departure?

Question 43.2

What is your initial pre-hospital plan?

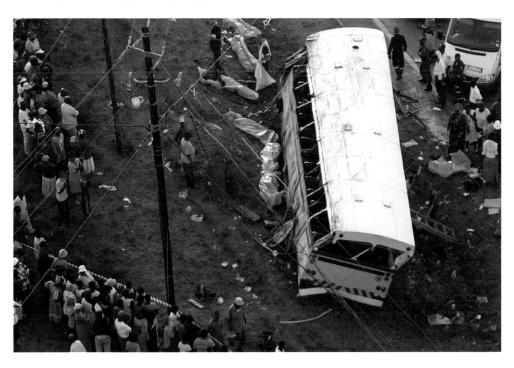

A picture of the scene has been made available to you via a local news network (above).

No additional information is received from the clinic prior to your arrival and you are able to land safely on a tarmac road nearby. When you arrive, you find the following:

- Five patients on stretchers in the reception of the clinic with one more due to arrive imminently.
- Six patients are said to be 'dead at scene'.
- Cardiopulmonary resuscitation is underway on a child.
- There are at least 10 unidentified people shouting and running around. Some are crying.

Question 43.3

Describe the scene in the picture.

Question 43.4

Describe your immediate actions on arrival at the clinic and thereafter.

Discussion 43.1

Additional PHRM team members and equipment may be assembled or immediately available. Taking appropriately packaged O-negative blood would also be highly desirable in this instance. Some retrieval services also have access to a major transfusion pack that can be taken on the retrieval (see Case 28). Discussions are needed with the pilot as to how many patients can be carried and whether aircraft modification is required to reduce weight (e.g. removal of seats, irrelevant equipment, etc.).

Travelling such a distance allows adequate time for planning. Plan to keep in touch with the tasking agency/coordinator for updates on numbers, ages and clinical condition of casualties. Discuss with them what potential local resources are available. How many nurses and paramedics are there? Where is the next nearest healthcare facility? Are additional regional air medical resources available? In essence, this is a modified primary tasking as patients are likely to have had little input into their care either before or in the clinic. You should discuss frankly the possibility of this becoming a major incident so the coordinator can look into extraordinary resource utilisation (e.g. military assistance). Most PHRM services will have a Major Incident pack (see Appendix 2) which should be taken by the team prior to departure. Finally, use the time en route to prepare by drawing up and labelling appropriate drugs, pre-priming fluid infusion lines and developing a pre-hospital plan with your team members.

Discussion 43.2

Safety

Patients are being taken to a clinic, which reduces (but does not eliminate) risk. It is likely that local resources will be massively overwhelmed and the environment in the clinic is likely to be chaotic.

Patients

The PHRM team should prepare themselves for multiple patients and should conduct a team briefing en route. Triage, as per major incidents (see Case 23), will be required early on. Initial use of the triage sieve will be valuable (Appendix 8). Consider splitting the team into two and doing a very quick assessment of, for example, three patients each over one or two minutes. Then regroup and discuss your findings and make a plan.

Destination

There is insufficient capacity for all patients on the aircraft. Some patients will need transfer to the nearest trauma centre.

Discussion 43.3

The bus looks unstable and may roll again. There is at least one person on the bus with minimal, if any, PPE. There is little crowd control. At least six victims are already in body bags. Pylons and wires make the scene potentially dangerous for any future emergency services teams, especially those who may arrive by helicopter.

Discussion 43.4

The team needs to try and gain some control over this difficult and chaotic scene. Even with your arrival, this incident has overwhelmed available resources and therefore fulfils the definition of a major incident. A major incident should be declared to the coordinator using the 'METHANE' approach (see Case 23). Each patient should then be triaged to try and establish the number of severely injured patients.

The key difference here is that even as the nominal medical incident commander (MIC), you will need to become directly involved in patient care. Extra resources, if available, will take a long time to arrive, so as MIC, there will be fewer resources to direct initially and more demand for direct clinical input.

Command and control is still of the highest priority and the scene will function much better if you can marshal the resources and allocate them in an orderly fashion. Being clear and decisive will encourage people to listen to you:

- Temporarily move all medical staff into one part of the room, and family, friends, etc. into another. Be prepared to utilise all suitable personnel.
- Following on from triage, you should be able to confirm exact numbers of casualties and their condition (e.g. using the P1, P2 and P3 technique from Appendix 8). In this scenario, you now know there are five patients.
- Try to allocate each patient a nurse/paramedic on a 'one-to-one' basis. Tell them to focus only on their own patient.
- Assess the arrested child. If the child is indeed dead, consider calling the CPR to an end. Be mindful that the parents may be in the room.
- Prioritise the other patients using triage sieve and give instructions to the carers.
- Begin treatment in priority order. Focus on haemorrhage control, securing airways and chest decompression.
- Utilise non-medical people as lifters or runners, etc.
- Remain in constant touch with the tasking agency/coordinator and find out what additional resources have been dispatched
- Work out the order in which patients will be dispatched to their destination. It is essential to document something (on regional major incident tags if carried), in case patients leave with another team.

If another resource is en route, you should prepare for two patients to go initially. Even then, you will be left with three or four patients and you only have room for two patients on your aircraft. Other options include sending your PHRM team member with two patients on the aircraft while you wait in the clinic with the remainder. There is also the rather onerous option of a halfway road meet. In this situation, a PHRM team travel by road towards the scene, and the local ambulance travels towards the trauma centre and they meet halfway. This may be the only option in remote locations with limited aeromedical assets.

There is no right answer for this difficult and complex scenario and the PHRM team, together with the tasking agency/coordinator will need to make the best decisions with the information available to them at the time. A detailed multidisciplinary debrief will be required.

Further discussion regarding multiple-patient scenarios occurs in Case 21 and an approach to major incidents is discussed in Case 23.

Key points

- Multiple patients in the resource-poor environment may constitute a major incident and the key principles of major incident management should be followed.
- Early triage is essential.
- In remote locations, be prepared for the original scene to be cleared and for patients to be located in nearby buildings or medical centres by the time the PHRM team arrives.

Additional reading

Advanced Life Support Group. Major incident medical management and support (MIMMS), 3rd edn. Wiley, 2011.

Incident

A rural doctor has called the PHRM service regarding a 53-year-old female under her care for the past 24 hours in a small community hospital. The patient presented with worsening shortness of breath over the previous 3 days.

The patient has a background history of type II diabetes and mild COPD. The working diagnosis presented by the rural doctor is an exacerbation of COPD and he has commenced treatment with some oral steroids, broad-spectrum antibiotics and regular bronchodilators. Despite this, the patient has become more short of breath and has now become tachycardic and hypotensive. She has never had a fever or any significant wheeze.

Clinical information

- Afebrile.
- GCS 15.
- P 108 regular.
- BP 90/52.
- RR 32.
- Sats 95% on 6 L via Hudson mask.

Relevant information

- **PHRM team transport options:** Choice of fixed-wing or rotary-wing aircraft.
- **Additional resources:** Small rural 6-bed GP-led hospital and nursing staff.
- **Retrieval destination:** Tertiary metropolitan hospital.
- **Other:** No radiology or blood tests available locally.

Question 44.1

What additional history and investigations would the PHRM team clinical coordinator specifically ask about?

Question 44.2

What specific portable investigation equipment and additional pharmacology should the PHRM team have available?

On arrival the PHRM team finds that the patient remains GCS 15, with an HR of 124 and a BP of 88/49. Respiratory rate remains elevated at 38 bpm and saturations are 95% on 15 L via an NRBM.

The PHRM team undertakes a point-of-care ultrasound (POCUS) exam (see images below).

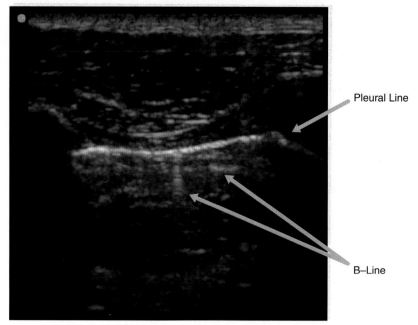

Pleural Line

B–Line

Figure 44.1 Lung window

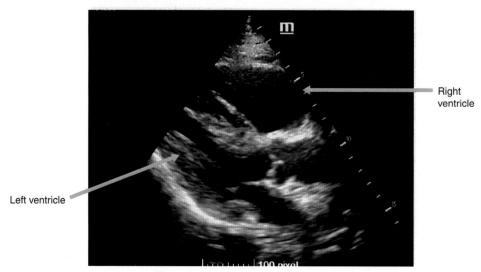

Right ventricle

Left ventricle

Figure 44.2a Parasternal long axis

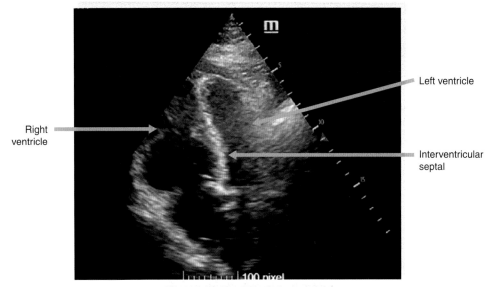

Right
ventricle

Left ventricle

Interventricular
septal

Figure 44.2b Apical 4 chamber

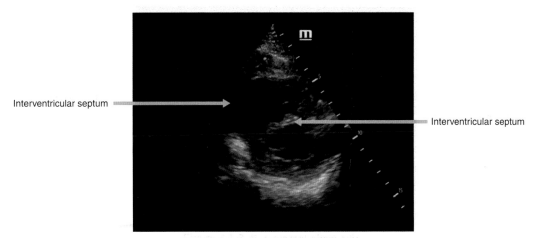

Interventricular septum

Interventricular septum

Figure 44.3 Parasternal short axis

Question 44.3

How might the PHRM team findings affect initial management and destination hospital response?

Discussion 44.1

Although the working diagnosis of an exacerbation of COPD may well explain the patient's clinical presentation, in the absence of both fever and/or wheeze it is important to maintain an open mind in respect of alternate diagnoses. Acute life-threatening pathology such as ischaemic heart disease and thromboembolic disease should be specifically considered, and a 12-lead ECG is required.

The local doctor confirms that X-ray facilities are unavailable, the patient has denied any chest pain or nausea but about a week prior to the onset of symptoms, spent time in a car travelling to visit her sister who lives a 3-hour drive away. The local doctor sends you the following ECG.

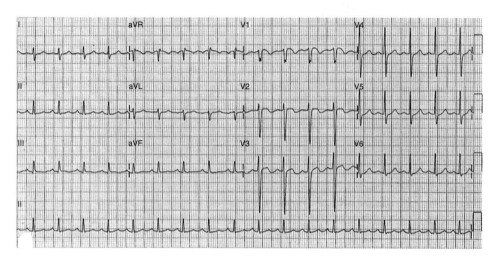

The ECG is abnormal with inverted or flattened T waves in the right precordial and inferior leads.

The differential diagnoses for this patient remains relatively broad. Respiratory tract infection, myocardial ischaemia +/− left ventricular failure and pulmonary embolism all remain diagnostic possibilities.

Discussion 44.2

Portable ultrasound utilised by the PHRM team may assist in helping establish the diagnosis. PHRM team members should be trained and accredited in the use and interpretation of POCUS.

Portable point-of-care (POC) testing devices giving blood gas, electrolyte, lactate and other laboratory markers (such as cardiac biomarkers like troponin) are also clinically useful.

If not part of the standard retrieval drug pack, then specifically sourcing and taking an intravenous thrombolytic agent should also be considered for this case.

Discussion 44.3

The lung fields (Figure 44.1) appear relatively clear with no consolidation, pleural effusion or excessive B-lines demonstrated and this is consistent with the clinical exam, which doesn't reveal any wheeze or crepitations on auscultation.

The point-of-care cardiac echo shows an obviously dilated right ventricle (right ventricle is bigger than left ventricle on the apical 4-chamber views – Figure 44.2a and 44.2b). Review of the dynamic images shows the right ventricular apex seeming to contract well, but the mid-right ventricular wall is hypokinetic (McConnell's sign). There is also paradoxical right ventricular septal wall systolic motion on the apical 4-chamber view (septal bowing – Figure 44.2b) with a 'D-shaped' septum in the short axis view (Figure 44.3).

While performing the POCUS exam, a point-of-care troponin is also carried out and reveals an elevated level.

The presence of a degree of cardiogenic shock, respiratory compromise with clear lung fields and an elevated troponin in conjunction with the POCUS findings are strongly supportive that this patient has a significant pulmonary embolus causing cardiovascular compromise.

This patient needs to be urgently retrieved to a cardiothoracic centre and if there is progressive cardiorespiratory deterioration en-route despite appropriate cardiovascular support, the PHRM team should consider the need for thrombolysis.

Prior to departure, invasive arterial access should be established and judicious fluid resuscitation commenced. Vasopressor or inotropic support may also be required to support the circulation. These can be temporarily administered via peripheral intravenous access. While central venous access is ideal, consideration should be given to the time required to place a central line safely prior to departure. As a general rule, invasive devices that are deemed absolutely necessary should be sited, under ultrasound guidance, prior to thrombolysis or formal anticoagulation.

The receiving hospital must be notified of the presumed diagnosis, the clinical condition and any significant deterioration via the PHRM clinical coordinator.

This should occur as early as possible to allow for consideration of extra-corporeal membrane oxygenation (ECMO) on patient arrival if clinically indicated.

Patients with massive pulmonary embolism have high morbidity and mortality. In addition to systemic thrombolysis, ECMO can be considered for ongoing support or as a bridge to surgical embolectomy or endovascular catheter-directed therapy/embolectomy.

Key points

- Portable ultrasound devices are valuable diagnostic tools for PHRM teams.
- An extended capability inclusive of point-of-care echocardiography is ideal.
- In clinical conditions that require significant respiratory or cardiac support, pre-notification to the receiving facility may allow the consideration of early ECMO.

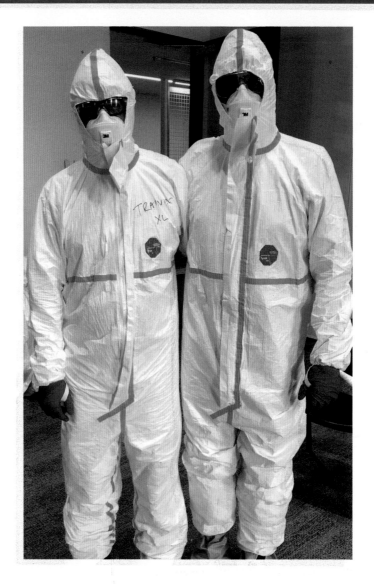

Incident

A highly infectious airborne respiratory virus is becoming more prevalent in your region. Case numbers of patients in severe respiratory distress, particularly those requiring intubation, are increasing on a daily basis.

You have been tasked to retrieve a 61-year-old male who has a productive cough, is febrile with a severe pneumonia. He is 250 km away in a rural hospital. He has a background medical history of ischaemic heart disease, congestive cardiac failure and suspected bowel malignancy. He is being managed by the local GP and his latest vital signs are as follows.

Clinical information

- BP 130/70.
- P 120 bpm.

- SaO_2 93% on 15L.
- RR 28 breaths per minute, tiring
- T 38.4°C (101°F).
- ECG: sinus tachycardia.
- Chest X-Ray: right lower lobe pneumonia and bilateral alveolar shadowing indicative of acute pulmonary oedema.
- ABG: pH 7.30, PaO_2 59mmHg (7.8 kPa), $PaCO_2$ 32mmHg (4.3k Pa), Lactate: 2.8 mmol/L

The rate of local community transmission of the virus is high. The hospital has sent a nasopharyngeal viral swab, but the result will take 24 hours to come back. A point of care rapid antigen test has come back positive.

Relevant information

- **PHRM team resources:** Fixed-wing.
- **Additional resources:** One land ambulance.
- **Retrieval options:** Nearest appropriate ICU is 250 km away.
- **Other:** Temperature is 30°C (86°F).

Question 45.1

How are you going to manage this retrieval?

This mission has subsequently been discussed in the weekly case review meeting and the PHRM clinical director has asked you to formalise a standard process of how the service will manage suspected and confirmed positive patients. The service utilises road, rotary and fixed-wing assets up to distances of 600 km round trip from the PHRM base.

Question 45.2

What are the important aspects in developing a PHRM service protocol on how to manage suspected or confirmed positive patients?

Question 45.3

How will you implement a new modified Rapid Sequence Induction (RSI) process and PPE protocol within the service?

Discussion 45.1

This management of this case can be divided into two categories: PHRM coordination and clinical management.

Coordination

The medical coordinator can help the local GP manage and resuscitate the patient (via telemedicine if available) until the PHRM team arrives. They can also be part of a discussion that may need to occur about the ceiling of care regarding treatment for this patient, in particular, depending on the grade and stage of his bowel malignancy. For example, does the patient have an advance care directive in place? Does he have the capacity to understand his condition and goals of care (see Case 41)? If not, who is his nominated surrogate decision maker? In this case, on the available information, it is clear that this patient is for full resuscitative measures including intubation and ventilation.

It is safe to assume that this patient has the airborne respiratory virus based on his symptoms and the high rate of local community transmission. Due to the infectious nature of this patient there are consequences for all the agencies involved in his transport, including local ambulance staff and pilots. In addition, the fixed-wing aircraft will not be available for several hours as it will need to be decontaminated after the mission has been completed. This may have an impact on the other planned patient transfers in the region.

The team will need to take appropriate PPE according to service and local guidelines. This patient is likely to need a negative pressure room in the receiving ICU, so an early phone call to alert the receiving unit is important.

There will be multiple occasions where the patient will be need to be transferred between different transport platforms during this long retrieval. A vacuum mattress may facilitate the multiple transfers in this situation. Consider extra equipment and additional batteries, given the prolonged nature of the retrieval time.

Given the high ambient temperature and the need to wear airborne PPE for an extended period of time, the team is likely to be fatigued and dehydrated after the mission. This will need to be managed and may impact any further missions the tasking agency has planned.

Clinical

This patient is in hypoxaemic type 1 respiratory failure and may benefit from non-invasive ventilation (NIV). There is a role of NIV in airborne respiratory viral illness similar to those in patients with a pneumonia or ARDS from other, non-viral aetiological causes. However, NIV is an aerosol-generating procedure and the risk of viral transmission is increased. In addition, there are few options for a negative pressure environment during the retrieval process, such as transfer isolation pods for single-patient carries. The use of isopods in cases such as this is described, and although not in routine use continues to be a developing area in PHRM.

In this case the patient has both features of acute pulmonary oedema and a pneumonia. Under normal circumstances, this patient may require NIV during the transfer. Depending on regional variation, some PHRM services would avoid the use of NIV in such a patient during transfer due to aerosolisation and the subsequent infection risk to others. A trial of NIV initiated at the referring centre (with appropriate local precautions) prior to PHRM team arrival may be of benefit to the patient. Should invasive ventilation be required, NIV may also be of benefit to optimise the patient.

Given the extent of his hypoxaemia and respiratory failure, and in the absence of NIV during transport, he will need intubation and invasive ventilation for the transfer. This will be a high-risk procedure, complicated by the need for strict respiratory precautions. A modified rapid-sequence induction in full PPE, will need to occur to mitigate transmission of the virus during the procedure. PHRM services should develop and train staff in this new protocol.

The following are the key differences between a standard and modified RSI:
- The team should remain away outside of the immediate patient-care area and set up RSI equipment, drugs and ventilator.
- An additional healthcare worker is designated as the outside (clean) runner.
- Donning of PPE should be done using a 'buddy' system to ensure it is performed correctly. Wearing two pairs of gloves allows the outer pair to be discarded immediately after intubation has occurred.

- BVM ventilation during the apnoeic period can be used to avoid critical desaturation.
- Video laryngoscope should be used to reduce the risk of viral transmission during intubation.
- The bougie should be removed carefully from the TT to prevent tracheal secretions being deposited on team members.
- The TT should be clamped before swapping from the BVM circuit to the ventilator circuit. Do not start ventilation prior to clamping TT or attaching the ventilator circuit.
- The TT should be clamped prior to all planned circuit disconnections.
- Inappropriate doffing of PPE poses one of the greatest risks to the PHRM team. The buddy system mentioned above should be maintained to ensure stringent adherence to doffing technique is maintained.

Lung ultrasonography can be a useful adjunct and should be performed at this time. Dynamic assessment before and after instituting respiratory treatment can offer the team information on the clinical effectiveness of the treatment. In this case, it can be used to demonstrate a resolution of B-lines resulting from acute pulmonary oedema (see Case 39). As a general rule, in airborne viral diseases, if bronchodilators are required, the use of metered dose inhalers in the ventilator circuit are preferred rather than the aerosol-generating effect of nebulisers.

Some patients may respond to being ventilated in a lateral tilt or prone position during transport. This presents significant logistical challenges and increased patient risk (see Case 30). Extracorporeal membrane oxygenation (ECMO) may be deemed necessary in some circumstances and a patient should be transferred to an ECMO-capable centre.

After the mission has been completed, a hot debrief with the extended team may provide both immediate and latent learning benefit and allow ongoing evolution of service protocols. Normally, where full PPE has been used and service policy adhered to, the team is not considered to be an exposure risk, and specific follow-up is not required unless symptoms develop.

Discussion 45.2

The aim is to focus on the priorities in the PHRM environment, which may differ from local health department or hospital processes. However, where possible, standardisation of processes should occur, and liaison between hospitals, the health department, the Ambulance Service and the PHRM service is recommended.

Having a multidisciplinary team with representatives from each of the professional groups within the PHRM service is of benefit. Topics should be divided into order of priority to maximise efficiency.

Retrieval and clinical coordination aspects should be approached separately. Examples may include the following.

Retrieval

- PPE: The levels of PPE and stock levels required, the donning and doffing procedures, methods of communication within the team, and staff wellbeing while wearing PPE for prolonged periods of time.
- Clinical interventions: Modifications to RSI and ventilation guidelines and how to create a 'clean or dirty' area in a rural or remote hospital. The risk benefit of

NIV in these patients (both for the patient and the team). The PHRM service will need to make a decision on whether NIV is to be used during missions.

- Transport platforms: Retrievals may require the use of a fixed-wing, rotary-wing, or road platforms, each of which will have specific considerations regarding infection control. In particular, the agencies providing pilots and ancillary staff may have separate guidelines or requirements. PHRM teams changing between different transport platforms will need to factor in these requirements.
- Equipment modifications: Staff PPE to be routinely added to packs, patient PPE requirements, additional airway equipment, additional equipment battery capacity.
- Implementation of new guidelines: how to train and assess all staff in a short timeframe (see below).
- Cleaning of medical equipment, decontamination of transport platforms, safe disposal of consumables.
- A weekly review of infectious retrieval cases as well as appraisal of recent research trials can assist with updating existing protocols.

Coordination

- Screening tools and PPE matrices to determine the risk to staff and therefore the level of PPE required for each individual patient. This tool should be based on local epidemiological guidance and be supported by the receiving hospitals.
- Discussion with the receiving hospitals, in particular emergency departments and ICUs, on how to transport the patients safely through the hospital.
- Liaising with external agencies to inform them of the PHRM services' model of care for these patients.
- Methods of communicating to all staff any updates to guidelines or testing regimens. Having a living document on a digital platform is the most preferable. Other options include email or a paper-based system.
- The PHRM service's capacity to replace staff who are either infected or in quarantine should be considered. Service resilience can be improved by having a peer-support framework in place for staff wellness and wellbeing. A vaccination program should be implemented for staff if available and according to local guidelines.

Discussion 45.3

The development and implementation of any new process requires multidisciplinary involvement and good intra-service communication to disseminate the information (such as a daily team brief – see Case 48 and Case 55). Two skill stations should be constructed; one on the modified RSI protocol and a second on PPE donning/doffing sequence. This will allow clinicians to 'drill the skill'. Consideration should be made for all relevant staff to experience these skill stations. Having demonstrated competence with these individual skills, they should now be integrated into a simulated clinical environment. This involves designing and setting up a simulation scenario which incorporates both protocols. Ideally both the skill stations and simulation scenario should be conducted on a daily basis. A method of tracking attendance and competence must be in place prior to commencement of training. Once competence has been assessed and confirmed, staff may incorporate these learned skills into the operational environment.

Key points

- Highly infectious airborne viral diseases pose additional risk to the extended PHRM team.
- The development of a pragmatic PHRM service model of care on how to manage patients with airborne viral disease is essential to mitigate risk to patients and staff.
- PHRM team members should have the dedicated time to acquire new skills and knowledge relevant to such high-risk situations.

SECTION C

Special Circumstances and Service Development

Foreword to the Special Circumstances and Service Development Section

The work of the Pre-Hospital and Retrievalist is both exciting and demanding, partly because the critically ill or injured patient may not present with something routine or familiar. One minute you may be en route to a HAZMAT scene, the next to a patient with snake envenomation, the next to an overseas destination on an international retrieval. And not only will your patients present with rarities that will have you reaching into the recesses of your cerebral catalogue, you will also find yourself working in environments you may have never imagined. And all of this as part of a small, high performing team with only the finite contents of your medical packs to get you through.

Prioritising team and personal safety, dealing with hazardous environments, seeing multiple patients and dealing with cases outside your area of expertise are *de rigeur* for the PHRM practitioner. The scenario training you commit to in your down time, and the rigour of clinical audit are solid investments in developing a systematic approach to the unprecedented or unfamiliar. The SOPS that have been developed for your service will have a sound basis in both current evidence and hard-won experience.

When the moment came for me to administer an intramuscular dose of ketamine to a 30kg child at the back of a cave in remote northern Thailand, it occurred to me that this was something I could never have conceived of during my years of medical training. But when I thought of my career in PHRM, I realised in many ways it was just another day at the office.

Prepare for the unexpected, and you can expect to feel prepared!

Dr Richard Harris SC OAM
BMBS, DA(UK), FANZCA, Dip DHM, Post Grad Cert Aeromed Ret, FFEWM, D. Univ (Flind), D. Univ (JCU)
Consultant Anaesthetist
Former Senior Consultant, MedSTAR Emergency Medical Retrieval Service, South Australia

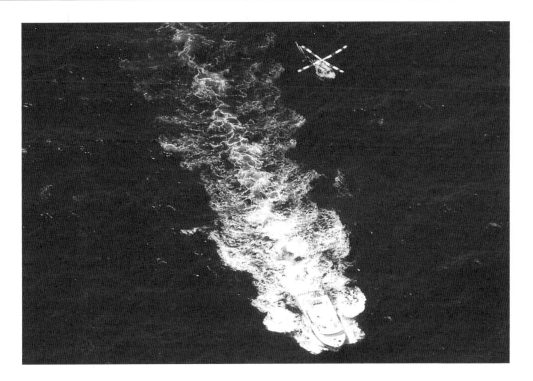

Incident

As the medical director of a pre-hospital and retrieval service, you are working a clinical shift in the emergency department of a major trauma hospital. A case involving one of your services' PHRM teams arrives by helicopter. At handover, the details are as follows:

- 28-year-old male tourist.
- Accredited open-water SCUBA diving course participant.
- No significant past medical problems.
- Rapid ascent from 15 metres (50 feet) to the surface.
- Waved for help before losing consciousness.
- Assisted from the water to the vessel distressed and short of breath.
- Oxygen applied.
- Ship's captain radioed for help.
- Winch rescue from vessel.

Relevant information

The PHRM team's handwritten on-scene notes record the following:

Complaining of generalised pain. Cool. Shut down.
GCS 13 (E3, M6, V4). P 118 beats per minute. BP 158/94 mmHg. RR 30. SaO$_2$ 94% on high-flow O$_2$.
Few crackles to both lung bases.

There is no documented neurological examination.
On-scene management:

- Intravenous access for analgesia. Morphine to total of 10 mg given.
- No intravenous fluid given in light of *'wet lungs'*.

In-flight (25 minutes over water):

- Increasing respiratory distress. Sat up.
- Became 'unresponsive' and proceeded to have a generalised tonic-clonic seizure.
- Intravenous diazepam 5 mg administered with good effect.
- Patient then apnoeic and vomiting.
- Difficult emergency in-flight intubation.

On arrival at the emergency department, the patient is unresponsive without further sedation. He has bilateral fixed and dilated pupils and is difficult to ventilate, requiring high airway pressures and 100% inspired oxygen. A chest X-ray reveals no pneumothorax. A head CT is requested, and the verbal report is as follows: 'Extensive intracranial intravascular air. Early loss of grey-white differentiation'.

The patient is admitted to the intensive care unit, where he deteriorates further and is declared brain-dead 24 hours following admission.

Question 46.1

Briefly outline the common diving-related emergency presentations.

Question 46.2

What is likely to have occurred in this case?

Question 46.3

Discuss optimal management of this patient. Is any team follow-up required?

Discussion 46.1

Common diving-related emergency presentations include: (a) those that occur on descent; (b) those that occur on or after ascent; (c) those related to diving at depth; and (d) other (incidental medical issues).

Those that occur on descent
- Facial, dental, sinus and middle-ear barotrauma

Those that occur on or after ascent
- Decompression illness (DCI) comprising cerebral arterial gas embolus (CAGE) and decompression sickness (DCS)
  - CAGE – Rapid ascent with barotrauma producing cerebral arterial gas embolism plus pneumothorax, pneumomediastinum, subcutaneous emphysema

- DCS – may be fulminant if decompression obligations have been omitted due to rapid ascent with missed decompression stops.

Those related to diving at depth and duration
- Nitrogen narcosis
- Hypothermia
- CNS oxygen toxicity
- Contaminated gas toxicity.

Other
- Exacerbation of pre-existent medical condition
- Immersion pulmonary oedema
- Salt water aspiration syndrome
- Envenomation or marine animal attack
- Boat injuries
- Drowning.

Discussion 46.2

The history of rapid ascent with initial loss of consciousness and latent deterioration at altitude and on changing posture is highly suggestive of cerebral arterial gas embolism (CAGE). In the absence of pneumothoraces, respiratory compromise may have been due to pulmonary artery involvement, aspiration during unconscious submersion or during the intubation attempt. The head CT confirms the diagnosis of CAGE, revealing extensive intravascular intracranial air.

Discussion 46.3

The management of diving-related emergencies in the pre-hospital and retrieval environment requires an understanding of the relevant pathophysiology and the likely differential diagnoses given the history. Frequently, however, information relating to the patient's past medical problems, dive profile or sequence of events is absent.

Clinical presentation following tissue space or intravascular bubbles, whether acute, as with CAGE, or more insidious, as with DCS, is highly variable. Bubble size, coalescence and distribution will dictate the presenting signs and symptoms. The brain is most at risk following the sudden introduction of large amounts of intravascular air in the setting of CAGE, or in the presence of a large shunting patent foramen ovale (PFO). Occlusion of the smaller end arterioles will result in distal tissue ischaemia and infarction. Furthermore, bubble movement along narrow vascular lumens may cause a secondary insult with latent endovascular injury, release of local inflammatory mediators, clotting disruption including disseminated intravascular coagulopathy [DIC], vascular occlusion and worsening end organ insult. Significant vascular leak occurs with resultant intravascular volume depletion and further hypoperfusion of downstream tissues. There are a number of simple therapeutic options that may minimise such tissue injury in the pre-hospital phase.

Application of oxygen in the highest concentration available
- May enhance nitrogen elimination (improved gradient for diffusion out of tissues) and reduce bubble size.

Fluid therapy
- Many divers are dehydrated while SCUBA diving, due to inadequate pre-dive hydration, sea sickness and immersion diuresis. Profound haemoconcentration is seen in severe cases of DCS. Fluid therapy will be crucial to restore intravascular volume and tissue perfusion and is essential even in patients who appear to have respiratory distress with signs of pulmonary oedema. The pulmonary 'filter' is overwhelmed by the bubble load in these cases and restoring blood flow becomes vital.

Patient positioning
- The head-up position can promote cephalad distribution of arterial bubbles. Full Trendelenburg seems attractive but may promote cerebral oedema. Hence level and supine is the best compromise. It is likely in the case presented that the change of position promoted the movement of bubbles to the cerebral circulation. The initial transit of bubbles through the brain produced the unconsciousness at the surface. Normal blood flow will usually move these bubbles on, but 'prime' the endothelium to which subsequent bubbles will stick and occlude.

Early advice and triage
- The tasking agency should facilitate early communications with a hyperbaric medical physician, and the patient should be triaged, primarily to a recompression facility if possible. The hyperbaric unit will also be able to provide up-to-date information on relevant regional or novel treatment strategies or potential adjuvant therapies. Geographical areas that are popular with divers may have local support and advice facilities in place (e.g. Diver Alert Network [DAN]), and the tasking agency can look into these for the PHRM team.

Transport considerations
- Altitude has a significant effect on gases (Boyle's Law) (see Case 27). Although trapped gas expansion is relatively minor in the operational altitude range of an unpressurised helicopter cabin, increasing altitude may prove detrimental to the patient in this setting. This information should be discussed with the pilots at the earliest opportunity so that the return flight path can be pre-arranged with air traffic control. The team should request the 'lowest safe altitude'. However, final decisions on aircraft altitude rest with the pilot. An alternative strategy is to request a fixed-wing aircraft, in which the cabin can be pressurised to ground or sea level. While not appropriate in this instance, a fixed-wing aircraft would be ideal for secondary retrievals or very long-distance primary tasks.
- Excessive vibration may promote bubble migration and alter the clinical picture. Vibration is a recognised and unavoidable problem in rotary-wing aircraft.

This case highlights a number of events that will require further review. Service-specific clinical governance processes, or quality and safety frameworks will dictate the exact response (see Case 52).

Key points
• Diving-related presentations are common but rarely of high acuity.
• The PHRM team should consider both acute and latent pathophysiology when managing high-acuity presentations.
• Recompression is definitive but movement of the patient to such a facility frequently presents logistic challenges.
• Good first aid, aggressive fluid resuscitation and oxygen in the supine position in the PHRM environment, followed by emergent recompression, can be life saving.

Additional reading

Mitchell SJ, Bennett MH, Bryson P, et al. Pre-hospital management of decompression illness: expert review of key principles and controversies. Diving Hyperb Med. 2018 Mar; 48(1):45–55.

Nutbeam T, Boylan M. (Eds) ABC of pre-hospital emergency medicine. Wiley Blackwell, 2013.

South Pacific Underwater Medicine Society (SPUMS): www.spums.org.au.

Trytko B, Mitchell S. Extreme survival: a serious technical diving accident. South Pacific Underwater Medicine Society (SPUMS) Journal 2005, 35.

The following questions relate to crew resource management (CRM) and the implications for the PHRM team. The terms crew resource management, team resource management, crisis resource management and human factors are often used interchangeably in this context.

Incident A

The team has just been activated to a 5-year-old child who has fallen from a height. The tasking agency tells you that the child is unconscious with grunting respirations. You are 10 minutes away from the scene by air (rotary-wing aircraft). The pilots are already on board with rotors running but, as you board the aircraft, you notice a puddle of pink fluid under the body of the helicopter (see below).

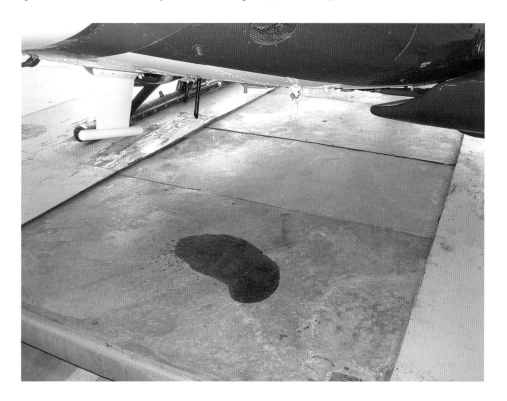

Incident B

The team has been tasked to a 'person under a train' and has arrived on the perimeter of the scene within 10 minutes of the incident. The patient has just gone into cardiac arrest. The team is unsure that safety protocols have been followed, and, despite being asked repeatedly by other emergency personnel to cross the tracks and enter the scene, the team follows protocol and first makes contact with the fire safety officer who confirms that the power is off and all train movements have ceased. Later, after an unsuccessful resuscitation, the local ambulance service paramedic team leader calls you aside and criticises your initial delay in entering the scene. He states that, as he and his team were already on the tracks, it was obvious that the scene was safe. He suggests that the death may have been preventable with earlier treatment.

Incident C

The PHRM team has arrived at scene following an incident in which a 7-year-old boy was hit by a car while crossing the road. The child has already been loaded into a land ambulance and packaged ready for transport. There is significant damage to the front of the car and there is a bullseye on the windscreen (see below). The nearest hospital is not a trauma centre and has no neurosurgery on site. The regional trauma centre is 20 minutes away by air. As you approach the rear door of the land ambulance, a crewman opens the door and firmly says that your team is not required, that they are now leaving the scene, heading to the nearest hospital, and that they can deal with the situation. Behind him you see the child having a tonic-clonic seizure inside the ambulance.

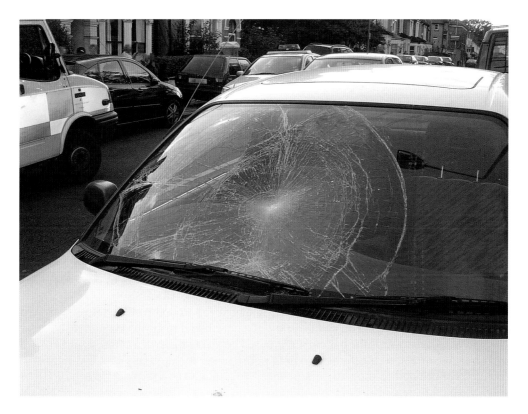

Incident D

The team is tasked by air to a multi-car road traffic accident with reports of three persons seriously injured and trapped. En route, 10 minutes from the scene, the weather closes in and the pilot states, 'I am not sure we are going to be able to land at scene – how sick is this patient?'

Incident E

The team has been tasked to a civilian helicopter crash that had four persons on board. On arrival, you link up with the Fire and Rescue Service team leader at the perimeter of the scene. The crash occurred 25 minutes ago. There is wreckage strewn around 40 metres (130 feet) in front of you, including an upside-down child safety seat. The scene smells strongly of aviation fuel and there is no noise or movement coming from the scene. The Fire and Rescue Service team leader tells you the scene is not safe and he is awaiting a specialist foam tender which will arrive within 10 minutes.

Question 47.1

Briefly describe how you will deal with each scenario.

Discussion 47.1

Incident A

There is fluid of unknown origin under the aircraft. Until proven otherwise, this should be considered to have resulted from a mechanical failure. In aeromedical pre-hospital and retrieval operations, each member of the team should recognise their role in team safety. That includes the operational base, aircraft and scene safety. System malfunctions, especially in rotary-wing aircraft, can be catastrophic for all crew and passengers, and no medical tasking is worth such a risk. In this instance, the fluid may be hydraulic fluid, and a leak of such fluid could lead to a major aviation system failure en route.

The safest course of action here is to don your helmet while outside the aircraft, connect to the aircraft internal communications system (ICS), and immediately tell the pilot what you have seen.

Incident B

In such a scenario, there is usually pressure for the team to enter the scene immediately once they arrive. As discussed in the railway scenario (Case 13), rail safety is paramount and carries high risks, especially on electrified tracks. The PHRM team must adhere to safety protocol. If other emergency services have followed the same protocol and the senior member of their team informs the PHRM team directly of this, then repetition is unnecessary. However, if any doubt is present, as in this case, then the protocol should be repeated.

The paramedic team leader is sufficiently aggrieved to confront you directly and a 'hot debrief' is indicated. You should allow the paramedic to air his concerns and steer the conversation towards the patient's injuries. The mechanism of trauma, together with early cardiac arrest, suggest unsurvivable injuries and it is unlikely that the extra few minutes contributed to the patient's demise. You should also explain that the PHRM service, like his, has protocols which must be followed. Citing a 'near miss' that you or your service were previously involved in may be useful. Finally, thank him and extend that thanks to his team for their efforts in this situation. Give him your contact details so that the two services can not only communicate about mutual improvements in managing these scenarios in the future but also be involved in the PHRM teams' review of the case at a later date.

Incident C

If the PHRM team is cancelled before arrival on-scene, then the situation is different. Ideally, only the tasking agency should cancel the PHRM team and only then after an accurate scene report (e.g. MISTO; see Case 18) indicating that the additional resource is not required.

The child is clearly unwell and has intracranial pathology until proven otherwise. The team must act quickly and decisively. Communicating what you have observed (i.e. a generalised seizure) may help. The child may have been alert and responsive until the very moment the doors were opened. Be honest and clear about your concerns (severe head injury). Shift the focus away from any perceived professional disagreement back onto the best possible outcome for the child. Offer assistance with transferring the patient (e.g. using the helicopter) voicing your concerns that the nearest hospital is unlikely to be adequate for such a patient.

As a two-person team, it is possible for one team member to be involved in this time-pressured but critical discussion while the other starts to assist with the assessment and management of the patient. Direct conflict (e.g. threats or shouting) must be avoided on-scene. If the land ambulance team categorically refuses access to the patient, the PHRM team should inform them that they will proceed to the nearest hospital as a secondary retrieval is almost guaranteed (this may also impact on their decision). Follow-up of the incident is then mandatory using service clinical governance and multidisciplinary audit processes. Remember, the issue is usually one of education and any action points generated by the follow-up should be positive, educational and ultimately drive improvements in PHRM/Ambulance Service (see Case 52).

Incident D

The pilot's comments reflect a concern for aviation safety. The pilot has complete authority over all aviation matters and could abort the mission without consulting the rest of the team. The fact that he has involved the team in discussion is good CRM. In support of the pilot, you should state quite clearly that the condition of the patients should not influence his decision regarding returning to base. It is reasonable to suggest alternatives such as landing at a nearby designated landing site and continuing by road.

Once it is clear that the team is not attending, liaise with the tasking agency by radio to discuss alternative arrangements. Following the return to base, the entire team (PHRM and aviation) should run a thorough debrief. Failure to debrief such a complex tasking can lead to misunderstanding, poor CRM and subsequent critical errors of judgement.

Incident E

The golden rule of pre-hospital medicine is scene safety (see Case 1). In this incident, the Fire and Rescue Service team leader has declared the scene unsafe and the PHRM team must not enter. The situation is made more complex by emotional factors including the potential presence of injured children. It can be very difficult to remain inactive at such significant incident scenes and this may take an emotional toll on the PHRM team as well as the Fire and Rescue Service team. Consider all the options in this scenario, including the likelihood of survival following such a high mechanism of injury. If clear signs of life are visible on-scene then the situation is different and inaction is likely to become untenable. In such a situation, a fresh plan should be made, perhaps involving a two-person 'extraction' team to rush in and bring the moving patient out as quickly as possible (see Case 4). This will require close liaison with the Fire and Rescue Service. In this scenario, no signs of life in the presence of such a mechanism should help all the emergency teams to stand back until the scene is safe.

Following such a job, a full debrief is essential. Peer support, wellness and wellbeing, and psychological support services should be available for all team members to consult if required.

Key points
• The PHRM team represents just one component of a multisystem PHRM response.
• An understanding of human factors as they relate to the PHRM environment is essential.
• Good CRM within the aviation and emergency services group improves scene management, team safety and ultimately patient outcome.

Additional reading

Bleetman A, Sanusi S, Dale T, Brace S. Human factors and error prevention in emergency medicine. Emerg. Med. J. 2012; 29(5):389–393.

Hearns S. Peak Performance under pressure: Lessons from a helicopter rescue doctor. Class professional publishing. 2019.

The following questions relate to crew resource management (CRM) and the implications for the PHRM team (see Case 47).

You have been asked to review the orientation program for new staff at your PHRM base.

Question 48.1

Outline key components of this program.

Question 48.2

Describe the roles of PHRM team members travelling in the rear cabin of a rotary-wing aircraft during the flight to scene (i.e. with no patient on board).

Question 48.3

What are the key components of the daily 'team brief' held at the crew base?

Discussion 48.1

- Identification and access:
  - Photo identification
  - Access to all areas of the PHRM base
  - Special access to the airside area of operational airports.
- Uniform and PPE: See Appendix 3.
- Base and equipment orientation:
  - Orientation to the base layout and facilities
  - Regular equipment packs plus specialist equipment packs
  - Monitors, ventilators and other biomedical equipment
  - Manual handling training
  - Access and routine for blood and blood products
  - Access and routine for drugs including drugs of dependence
  - Familiarisation with base daily routine
  - Familiarisation with vehicles on base, e.g. rapid response vehicles (including advanced lights and sirens driving if required).
- Aviation currencies
  - Helicopter familiarisation including formal safety brief (eg Civil Aviation Orders 20.11 - Australia).
  - Helicopter Underwater Escape Training (HUET)
  - Fixed-wing orientation, including formal safety briefing
  - Other aviation platforms (e.g. jet).
- Clinical skills and currencies
  - Core skills stations (e.g. traction splint, finger thoracostomy)
  - Special skills stations (e.g. use of fibre-optic equipment, transvenous cardiac pacing)
  - Major incident training
  - Scenario training to provide an opportunity for:
    - Application of core and special skills into a high-fidelity simulation
    - Inclusion of human factors training into clinical practice
    - Escalating scenario complexity:
      - Simple scenario, simple environment
      - Complex scenario, simple environment

- Simple scenario, complex environment
- Complex scenario, complex environment.

○ Familiarisation with clinical coordination
  - Visit to clinical coordination centre
  - Importance of on scene communication (e.g. sit reps – see Case 9)
  - Radio etiquette.

○ Broader service orientation
  - Local Ambulance Service resources including familiarisation with land ambulance vehicles
  - Local Fire and Rescue Service
  - Local Police service
  - Local hospital and health facility resources.

○ Audit and clinical governance arrangements, including debriefs and data entry.

○ Wellness and wellbeing, peer support and psychological support arrangements (see Case 67).

○ Assessment and sign-off
  - Initial competency assessment
  - Ongoing assessment (e.g. 'buddy shifts' with a senior PHRM clinician).

Discussion 48.2

The medical team has a dual role on aeromedical taskings, especially rotary-wing. Their primary duty is to the patient, but they also have a key role as air crew members. One member of the team should take the lead in the back of the cabin. Initial duties include making voice contact with the pilot and then securing the cabin pre-take-off. Make sure all cabin personnel have helmets on and chin straps fastened. Seatbelts should be fastened, and the aircraft doors should be in the locked position. The pilot will ask whether the rear cabin is secure, and the team leader should confirm this. During take-off and landing in both fixed-wing and rotary-wing platforms, the team in the cabin should avoid speaking. This 'sterile cockpit' allows the pilot to focus attention during these periods of higher risk. The exception to this is the requirement of all air crew to look out for hazards to the aircraft. This can be anything from unsecured objects on the ground, to wires and air traffic. Do not hesitate to alert the pilot to these potential threats and never assume that they have already been identified (see Case 1). Once airborne and, with the pilot's permission, the team can discuss relevant aspects of the tasking, including equipment required and drug doses. Contact should be made with the tasking agency for updates, arrival information and the proposed destination hospital. The team should keep observing for air traffic at all times and should listen to the air-traffic control frequency for traffic updates. On arrival at the scene, assist the pilot with identifying potential landing sites if required and follow the same rules for landing as for take-off (see Case 1, HEMS acronym). For emergency landings in non-designated landing sites, pay particular attention to members of the public and warn the pilot if you see any people (including emergency services personnel) heading to the rear of the aircraft. Note that many aircraft have a rear-facing seat in the cabin, and this will afford the best view of this part of the aircraft. After landing, await clearance from the pilot and safely leave the aircraft and the rotor disc area. Discussion with the pilot prior to landing is required if you plan to leave the rotor disc area immediately on disembarking the aircraft and prior to engine shut-down ('hot deplane').

Discussion 48.3

The daily brief should occur just before the team goes operational and must be attended by all members of the team. The brief should be divided into aviation and medical matters. A sample daily brief includes:

Aviation

- Weather
  - Formal reports including TAFs (terminal aerodrome forecast) and METARs (meteorological aviation reports) are consulted.
- NOTAMs (notice to airmen).
  - Up-to-date information on hazards that the air crew can expect in their area during the shift.
- Aircraft serviceability.
- Team composition, tasks and crew duties.
  - Include any aviation training required.
- Questions.

Medical

- Equipment.
  - To notify the team that equipment is checked and ready to be used.
- Information relevant to the day (e.g. drugs to be collected or updates to service guidelines).
- Crew training needs.
  - Including the need for simulations, familiarisation with kit or mission debriefs.
- Observers and visitors.
  - People who may visit the air base include previous patients or other emergency services teams.
- Questions.

For both medical and aviation matters, the brief can occasionally end with a simulated emergency so the team can rehearse the corrective measures together. Such emergencies may range from an aircraft warning light to an accidental extubation in flight. Finally, the meeting should be documented (a simple checklist with notes is sufficient) and the documents filed. A complete team brief is required after each shift change. Notes from the previous shift's team should be reviewed.

Key points
• Service orientation should be detailed and accurately reflect service operations allowing for assessment of competency.
• Medical personnel who form part of the PHRM team will have numerous responsibilities outside the medical sphere.
• Equipment, standard operating procedures and protocols will vary between aeromedical bases.
• The team brief is an essential part of the operational shift.

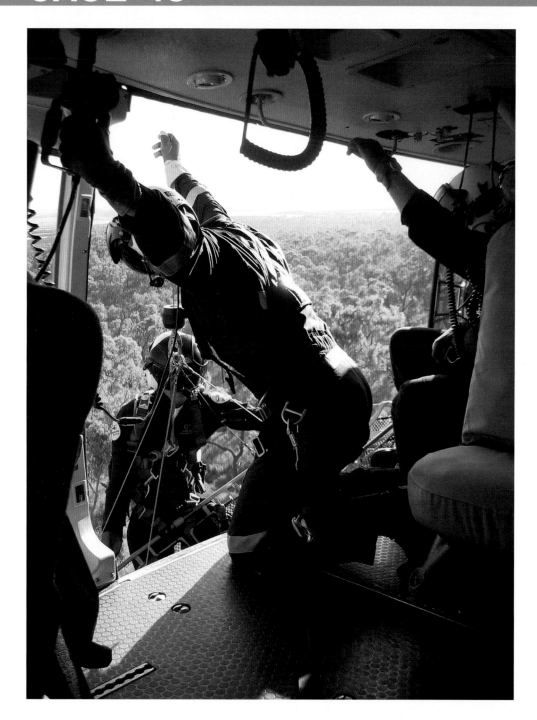

Incident

A 25-year-old male has fallen 3 metres (10 feet) from a hiking track in an isolated, mountainous and heavily forested national park. He is unable to walk due to a suspected lower limb fracture and is complaining of neck, abdominal and lower back pain. His only companion is uninjured and has notified emergency services via a satellite phone.

Relevant information

- **PHRM team transport options:** Rotary-wing capable of winch rescue.
- **Additional resources:** Hiking companion on-scene. Voluntary land ambulance and national parks personnel at nearest access road 2 km (1.2 miles) from scene.
- **Retrieval options:** Regional hospital 50 minutes by air.
- **Other:** Temperature 35°C (95°F). Wind at 3 km/h (2 mph). Local time 13:20 hours.

Question 49.1

Outline the possible options for patient access and egress in this situation.

Question 49.2

What factors should be considered when formulating the plan?

Question 49.3

A winch rescue is planned. Outline the key components in this process.

Question 49.4

What common problems and rare emergencies associated with winch operations should the PHRM team be aware of?

Discussion 49.1

Any combination of the following is possible. A brief overview is provided for each in the table below.

Options for patient access and egress	
Patient access	**Patient/team egress**
Winch-in A winch-in will allow at least one member of the PHRM team to be with the patient as soon as possible. Additional medical and rescue equipment can also be winched in. In combination, this will facilitate early patient assessment and treatment.	**Winch-out** A winch-out will see the patient en route to the nearest medical facility relatively quickly. In addition, patient movement may be minimised when compared with a prolonged stretcher carry or road transfer over uneven terrain. Due to the inherent risk of winch operations, a risk–benefit analysis must be considered.
Walk-in The PHRM team and required equipment may be dropped at the nearest safe landing site and then (ideally with the assistance of ground resource personnel) proceed to the scene by foot.	**Walk-out** Following the winch-in, the aircraft may reposition to the nearest available safe landing site. The plan may then be to rendezvous with the PHRM team and patient or return to base and allow the team and patient to proceed by road ambulance.

Options for patient access and egress—cont'd

Patient access	Patient/team egress
Other Rarely, PHRM team members or other personnel may access a scene by being lowered to a patient in a controlled manner by a rescue team or via rappelling techniques (abseiling down a static line while controlling descent with a variable friction device) or via hover exit from the aircraft. These techniques are not discussed further here.	**Other** A rescue strop (harness) or rescue body sling is frequently used for uninjured persons or if a stretcher is unsuitable due to the environment (cliff face or marine), requiring a hoist rescue. This technique would not be appropriate in this setting and is not discussed further. An off-road vehicle may be available for team and patient transport to and from a rendezvous point with either the aircraft or road ambulance vehicles. Regional variation will dictate both availability and capability in this regard.

Discussion 49.2

The key decision here is whether a winch rescue is appropriate. A risk–benefit analysis is required, often at a time when relevant factors are either not entirely clear or variable. The key to any dynamic mission planning in this setting is a shared mental model involving the entire mission team (aviation and medical). Pre-mission briefing and regular team training, operational exposure and debriefing will maximise the team's ability to respond safely and effectively in such situations. Ultimately, the pilot is the mission commander and final decisions regarding any aircraft movement rest with them.

A non-exhaustive list of factors that should be considered includes:

Aviation
'WINCHES'

- W – Weather and wind.
  - Inclement weather and poor visibility clearly increases the aviation risk. In addition, extreme heat and minimal wind will increase the power requirements of a rotary-wing aircraft in the hover position.
- I – In and out (approach and exit).
  - A flight path into and out of the hover/winch position should be clear of hazards.
- N – Night or day? Is the aircraft NVG (Night Vision Goggle) equipped?
  - Night or twilight winch operations increase the complexity and risk of such missions.
- C – Capacity (load) and endurance of aircraft.
  - Rotary-wing aircraft will vary in terms of engine number and performance. The load capacity of any one aircraft will also vary between missions. Large numbers of personnel and equipment, high ambient temperatures, minimal wind speeds and high fuel requirements will significantly limit both the range (distance travelled) and endurance (engine time) of the aircraft for a given mission.
  - In this case, there may be very little time on the ground for the PHRM team should a winch-in/winch-out plan be made. Consider staging the helicopter at a helicopter landing zone (HLZ) until the PHRM team is ready to extricate.

- H – Hazards and height.
  - Hazards including wires, trees and towers are described further in Case 1 and Case 48.
  - High winch operations add complexity to the practicalities of performing the winch and minimise the benefit to the aircraft of 'in-ground effect' when in the hover position (it takes more power to hover at height than close to the ground). Additionally, high winch activities may provide limited points of reference for the pilot who is required to maintain a very static hover. However, there is a considerable reduction in downwash, reducing the risk of the load being struck by tree branches or loss of visibility due to dust, sand or snow.
- E – Emergency options.
  - An in-flight emergency such as an engine failure may require the pilot to land the aircraft urgently. When this occurs close to the ground, there is limited time to steer the aircraft to a suitable area and the aircraft's autorotation capability (ability to fly forward on descent with no power to the main rotors) will be limited. If there is a load on the winch hook during an aircraft emergency, every effort will be made to recover the load on the hook into the cabin. The pilot will determine if the cable is to be cut in order to save the aircraft and crew onboard.
- S – Surface and terrain.
  - The scene topography is an important consideration for both the responding team and the pilot. Steep, uneven or loose surfaces pose a significant challenge to personnel winching down. This, and the heavily forested area, will also add to the challenge of grounding the aircraft safely in an emergency.

Team
Training and familiarity
- Safe and effective winch operations require a team with a high level of current skill and knowledge. In addition, the team should be familiar with each other's abilities and roles, having regularly trained for and performed winch activities.

Fitness
- Winch rescue demands a higher level of physical fitness than standard PHRM operations.

PPE
- In addition to standard PPE for all PHRM crew members, personnel involved in on-ground winch rescue activities should be prepared for unexpected mission variations. The most extreme of these may include the need to spend a prolonged period of time in a wilderness environment awaiting your own rescue.

Patient
Acuity
- A winch-in/winch-out scenario provides the swiftest delivery of a higher level of care to the patient and the swiftest movement of the patient to the receiving facility. Patients with time-critical injuries are therefore ideally retrieved from such scenes utilising this technique. Less acute patient groups may tolerate longer pre-hospital times resulting from non-winch egress.

Complexity
- Patients with complex injuries who require careful assessment, initial treatment and packaging may benefit from the relatively swift and smooth egress provided

by winch extrication. It should be remembered, though, that time on-scene may be profoundly limited when an aircraft is operating at the limit of its endurance. This will limit what can be done by the PHRM team on-scene, unless the aircraft can be staged nearby.

Discussion 49.3

Roles

Ideally, a minimum of four people are required for the winch rescue of a rescue litter and patient. These are:

- The pilot dedicated to maintain flight and reference, who is also responsible for safety of the aircraft and all crew
- A winch operator, who remains in the aircraft
- A rescue crew person (who may also be part of the PHRM team)
- A member of the PHRM team dedicated to the patient.

Communications

In-cabin communications are facilitated by the internal communications system (ICS) of the aircraft. Once outside the aircraft, mobile radio devices are required should the rescue crew person or PHRM team member be required to communicate by voice with the pilot or winch operator. In general, the winch operator remains in constant voice contact with the pilot, who may be unable to visualise the winch target area or crew outside of the aircraft. The winch operator will often guide the pilot to move into the correct position, notify them of any hazards and inform them of the mission progress. Communications between the crew outside the aircraft and the winch operator are also facilitated by hand signals.

All stages of the plan, including potential or actual difficulties, role variations and contingencies should be verbalised before separation from the ICS.

Preparation

Cabin

- All equipment should be stowed or adequately restrained before the opening of cabin doors. Even small items can cause serious damage or injury to either the aircraft or unsuspecting people below if they are not secured. Ensure that stretcher and equipment restraint straps or mechanisms are in place during cabin preparations. Stretchers and equipment must be immediately secured when recovered.

Personnel

- All personnel must be secured prior to the opening of doors. Personnel will either be in their seat with seatbelt fastened, in an air-crew safety harness attached to the aircraft floor via a 'wander lead', or in the winch harness, which is attached to the winch cable hook, awaiting egress from the cabin. All crew that operate on a wander lead must be competent in the quick-release mechanism in the event of an emergency.

Equipment

- Equipment required for patient assessment, treatment and packaging (including the rescue litter or stretcher) must be identified and prepared for winch. Like personnel, all equipment must be secured at all times, either to the aircraft or on the winch cable. Remember, anything that goes down will need to come back up. A standard operating procedure detailing equipment for such missions should aim to avoid carrying too much gear, making last-minute decisions or being without the required gear on ground.

• Check external down-the-wire communications and radio frequencies prior to exiting aircraft.

Patient access

The rescue crew person is usually first to descend, often accompanied by some or all of the equipment required. The PHRM team member will usually follow. In basic terms, the procedure for each is as follows:

On-hook

• The winch hook will be attached to the main harness karabiner while the team member remains secured in their seat. Once attached and checked by the winch operator, the team member can come out of their seat and proceed to the open cabin door. Ensure there is minimal slack in the winch cable to prevent a 'shock load' if the person attached falls unexpectedly.

Egress from cabin

• The winch operator will again check the team member's harness, attachment to the winch hook and security of any equipment planned to be winched down. They will then take up any winch cable slack to take the weight of the team member in the harness as they move out onto the aircraft skid or outer body. The team member will indicate that they are ready to be winched. The team member may need to fend off the skid or aircraft body, as they negotiate this movement, and they must attempt to ensure that the winch cable is plumb to the winch drum. The cable must be respected and cared for and not shock loaded or bent due to negligence.

Descent

• A brief stop under the aircraft to ensure correct winch functioning is common practice. This may be repeated at other points during descent and ascent (see 'Rare emergencies' over the page).

• The team member may need to fend off trees, etc., during the descent and will assist the winch operator by using standard hand signals to identify hazards or appropriate access points.

Grounding

• This can be hazardous as it is difficult to judge the landing site topography from the air. Look for shadows and orientation of trees. Hand signals should be used to communicate with the winch operator. The team member should never come off the winch hook until secure on the ground. Equipment is usually slung under the team member on descent. Be careful that this does not result in equipment damage or injury to on-scene persons. Once unhooked, continue maintaining control of the winch hook to prevent fouling until the hook has been recovered to the aircraft.

Patient and team egress

Packaging

Therapeutic patient packaging has been addressed in Case 8. Additional considerations here relate to movement of the patient, and securing into the rescue litter, patient head, eye and ear protection, and the need for explanation and reassurance for awake patients.

Before indicating 'ready to winch', both team members are to complete a challenge and response check using the following acronym **SPECTRE**:

- **S**tretcher assembled correctly
- **P**atient secured and briefed
- **E**quipment secure, i.e. monitors, IVs, etc.
- **C**arabiner gates closed and position checked
- **T**agline attendant ready
- **R**isk assessment complete and radio call to aircraft identifying patient weight, wind direction and hazards identified
- **E**nvironment concerns, i.e. tree branches, dust, lighting.

On-hook

- Both the PHRM team member with the patient and the rescue litter are required to be attached to the winch cable hook. It is critical that the winch cable is free of snares or entanglements during this time. Equipment not required for the patient should be left to come up in a separate winch wherever possible. When loading the hook, the attendant is always first on and last off. Hold the cable with both hands to maintain control of the cable slack at all times.
- The rescue crew person on the ground will attach a tag line to the foot end of the rescue stretcher. This will stop the stretcher and patient rotating on ascent.

Ascent

- Use hand signals indicating readiness to winch. The PHRM team member may need to fend off trees and other obstacles, the tagline operator may be able to assist by rotating the stretcher to avoid hazards. Expect a brief control stop under the aircraft to ensure there is time to isolate a runaway winch cable and also to negotiate the stretcher over the skids or the lower aircraft body and orientate the stretcher to slide into the cabin appropriately. The tag line will need to be released, either by the PHRM team member or winch operator.

Off-hook

- Once the stretcher is secured in the cabin and the PHRM team member is secured to the aircraft floor or back in a seat, the winch hook can be removed and stowed by the winch operator.

The rescue crew person responsible for the tag line on ascent will now be winched into the aircraft with any remaining equipment.

Discussion 49.4

Common problems

Rotor wash spin

- Team members suspended on the winch cable without tag-line stabilisation are prone to develop rotational movement. Holding arms and/or legs extended will slow rotation because of both reduced centrifugal force and increased air resistance.
- Pendulum movements may also be problematic, particularly in high-wind situations.

Winch harness pressure

- A poorly fitting harness can cause considerable discomfort when full body weight is suspended. This is particularly the case about the perineum. Care should be taken to ensure appropriate positioning of harness straps.

- In addition, if the winch cable is attached to the harness above the navel, vertical rotation about this point may lead to inversion.

Static electricity and earthing

- Airborne aircraft generate static electricity. The winch cable provides a conduit for earthing. When personnel receive the hook and cable while on the ground, a small 'electric shock' is not uncommon. A static-discharge pole may be used to prevent this or touch the hook with the back of the hand before grabbing the hook.

Avoidance of holding the winch hook

- Jamming of fingers around the winch hook and karabiner is a risk. When suspended on the winch cable, team members should avoid holding the hook/karabiner connection.

Rare emergencies (excluding aircraft emergencies)

HFIRES is an acronym commonly used to brief inflight and winching emergencies.

- **H**eight
- **F**ouling
- **I**ntercom failure
- **R**unaway winch
- **E**mergencies – Cable 'CUT CUT CUT' major and minor aircraft emergency actions
- **S**toppage

Winch failure

- Power failure: may occur at any time before or during the winch operation. If a team member is suspended, they may need to remain so while the aircraft repositions and places them onto the ground. If awaiting retrieval from the ground, the team may need to remain at the site or walk out for assistance.
- Jamming of winch cable: as per 'power failure' above.
- 'Run in': the braking mechanism on the drum of the winch may fail. Continuous winching in may ensue. This is a critical event as the winch cable, once fully winched in, will eventually be stretched to breaking point.
- 'Run out': the braking, drive or gearing mechanism may also fail resulting in uncontrolled winch-out. The winch operator will usually perform a stop at various points during the winch-out/winch-in process to ensure proper winch function in this regard.

Cable cutting

- The winch operator and the pilot have the ability to cut the winch cable at any time. A small explosive charge activates a cutting device located at the entrance of the winch cable into the drum housing. Catastrophic aircraft failure or cable snares threatening the aircraft are some examples of incidents requiring emergency winch cable cutting.

Quick-release mechanism

- A team member on the winch cable is also able to disconnect themselves in the event of an emergency. A quick-release device located between the harness and winch hook can be activated with one free hand.

Key points

- Helicopter winch rescue allows patient access, delivery of medical care and patient egress from areas where ground access is limited.
- Safe vertical rescue missions require a highly trained aviation and medical team.
- Medical personnel involved in such missions must have a clear understanding of the winch rescue process (including operational limitations and potential emergencies), their role and the roles of other team members.

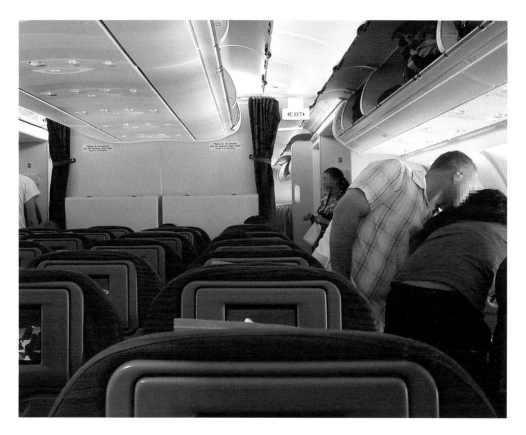

Incident

You are an 'off-duty' PHRM doctor travelling with your family on an international flight when you notice a commotion in the seat just ahead of you. Two passengers are attending to a fellow passenger.

Shortly afterwards, a request is made over the public announcement system for a doctor.

Question 50.1

What are the issues associated with offering assistance?

A 56-year-old gentleman in economy class is complaining of central chest pain. He has known ischaemic heart disease and has had a previous myocardial infarction. He is clammy and pale and has vomited once. The aircraft is 9 hours into a 13-hour flight.

Question 50.2

Describe your initial actions.

Question 50.3

What equipment can you expect to find on board?

Question 50.4

Describe your management plan and further course of action.

Discussion 50.1

Personal

Many doctors feel an obligation to offer assistance in such circumstances but, for most, there is no legal requirement to do so. However, it is widely accepted that physicians do have a humanitarian requirement to offer assistance in an emergency to the best of their ability. It is important that the doctor offers to help or is invited to help rather than simply 'taking over' the situation. As in all aeromedical situations, the pilot is in overall control of aircraft movements and safety.

Legal aspects

Offering assistance in such circumstances is infrequent and industry experts calculate that a doctor may encounter such an emergency only once or twice in a lifetime. In addition, they estimate that the chance of litigation is close to zero. However, this is a complex area and there is no guarantee of indemnity. Legal issues will also vary considerably from country to country. It is best to state at the outset that you are volunteering for this role and that, although you have pre-hospital experience, you do not have any of your equipment with you and that you will do your best for the patient considering the situation, the environment and the equipment.

Many major airlines have insurance policies which will indemnify doctors who come forward to assist in an emergency. If desired, doctors should seek written confirmation of indemnity from the aircraft captain. The US *Aviation Medical Assistance Act 1998* protects doctors who provide assistance on aircraft registered in the US.

Alcohol

Having taken an alcoholic beverage does not preclude the doctor from assisting. However, the doctor should take into consideration how much alcohol they have consumed and make this clear to the cabin crew and patient before becoming involved in patient care. In some jurisdictions immunity will not apply if your ability to perform is significantly impaired by the consumption of alcohol or drugs.

Other doctors

It is possible that other doctors are on the same flight, and it is worthwhile for the available clinicians to decide among themselves who is most appropriate to lead the care. Factors such as specialty, alcohol or drug consumption and fatigue should be considered. Other clinicians may be better placed to assist the lead clinician with specific roles or advice.

Discussion 50.2

ABC

A brief assessment of the patient's vital signs is required. It should be possible to assess the severity of the situation within a few minutes. Record your findings.

Crew communication

The cabin crew will be looking to you for a plan and you should voice clearly and concisely your concerns. Avoid medical jargon. The space constraints in economy class are marked and an immediate request to move the patient is appropriate. More space and an ability to lie the patient flat makes first or business class ideal, but there may be better 360-degree access in the galley area. However, it may be easier to move other passengers to make room rather than moving the patient. If there are other medical personnel (e.g. nurses or paramedics) on board then try to create the 'two-person team' with which you are familiar. Alternatively, utilise a member of the cabin crew. Ask for all the medical equipment to be brought to your location.

Discussion 50.3

There is a wide variation in medical equipment carried by passenger airlines. The Aerospace Medical Association has a regularly updated list offering guidance in this area. The box below shows the 2019 recommendations for this kit list. There is also a First Aid Kit listed which contains essential basic equipment (e.g. gloves, dressings, etc.).

Some aircraft have access to advanced monitoring devices, which can monitor heart rate, blood pressure, oxygen saturations and even 12-lead electrocardiograms. Certain monitors allow the information to be transmitted to a dedicated medical team on the ground (e.g. MedLink). Other aircraft will have an automatic external defibrillator (AED) device on board, which will allow cardiac monitoring and defibrillation.

Recommendations for kit list

Emergency Medical Kit (EMK)
The equipment contents of an aircraft emergency medical kit would typically include:

- Sphygmomanometer
- Stethoscope
- Airways, oropharyngeal (appropriate range of sizes)
- Supraglottic airway. (They serve the same function as the oropharyngeal airways, but in addition can be used to ventilate a patient, when necessary)
- Syringes (appropriate range of sizes)
- Needles (appropriate range of sizes)
- Intravenous catheters (appropriate range of sizes)
- System for delivering intravenous fluids
- Antiseptic wipes
- Venous tourniquet
- Sharp disposal box
- Gloves (disposable)
- Urinary catheter with sterile lubricating gel
- Sponge gauze
- Tape adhesive
- Surgical mask
- Emergency tracheal catheter (or large-gauge intravenous cannula)
- Umbilical cord clamp
- Thermometer (non-mercury)
- Torch (flashlight) and batteries

Recommendations for kit list—cont'd

- Bag-valve mask
- Basic life-support cards

The drug contents of an aircraft medical kit would typically include:

- Epinephrine 1:1000
- Epinephrine 1:10,000
- Antihistamine injectable and oral
- Anti-psychotic drug (e.g. haloperidol)
- Dextrose, 50% injectable, 50 mL (single-dose ampoule or equivalent)
- Nitroglycerin tablets or spray
- Mild to moderate analgesic/anti-pyretic
- Major analgesic, injectable or oral
- Anticonvulsant, injectable and oral
- Antiemetic, injectable and oral
- Bronchial dilator inhaler with spacer
- Atropine, injectable
- Adrenocortical steroid, injectable or similar oral absorption equivalent
- Diuretic, injectable
- Sodium Chloride 0.9% (1000 mL recommended)
- Acetyl salicylic acid (aspirin) for oral use
- Oral beta blocker
- Anti-diarrheal
- Opioid antagonist

Aerospace Medical Association, 2019

Discussion 50.4

Treatment

From the history and symptoms, acute coronary syndrome (ACS) is the most likely diagnosis but the list of differential diagnoses is extensive. The ability to perform a 12-lead electrocardiogram will be of diagnostic benefit in this regard. Supplemental oxygen is important in the aircraft cabin (see Case 27 and Case 53). There is a limited supply of oxygen on the aircraft and low-flow oxygen should be used if possible to preserve supplies. Oxygen delivery should be titrated to oxygen saturations if available. Other treatments should follow in-hospital emergency guidance for ACS and include aspirin, glyceryl trinitrate and analgesia. Do not forget to discuss treatment with the pilot, the crew, the patient and his relatives (if present).

Advanced communication

Continued discussions with the cabin crew are essential throughout the incident. At some point, the doctor should speak directly to the pilot or first officer and it is likely one of them will already have approached the doctor. The pilot and the doctor should broach the subject of the aircraft diverting and what options are available. The final decision on diverting lies with the captain but he/she may rely heavily on the medical report. Note also that diverting may not be in the patient's best interest depending on the current location of the aircraft. It will be of greater benefit to the patient to have initial treatment in flight and arrive a few hours later in a country with advanced healthcare facilities than to be diverted urgently to a country with a less robust healthcare system and then left there. There are also cost and safety issues that will arise with diverting, and the decision requires thought and discussion.

The airline may have access to a telemedicine arrangement (including the telemetry- enabled monitors as described earlier) in which case the treating doctor will have the ability to discuss the case with a ground-based medical team. If available, this should be utilised not only as a valuable second opinion but also as an additional layer of medico-legal protection. This facility will also be of help with decisions regarding the need to divert the aircraft.

Documentation

The doctor should keep contemporaneous notes of the incident, particularly of key medical decisions. This is useful in the unlikely event of medico-legal issues arising, but is also good practice.

Landing and handover

Most incidents on commercial aircraft do not require a change to the flight plan and it is likely the aircraft will continue to its destination. Unless there is complete resolution of the problem, the doctor should request to stay with the patient for the remainder of the flight. This is certainly the case in this scenario. Ensure that the pilot has radioed ahead to notify the receiving airport of the medical emergency. Request an appropriately staffed land ambulance to meet the aircraft, preferably on the tarmac. Unless the situation deteriorates significantly, try to allow the other passengers off the aircraft first and consider using a wheelchair to facilitate extrication (see Case 53). Do not leave the patient until he is handed over to the ground ambulance team. If time allows, try to provide a written summary of your actions for the land ambulance team as well as one for the captain.

Key points

- Doctors have an ethical duty to provide assistance in an emergency.
- When providing aid to a passenger during an in-flight emergency, medical practitioners are protected from liability by a combination of legislation, indemnity by the airline and their own professional indemnity.
- Airline medical equipment is variable, but monitoring and communication equipment is becoming increasingly sophisticated.
- Regular updating of the air crew is good CRM and will allow an unfamiliar group to function as a team.

Reference

Aerospace Medical Association. Air transport medicine guidance document 2019. Online. Available: https://www.asma.org/asma/media/AsMA/Travel-Publications/FAA-med-kit-Guidance-Document-June-2019.pdf.

Additional reading

Gulam H, Devereeux J. A brief primer on Good Samaritan law for health professionals. Aust. Health Rev. 2007; 31(3):478–482.

Martin T. Judging jurisdiction. Medical Protection Society United Kingdom Casebook 2008; 16(1):27.

Medical Board of Australia. Good medical practice: a code of conduct for doctors in Australia. Section 2.5. Online. Available: medicalboard.gov.au/Codes-Guidelines-Policies/Code-of-conduct.aspx.

Peterson DC, Martin-Gill C, Guyette FX et al. Outcomes of medical emergencies on commercial airline flights. N. Engl. J. Med. 2013; 368:2075–2083.

Thibeault C, Evans A. Air Transport Medicine Committee, Aerospace Medical Association. Emergency Medical kit for commercial airlines: an update. Aviat. Space Environ. Med. 2007; 78(12):1170–1171.

Tibballs J. Legal liabilities for assistance and lack of assistance rendered by Good Samaritans, volunteers and their organisations. ILJ 2005; 16:254–280.

Tonks A. Cabin fever. BMJ 2008; 336(7644):584–586.

Wallace WA. Managing in flight emergencies: a personal account. BMJ 1995; 311(7001): 374–376.

Williams S. Flying doctors: is protection plain? Medical Protection Society United Kingdom Casebook 2008; 16(1):8–11.

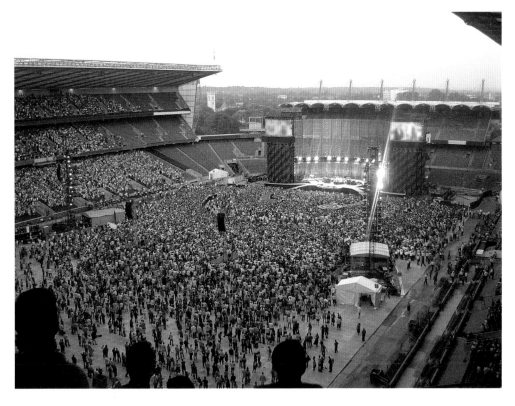

Incident

You have been asked to oversee medical and major incident cover at a music concert in a large capital city. The organisers expect 50,000 people to attend.

Question 51.1

How will you plan for the event? Present a broad outline for managing mass-gathering events, focusing on a venue such as that in the picture.

Question 51.2

What are your priorities on the day?

Discussion 51.1

For mass-gathering and event medicine, preparation and planning is key and should begin well before the event.

Safety

Safety is the number one priority, and most plans are put in place to protect the emergency services personnel as well as the crowd.

The venue

Accurate information about the venue is essential and, ideally, the clinician should visit the location in advance. Considerations that should be addressed include the following.

- Geographical location.
- Nearby hospitals and available medical specialties.
- Open-air or closed venue?
- Seated, standing or both?
- Access and egress to all locations within the venue.
- Access and egress to local hospitals and estimated timeframes.
- Local and national guidelines for stadiums and events.

The population

- There is a reasonable estimate of the number of persons attending based on ticket sales, but for free events, such as street parades, there is no accurate way of predicting attendance.
- The nature of the event will define certain aspects of the population attending. This event, being a music concert, suggests a young crowd with a high risk of alcohol and drug use. It is very likely that alcohol will be available in the venue, albeit with certain restrictions.

The medical team

- This is an event requiring several medical personnel and, as lead clinician, you must establish what medical personnel are available.
- National guidelines may dictate how many physicians are required at such an event, but there are rarely guidelines as to the training and experience of such doctors. In some situations, you may be the only doctor.
- The venue may have a medical centre, which can resemble a hospital or clinic, but the environment outside the medical centre will also need medical cover.
- The lead clinician must have experience in pre-hospital and retrieval, event medicine and major incident management. If other physicians are available, they should also ideally have experience in one or more of these fields. There will also be nurses, paramedics and volunteer first aiders available. A suggested approach is as follows:
  - The medical centre forms the nucleus of medical care for the venue and the plan should be that all seriously ill or injured patients should be taken there for advanced management. All retrievals to local hospitals should occur from this clinic, which should have rapid trolley access to outside the venue where ambulances are parked.
  - Satellite centres should be strategically positioned around the venue and should be staffed by a physician and nurse/paramedic team. Patients can either walk in to these locations or be brought in.
  - Mobile medical teams should move around the venue with equipment and a foldable stretcher. The team should comprise at least a nurse/paramedic, but should always include two persons as a minimum. Physicians can join the team to bring advanced skills and equipment if needed. It should be feasible

for a defibrillator, if required, to reach any part of the venue within 5 minutes. Most stadiums will have several defibrillators placed at various locations on-site which you should be aware of.

- Medical 'snatch' squads in high-risk areas are appropriate for certain events. At some music concerts, crowd surges towards the stage are common and people occasionally need extrication from the crowd at this point. Safety issues must be highlighted to the snatch teams.
- A full major incident plan has to be in place before the event, and major incident roles should be allocated and fully explained before the venue opens. Some personnel may have dual roles (i.e. treating of routine patients unless a major incident occurs), but be aware that medical personnel with dual roles run the risk of being drawn into prolonged patient care and, therefore, may be unable to respond rapidly in the event of a major incident. Certainly the lead clinician should avoid patient contact if at all possible.

Medical equipment will be available on-site, but a breakdown of the kit and its location should be studied in advance. There will always be limitations on available kit and efforts should be made to work with what is available. Remember this is unlikely to be the first event catered for at this location and other members of the team may be familiar with the kit. If you feel there is anything crucial missing, then it can be requested in advance from the organisers or brought as personal equipment.

Inter-service liaison

This is a multidisciplinary arrangement and will not be functional without close liaison between the emergency services:

- Overall, the Police are in command and the lead clinician should link up with the Police service commander and, likewise, with the Fire & Rescue Service commander. Both these services have responsibilities for public safety, and medical personnel must be aware of their plans. The Police and Fire & Rescue Service commander along with the local ambulance control and yourself, as the medical incident commander, would usually be co-located in a security room with the stadium security commander. This will act as either a gold or silver command room in the event of a major incident.
- Some mass-gathering venues have coded warnings to alert members of the emergency services to a potential major incident without generating panic in the crowd. Make sure you know these warnings, which will usually be broadcast over the public address system and will sound very benign (e.g. 'Will the stadium manager please report to Gate A' could be the coded warning for a credible bomb threat). It should be noted that large scale public events such as this have been targeted internationally by terrorist organisations.
- Local ambulance control should already be aware of the event and will have their own plans in place for hospital transfers and major incidents. These should conform to national guidelines. Speak to the Ambulance Service commander and run through medical evacuations, number of ambulances available and major incident roles. Make sure ambulance control have made plans with the Police for traffic flow in the event of an evacuation to hospital. This can be particularly difficult in the hours after the event when the roads are full of people exiting the venue. There should also be a plan for persons calling for an ambulance from inside the venue on mobile phones whereby details and location are forwarded to the mobile medical teams.

- Local voluntary organisations (e.g. the Red Cross) or paid medical companies are often the core providers of healthcare in mass-gathering events. Make sure that contact is made with the commander of these organisations early on. All plans, including major incident plans, should be discussed with this provider.

Discussion 51.2

Check weather reports a few days in advance as this will help with planning. Clothing should be practical but protective and you should receive appropriately labelled reflective tabards at the venue. Arrive early on the day and obtain your security pass.

Walk through as much of the location as possible, noting exits and choke points (e.g. the stairwells). Visit the control room (all venues will have a central command position) and introduce yourself to the people inside. There is likely to be an impressive array of closed-circuit television and this can help to generate a mental image of the location. In addition, these cameras can be the first to spot a casualty in the crowd and your mobile medical teams may be directed to the site by the camera operators.

Make sure local hospitals are aware of the event and the potential of extra work, especially after the event. Visit the medical centre, introduce yourself to the medical personnel and check the equipment. For large events, many of the above tasks should be done in the days prior to the event to maximise efficiency.

Communications at such events are usually excellent and each team should have a radio and a call sign as well as a back-up mobile phone. Run through radio etiquette before the event to make sure everyone is familiar with procedures. Stress the importance of describing a location accurately. Labelled miniature maps of the location utilising grid reference systems may be of help.

A briefing of all medical and voluntary services personnel should occur before any member of the public enters the venue and the chain of medical command must be highlighted. Medical staff must be aware of the importance of documenting all patient contacts and a standardised patient documentation form should be provided.

Finally, make sure medical staff are not distracted by the event itself or by the celebrity performers. Many performers provide their own medical cover (personal doctor, etc.) and this should be established early on. In the absence of personal medical cover for the performers, a specific 'backstage' team needs to be formulated. As lead clinician, do not disappear backstage as this will leave the remainder of the venue 'uncovered'.

After the event

Thank all the staff and emergency personnel whether they were busy or not.

Provide feedback to the organisers regarding things that went well during the day, as well as offering suggestions for improvement. A full written report, including a critical appraisal of the event is ideal. Offering to help at any future training events held at that and other locations will improve crew resource management.

Key points

- Careful planning in the days and hours before the event will improve clinical risk management.
- The lead clinician should not be involved in direct patient care.

Incident

During a regular pre-hospital and retrieval service clinical governance meeting, a number of recent incidents and events were discussed. Included were:

- The death soon after arrival at hospital of a young SCUBA diver retrieved following a diving emergency
- A 'near-miss' drug error that could have resulted in a potentially fatal dose of midazolam being given by one of the PHRM team to an 18-month-old child in status epilepticus
- A complaint from one of the helicopter air crew who found a blood-filled syringe and needle in a rear, side pocket of the aircraft
- A vital piece of equipment missing from one of the sealed equipment bags, causing a clinically significant change in the medical plan
- Repetitive equipment malfunction involving one of the monitors after it fell from a stretcher during a retrieval mission
- Ongoing delays in the response for time-critical, pre-hospital trauma tasks caused by 'communication failures' in the coordination centre
- A complaint from one of the receiving ICUs regarding both the clinical care given to a patient during retrieval and the behaviour of the PHRM team.

Question 52.1

What processes can be applied to both monitor and manage such incidents and events?

Question 52.2

How can the quality of clinical care and the safety of the service be improved?

Discussion 52.1

Modern PHRM services are expected to ensure that the right patient receives the right treatment in the right time and is then transported to the right destination via the right transport. There are subsequently a number of opportunities for adverse clinical and operational incidents to occur. These may vary both in terms of severity (potential or actual outcome) and frequency.

Incident monitoring and the management of incidents or adverse events is an important component of overall risk management. However, when compared with an in-hospital clinical unit, risk management and incident monitoring may be more challenging for a pre-hospital and retrieval service for the following reasons:

- The selected patient cohort is generally of high clinical acuity and complexity. Morbidity and mortality may, therefore, be high, regardless of any potentially avoidable incidents or events.
- The clinical environments are variable, complex and potentially dangerous to both patient and team.
- The clinical and logistical (e.g. aviation) components of the service must closely interact, and service delivery is unavoidably multidisciplinary.
- The delivery of clinical care frequently occurs across differing healthcare facilities, healthcare sectors, state boundaries and even national borders.
- The PHRM team often works in relative clinical isolation.

- The key stakeholders involved in service delivery are broad and may include clinical, political, financial and patient advocacy groups.

Key incident and event monitoring and management tools include the following:

- Incident and adverse event reporting. This incorporates activities such as:
  - Learning from incidents or patterns of incidents occurring regionally and in other jurisdictions
  - Reviewing both aviation and medical 'near misses' (also referred to as 'near hits')
  - Managing serious adverse events
  - Maintaining a contemporaneous risk register
  - Monitoring aviation events or medico-legal cases
- Sentinel event reporting (see below), including:
  - Defining relevant events to be classified as 'sentinel'
  - Monitoring, investigating and reporting of such events.
- Risk–profile analysis, including:
  - Identification, investigation, analysis and evaluation of clinical risks
  - Risk stratification in terms of both severity and predicted frequency
  - Selection of the most appropriate method of correcting, eliminating or reducing identifiable risks.

A sentinel event may be defined as a reportable incident that potentially or actually caused serious harm. While regionally variable, an example for a PHRM service may be the death of a patient while in the care of the PHRM team. Sentinel events may signal serious breakdowns in healthcare systems. They therefore require immediate investigation and response. The investigation process for a sentinel event should identify root causes and contributing factors so that strategies can be implemented to minimise the occurrence of similar events in the future. Root cause analysis (RCA) is one method of investigating sentinel events. RCA is a comprehensive and systematic methodology conducted by relevant multidisciplinary teams to identify the gaps in a system and the systemic processes that may not be immediately apparent and that contributed to an event occurring. The RCA team will recognise that most errors are made by competent, careful and caring providers of clinical care and that preventing such errors (thereby reducing the severity and frequency of incidents and events) involves embedding the providers in a robust system and a 'culture of safety'.

An RCA will:

- Ask what happened, why it happened and what can be done to prevent it happening again
- Focus on the system as a whole rather than on an individual performance
- Look closely for underlying contributing factors and root causes
- Identify changes that could be made to improve systems and processes to prevent similar events recurring
- Provide recommendations regarding safer, more-efficient ways to provide clinical and operational service delivery.

Discussion 52.2

Quality of care is a multifaceted concept, which can be defined in different ways. In broad terms, quality reflects the extent to which a healthcare service produces a desired outcome. The components of quality include safety, effectiveness, patient-centeredness, timeliness, efficiency and equitability. Of note, safety and the reduction of risk is, in fact, a component of quality. However, safety may be more difficult to measure as monitoring of incidents and events (as detailed above) often requires voluntary reporting.

Clinical governance is a term used to describe processes, activities, systems and tools applied to clinical service delivery with the expressed aim of improving the quality of service and, ultimately, patient outcome. Clinical governance provides the framework for both the measurement and improvement of service quality. There is no single 'tool' that provides complete measurement and improvement of quality. Examples of available tools are detailed below.

Tools to measure quality

Measures of service structure
- How is service delivery organised (e.g. funding models, corporate governance arrangements, numbers of senior staff available, interagency relationships, etc.)?

Measures of operational service performance or process
- Usually measured against accepted key performance indicators (KPIs) and service standard operating procedures (SOP) (e.g. response times, scene times, performance of critical interventions, etc.).

Measures of clinical outcome
- Follow-up of patient outcomes and analysis of actual versus predicted (based on severity of injury or illness) clinical course.

Measures of complaints and praise
Measures of adverse incidents and events (as detailed above)

Tools to improve quality

Human factor tools
- Team briefs and time outs
- Challenge and response checklists
- Sharing mental models
- Leadership behaviours
- Communication and handover

Clinical audit
- May include week-to-week (all tasks), month-to-month (selected clinical tasks), quarterly, biannual and annual (service activity reporting) processes.
- Regular (e.g. weekly) morbidity and mortality meetings are an excellent forum for identifying and following up areas amenable to audit.
- May involve more in-depth review of a series of cases in a multidisciplinary, longitudinal forum less frequently.
- Should cover documentation and data recording on a regular basis. This includes base documentation as well as patient documentation. Checks of the medical equipment, stock and transport platform should be in 'tick box' format and should be done and signed off as a two-person exercise (e.g. challenge and response).
- Should drive service training and teaching requirements so as to provide a 'closed- loop' process of quality improvement.
- Should aim to develop and enhance the service 'culture'.

Advisory groups
- Multirepresentative of relevant clinical and non-clinical disciplines (e.g. emergency medicine, ICU, anaesthetics, Ambulance Service, aviation personnel, patient representatives, etc.).

Clinical practice improvement projects
- Variations on the 'Plan-Do-Study-Act' (PDSA) project cycle.

Service SOP development and regular review
- Clinical advisory group input is recommended.

Research and evidence-based review
- Good research requires relevant and accurate data collection.
- Non-clinical time should be protected for staff to develop and complete research projects.
- Service staff should have access to relevant clinical journals, and regular journal review meetings are encouraged.

Teaching and training
- Programs should be driven by the outcomes of clinical governance processes.
- Need to reflect the multidisciplinary nature of service delivery.
- Ideally standardised and embedded in postgraduate educational institutions.

Key points

- Providing a high-performing, safe, efficient and outcome-driven service is challenging.
- Clinical governance tools provide a framework for both the measurement and improvement of service quality and safety.
- Services should aim to explore systems issues in a culture of operational and clinical safety, mutual support and continuous learning.

Additional reading

Association of Air Ambulances. A framework for a high performing air ambulance service. Online. Available: http://aaaframework.co.uk/. 2013.

Australian Commission on Safety and Quality in Health Care. Patient safety and quality systems. Online. Available: www.safetyandquality.gov.au/standards/nsqhs-standards/clinical-governance-standard/patient-safety-and-quality-systems.

Gawande A. The checklist manifesto: how to get things right. Picador, 2010.

Hearns S. Peak performance under pressure: lessons from a helicopter rescue doctor. Jones & Bartlett Learning, 2019.

Wachter RM. Understanding patient safety, 3rd ed. McGraw Hill, 2017.

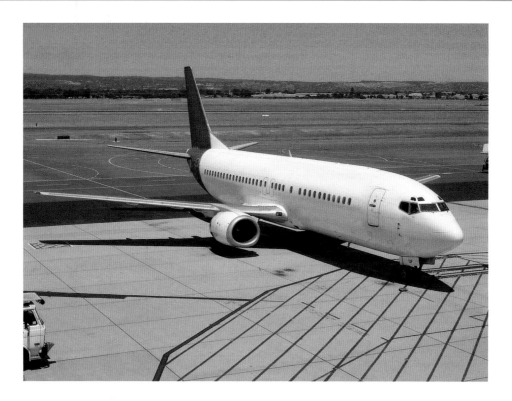

Incident

A 67-year-old male developed chest pain while on holiday in Bali. He was diagnosed with an anterior myocardial infarction and thrombolysed at the local hospital. He is now 6 days post-infarction and has been discharged that day from hospital. He is an Australian citizen who now needs repatriation. You have been asked to be a medical escort for the patient, who is currently in a local hotel.

Medications:
- Aspirin.
- Clopidogrel.
- β-blocker.
- Angiotensin-converting enzyme inhibitor.

Shortly after arrival, you locate the patient who is ambulant and looks very well.

Clinical information

- P 52.
- BP 110/60 mmHg.
- SaO_2 95% on air.

Physical examination reveals sparse bibasal crepitations and a soft ejection systolic murmur.

Relevant information

- **Aircraft:** Commercial jet airliner (as per picture). Return flight (5 hours' duration) is booked for the next day.

■ **Resources:** Travelling as a solo physician, no other team members. Extensive, portable medical kit including drugs, monitor and defibrillator.

■ **Transporting to:** Patient's home address in Australia.

Question 53.1

Is the patient safe to fly commercially? Give a balanced argument.

Question 53.2

Describe, in detail, your plan for the journey home from start to finish.

Question 53.3

After boarding, a member of the cabin crew tells you the supplementary oxygen cylinder has been 'delayed' and asks if you are happy to travel without it. Are you?

Discussion 53.1

Most medical repatriations are done through insurance companies and most of the paperwork and initial telephone assessment will have been done by experienced company staff (usually nurses with physician input). The role of the doctor 'on-scene' is to assess the patient clinically and ensure the information given to the insurance company is accurate. For this reason, the doctor is often flown out the day before the scheduled return. It is unusual to find that the patient is clinically worse than expected.

There is clinical risk involved in the transfer of such patients and, for this reason, a physician escort has been arranged. Options are limited (see box below) and a careful risk–benefit analysis is required. A dedicated air ambulance may be the lowest risk for transfer but resource allocation and cost make this a poor choice under these circumstances.

Transfer options (with increasing illness severity)
Patient travels alone commercially.
Patient travels with nurse escort commercially.
Patient travels with physician escort commercially.
Patient travels with doctor and nurse on a commercial flight with special arrangements (e.g. rear of cabin converted to carry stretcher).
Patient travels with doctor and/or nurse on an air ambulance.

On the evidence available, this patient seems safe to fly commercially with a physician escort. Consider delaying or cancelling the transfer if you find that the patient is not as has been described.

Discussion 53.2

Patient contact

● Meet the patient at the hotel, allowing enough time to examine the patient again and to arrive at the airport over three hours prior to your departure.

● Record a set of observations and ensure the patient is pain free.

● Travel to the airport in a comfortable, pre-booked taxi.

Extra checks

- Contact the company for whom you are working and check the following.
  - Flight is on schedule and expecting a medical passenger.
  - A wheelchair has been requested at the airport.
  - Supplementary oxygen has been ordered for the flight.
  - Any transfers or meeting arrangements at the destination are confirmed.

Arrival at the airport

- Contact a representative of the airline and collect the wheelchair. In order to avoid excessive fatigue and potential exacerbation of the underlying illness, the wheelchairs should always be requested and utilised. In addition, a wheelchair should allow priority at check-in, customs, passport control and during boarding.
- Check with the airline representative that supplemental oxygen is available on your flight.

Check-in

- All the medical kit in your possession is for an emergency and should not be stored in the aircraft hold. You may have to compromise and allow sharp items and defibrillators to be stored in the cockpit until required. As in all aeromedical situations, the pilot has the final say and can refuse to fly you. Note also that this medical repatriation has been arranged in advance and you should contact the company for whom you are working if a balanced solution cannot be found. However, you should not fly the patient without access to your kit, as an avoidable medical deterioration would be hard to justify.
- Ensure that you and your patient are in business class or have extra empty seats next to you and that you have airport lounge access. Wait in the lounge until boarding is called.

Boarding

- The two options are either to board with everyone else, taking the wheelchair to the main door of the aircraft, or via a hydraulic platform on the other side of the aircraft. Either way, the patient should be one of the first to board.
- Introduce yourself and the patient to the cabin crew, tell them you are a doctor and explain to them what kit you have. Request the supplemental oxygen as soon as you board.
- Bear in mind that you may be required to provide medical assistance to other passengers in the event of an emergency.

During flight

- Take a set of observations, including saturations, while in the aircraft cabin prior to take-off. Set up the oxygen (usually via nasal prongs) and start at a low-flow just prior to take-off.
- Avoid alcohol and ensure you have managed your fatigue proactively.
- Make sure the patient takes medications that are due during the flight.
- Observations should be repeated at appropriate intervals. The absolute minimum for observations should be at take-off, peak altitude and landing.

Arrival

- Wait for everyone else to leave the aircraft and make sure a wheelchair is available for your use outside the aircraft door. The hydraulic platform option, if required, should be arranged with the cabin crew during the flight.
- Consider the patient's destination. Having come from a hotel, it is likely that he is suitable to go to his home, especially if relatives are already there. If you are not happy for him to go home, you will need to arrange a suitable hospital bed via the company arranging the repatriation. As a minimum, the patient should consult his family doctor in the next day or so.
- Travel with the patient to his house and escort him inside. Perform one final set of observations and ensure all documentation and notes are completed. Leave a brief summary letter with the patient for his family doctor.
- Notify the insurance company of your arrival and patient handover.

Discussion 53.3

Occasionally, the pre-requested oxygen is sent to the destination on a different flight. Any delays to this flight may result in the oxygen being unavailable. Unfortunately, there are no alternatives and you cannot use the aircraft 'emergency' oxygen. On a commercial airliner at peak altitude, the cabin pressure will be around 6000–8000 feet (1800–2500 metres) and oxygen saturations in a healthy adult will be around 94% (see Case 27). This patient started with saturations of 95% and these will probably drop to around 90% in flight. This level of hypoxia for a prolonged period may compromise patient recovery, and flying the patient should be delayed until oxygen is available. Contacting the insurance company may allow other sources of oxygen to be sought in time for the flight.

Key points

- Certain patients are appropriate for commercial flights with a suitable escort.
- Careful planning and preparation for the journey will reduce the chance of unexpected in-flight problems.
- Supplemental oxygen is recommended in the commercial aircraft cabin.

Additional reading

Aerospace Medical Association. "https://protect-au.mimecast.com/s/ZuuMCROAGQimKkY PI9V5Un?domain=asma.org" http://www.asma.org/publications/medical-publications-for-airline-travel/medical-considerations-for-airline-travel

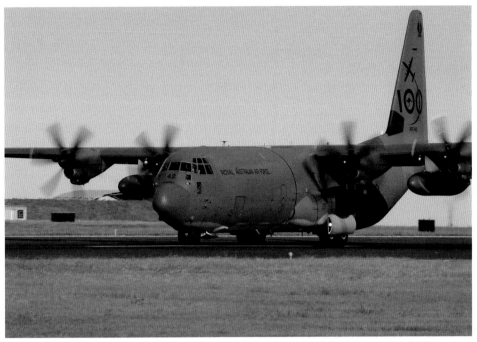

Image 1 With kind permission from Department of Defence - Australia.

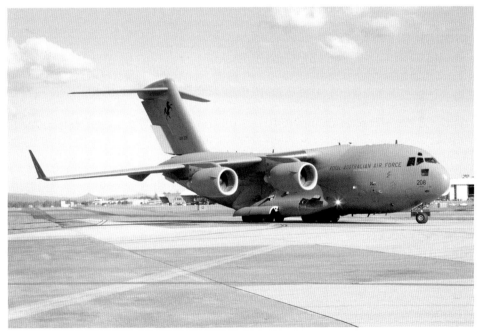

Image 2 With kind permission from Department of Defence - Australia.

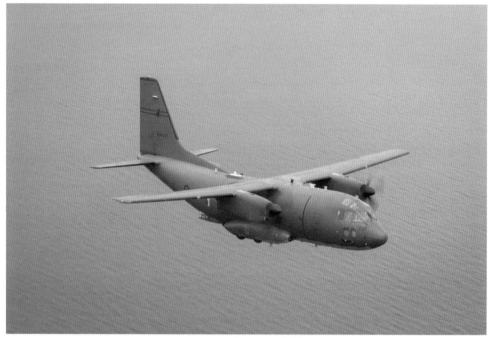

Image 3 With kind permission from Department of Defence - Australia.

Incident

Following battlefield care and forward air medical evacuation (AME) to a surgical facility, a number of service personnel involved in an overseas conflict now require transfer from the military theatre of operations to their home country for ongoing care – a distance of 8200 km (5095 miles).

As the AME officer-in-charge (OIC) of this operation, you are provided a patient manifest, which includes three soldiers from an anti-personnel device explosion and a number of other ill and injured military personnel. In total, there are two very seriously ill (VSI) patients who are mechanically ventilated. One has an open abdomen and the other has undergone craniotomy and clot evacuation. A further 15 patients are immobile and stretcher-bound and 10 are ambulatory. No non-medical personnel (other than the air crew and patients) or equipment are planned to be transported.

Relevant information

- **Aircraft:** As pictured on the previous page.
- **Local resources:** Military land ambulance (capable of dual patient carriage). Multiple AME teams (medical officer, nursing officer and medic), including 2 critical care AME teams (critical care medical officer and nursing officer).
- **Retrieval options:** Civilian ICU and large military hospital.
- **Other:** Nil.

Question 54.1

Outline the various categories of military AME. Into which category does this mission fit?

Question 54.2

In general terms, what is the role of the OIC in this mission?

Question 54.3

How will the composition and number of AME teams be decided?

Question 54.4

Compare and contrast the three aircraft pictured above. Which would be utilised for this mission and why?

Discussion 54.1

Forward AME

The evacuation of casualties from point-of-injury within the battlefield to a forward medical facility for initial assessment, resuscitation and stabilisation.

Tactical AME

The movement of patients between medical facilities within an area of military operations.

Strategic AME

The movement of patients from an area of military operations to a non-operational area.
Military AME is further defined into three specific categories.
- Opportunity AME: the movement of patient/s on a non-AME dedicated aircraft.
- Special AME: an AME which is conducted on an aircraft that has been dedicated to that mission.
- Scheduled AME: the regular performance of AME missions (occurs particularly when demand is high).

This particular task would fall into the 'special AME' category and classed as a strategic mission.
Patient movement priority should also be defined for each category of AME:
- Urgent – (priority 1): immediate threat to life, limb, sight.
- Priority – (priority 2): serious threat to life or limb.
- Routine – (priority 3): patient transported when appropriate transport option available.

Discussion 54.2

The OIC AME has overall command and control for the conduct of the mission, noting the pilot-in-command controls the entire mission and aircraft. The OIC AME oversees and coordinates clinical and logistic aspects and ensures that the aircraft is configured, staffed, equipped and prepared to accommodate the requirements of all patients and attending AME team members. Effective communication, clinical and logistic organisation and leadership are key requirements for this role. The OIC AME may not be the medical or nursing officer with the most medical or AME experience or with the highest rank. The OIC does not become directly involved in patient care, but can provide advice as required.

A non-exhaustive list of OIC AME roles may include the following.

Communication

- With air crew (particularly load master) and aircraft captain.
  - Flight plan, originating medical facility (OMF), in-transit medical facility (IMF) and destination medical facility (DMF).
  - Refuelling requirements (e.g. will the patients need to be unloaded during refuelling?).
  - Weather.
  - Other cargo/passengers.
  - Any anticipated clinical or aviation problems.
- Regular communication with the mission coordination centre with specific regard to clinical issues, transport waypoints and mission progress (estimated time of departure/arrival).
- With AME team members.
  - Determine patient and AME team requirements.
  - Complete all necessary paperwork.
  - Mission report.
  - Equipment manifest, etc.

Clinical and logistical organisation

- Allocate AME team positions and duties.
- Clarify patient numbers and classifications.
- Allocate patient loading positions on aircraft.
- Facilitate AME team and patient requirements:
  - Land transport.
  - Medical equipment.
  - Oxygen requirements.
  - Cabin pressure.
  - Comfort (e.g. on-board toilets and food for AME team and patients).

Leadership

- Assumes responsibility for AME team and patient safety.
  - Checks PPE.
  - Oversees enplaning/deplaning and patient loading with load master.
  - Ensures management of AME team fatigue.
- Gives briefs to AME team.
  - Mission profile and plan and post-mission debrief.
  - Aircraft safety.
  - Predicted problems.
- Addresses medical implications of unexpected challenges.
  - Changes to patient requirements or numbers.
  - Unexpected stopovers.
  - AME team welfare, illness or injury.

Discussion 54.3

The composition and number of AME teams will depend on patient load, patient classification (see below), duration of mission and anticipated in-flight care requirements.

Generally, patients are classified into passenger (no predicted medical requirement), ambulatory (may need assistance during the flight or with aircraft egress) and 'litter' or stretcher (may be immobile or mobile with assistance). Psychiatric patients commonly receive a separate classification. Few psychiatric patients should require a litter, and those at high risk must have adequate AME team members allocated should intervention be required.

As above, patients will also be classified by movement priority.

Seriously ill (SI) and VSI patients usually require a specialist AME team, dependent on the level of care required. Each military organisation will have a different approach with variations of a standard AME team able to provide critical care in the military aeromedical environment. Critical care teams are added to augment strategic AME teams when SI or VSI patients require transport. Each team usually consists of a medical officer and nursing officer, both with critical care specialist skills with the ability to care for 1–2 patients per team (level of care dependent). The team will also be used, where able, to assist with the general AME mission, particularly if patients deteriorate unexpectedly in flight. The critical care team usually will elect an OIC for its team. The OIC AME and the critical care OIC must liaise closely at all times.

Total patient numbers will be limited by aircraft load capacity, which may vary at short notice if the movement of non-medical military equipment and personnel take precedence over the AME mission.

Discussion 54.4

Image 1 shows a Lockheed Martin C-130J Super Hercules. The Hercules has the longest continuous production run of any military aircraft in history. It is a partially pressurised and air-conditioned military transport aircraft with short take-off and landing (STOL) characteristics. It is designed for the carriage of personnel and cargo, dropping supplies or personnel by parachute, and AME. It continues operations with a large number of military services worldwide. During more than 50 years of service, these aircraft have proved to be very capable in innumerable military, civilian and humanitarian aid operations, including AME missions.

Image 2 shows a Boeing C-17 Globemaster III. The C-17 is currently operated by the United States Air Force, the British Royal Air Force, the Royal Australian Air Force and the Canadian Forces to provide rapid strategic airlift of personnel and cargo. It also provides an AME platform with global standardisation of medical equipment across all services. The C-17 also has STOL (3500 feet, 1065 m characteristics and is designed to operate from runways as short as 1000 m (3280 feet) and as narrow as 27 m (90 feet). In addition, the C-17 can operate out of austere environments and unsealed surface landing strips. The thrust reversers can be used to reverse the aircraft, change direction and perform a multipoint turn.

Image 3 shows an Alenia C-27J Spartan Battlefield Airlifter. The C-27J is the most recent addition to the Royal Australian Air Force medium–heavy-lift aircraft fleet and is also available in other countries. It is able to access more runways (sealed and unsealed), combining its STOL (when applying full reverse thrust on landing, it can stop in 300–450 m) characteristics and its weight, speed and range. It provides an effective multi-mission profile that can be configured to support personnel, air-drop, cargo and AME operations. The C-27 can operate in the forward, non-permissive environment due to its suite of defensive systems and battlefield armour

Comparison of C-130J, C-17 and C-27J aircraft

Characteristic	C-130J (Hercules)	C-17 (Globemaster)	C-27 J (Spartan)
Air crew	3 to 6	3	3
Capacity	Potential for 94 litters	36 litters	21 litters
AME implications	• Relatively poor lighting • Relatively limited cabin climate control • High noise (difficult in-flight communications without internal communication system [ICS]) • Variable medical equipment and ability to secure the equipment across services • No instrinsic therapeutic oxygen supply – must be brought on-board • Cabin pressurisation to 5000 feet (1500 m) at 28,000 feet (8500 m) • Low level of comfort for AME team and passengers on long missions	• Excellent lighting • Excellent cabin climate control • Medium noise (easier in-flight communications without ICS) • International standardised medical equipment and equipment bridge across services • Intrinsic therapeutic oxygen (maximum 60,300 L, including liquid oxygen) • Sea-level cabin pressure available • High level of comfort for AME team and passengers (comfort pallet on long missions)	• Relatively poor lighting • Relatively limited cabin climate control • High noise (difficult in-flight communications without ICS) • Variable medical equipment and ability to secure the equipment across services • No instrinsic therapeutic oxygen supply • Cabin pressurisation to 5170 feet (1570 m) at 30,000 feet (9140 m) • Low level of comfort for AME team and passengers on long missions – single airliner toilet on-board

Continued

Comparison of C-130J, C-17 and C-27J aircraft—cont'd			
Characteristic	C-130J (Hercules)	C-17 (Globemaster)	C-27 J (Spartan)
Payload	19,090 kg (42,000 lb)	77,519 kg (170,900 lb)	11,600 kg (25,574 lb)
Loading	Rear ramp (narrow)	Rear ramp (broad)	Rear ramp (narrow)
Engines	Turbo-prop	Jet	Turbo-prop
Cruising speed	643 km/h (400 mph)	830 km/h (515 mph)	602 km/h (374 mph)
Range	3313 km (2059 miles)	Unlimited with in-flight refuelling	1700 km 1056 miles
Availability for AME	High level of availability	High non-AME military demand	High level of availability
Cost (purchase)	2 units	8 units	1 unit

The choice for this mission, if available, would be the C-17 due to:
- Length of mission versus range of aircraft
- Demands of VSI patients
  - 360-degree access to patient.
  - Less noise (team communication easier).
  - Better lighting (can be tactical/night vision as needed).
  - Better climate control.
  - Easier loading and unloading.
  - Cabin pressurisation is likely to be required.
  - Oxygen requirements versus oxygen availability.
  - Avoidance of refuel stops.
  - Better endurance and reach.
  - Faster: so less time in transport environment.
- Comfort requirements for AME team and ambulatory patients (toilets, etc.).

Key points
• Modern military strategic AME provides significant long-distance air medical transport capacity for large numbers of patients. • The concepts applicable to civilian retrieval and AME are equally applicable to the military environment.

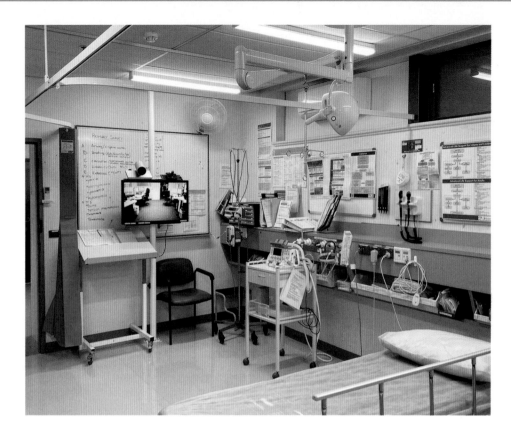

Incident

A case is discussed at the PHRM service clinical case review meeting. A 50-year-old female was involved in a house fire at 2 a.m. and was taken to the local rural hospital, 250 km away from the nearest major trauma and burns centre. The patient had a reduced conscious state with a swollen face, hoarse voice and carbonaceous sputum along with severe partial- and full-thickness burns to the chest and abdomen.

The attending local doctor and nurse had inserted a supraglottic airway device and two intravenous cannulas through which they had given some intravenous analgesia and fluid. The doctor had contacted the PHRM service medical coordinator via the tasking agency requesting a retrieval team to transfer the patient. The medical coordinator had used telemedicine to lead the trauma resuscitation and guide the PHRM team through a fibre-optic airway exchange from a supraglottic airway device to a tracheal tube. An example of the environment in which this telemedicine consult occurred is shown in the image above.

Following the case review, it is decided that this case will be used as the basis for a teaching and training simulation scenario. You are tasked with writing the scenario, with the aim of training PHRM clinicians how to use telemedicine to manage a remote resuscitation. The emphasis should be on clinical coordination, communication and teamwork.

Relevant information

- **PHRM team transport options:** Fixed-wing aircraft.
- **Additional resources:** One road ambulance and crew. Local GP and nurse

- **Retrieval options:** Major trauma and burns centre 250 km away and a 90-minute fixed-wing flight
- **Other:** 2 a.m., dedicated additional pack for difficult airways containing fibre-optic scope and monitor available (see Case 29).

Question 55.1

What are the steps required to write and prepare a simulation scenario?

Question 55.2

How would you ensure that all clinicians in the service have undertaken the simulation and achieved the outcomes set?

Question 55.3

How would you ensure that a clinician's competencies are maintained?

Discussion 55.1

Developing a successful simulation scenario can take a significant amount of time and preparation. The scenario needs to be valid (i.e. based on a pre-hospital and retrieval curriculum) and reliable (i.e. it is easily reproducible, by different personnel, to achieve the same learning outcomes).

1. Identify no more than three to four key learning objectives. Using this case, the key learning objectives could be:
   - Proficient use of the telemedicine system
   - Appropriate burns management
   - Demonstration of a good standard of communication, leadership and teamwork (non-technical skills).

     The number of key learning outcomes may also depend on the time available to run the scenario – generally, the shorter the scenario running time, the fewer learning objectives can realistically be achieved.
2. Create a checklist of benchmark or Gold Standard *behaviours and actions* for each learning objective. These need to be objectively measurable; for example:
   - **Objective**: *Proficient use of the telemedicine equipment*. The **performance criteria** may include:
     - Demonstrates ability to dial referring hospitals' telemedicine unit.
     - Demonstrates ability to adjust and manipulate the camera(s) to gain the best viewpoint to perform a history and assessment of the patient.
   - **Objective:** *Appropriate burns management*. The **performance criteria** may include:
     - Demonstrates comprehensive history taking of how/where/when burn injury occurred.
     - Demonstrates appropriate A→E assessment of patient or requests this history from the attending staff.
     - Suggests treatments and interventions consistent with local burns management guidelines, in a timely and well prioritised manner.

- **Objective:** Demonstration of a good standard of communication, leadership and teamwork (non-technical skills) in a high cognitive load environment. **Performance criteria** may include:
  - Introduces themselves (and the PHRM clinical coordination team, if applicable) to the local team.
  - Provides reassurance that a retrieval team has been tasked, and their estimated time of arrival (ETA).
  - Requests information to obtain the history of the burn injury (as described above).
  - Encourages input from team members, both at the referring end and in the coordination centre.
  - Demonstrates ability to share the mental model.
  - Demonstrates closed-loop communication techniques.
  - Demonstrates ability to summarise and update the team.
  - Demonstrates effective conflict-resolution techniques.
  - Demonstrates effective graded assertiveness techniques.
  - Demonstrates supportive guidance to the retrieval team to use the fibre-optic videoscope to exchange the laryngeal mask airway (LMA) for a tracheal tube.

    The essential minimum performance criteria required to demonstrate competency must be clearly defined as distinct from non-essential but important additional criteria.

    When writing the performance criteria, use words like 'describes, demonstrates, checks, confirms, explains, outlines, listens, addresses, shares'.

3. Choosing a vignette. Successful simulations tend to be based on real-life cases. Use vignettes to form the basis of the scenario and make necessary alterations that allow the participant the potential to achieve the desired goal.

4. Instructions and scripts: There are numerous scenario templates available. To allow multiple assessors to run the same scenario while following a predetermined timeline, there needs to be sufficient but concise written information available.

5. It is often easier to have one assessor running the scenario and another writing notes for the debrief and/or 'marking off' the performance criteria/assessment framework. The scenario template needs to outline the key learning objectives and provide details of the case.

6. The scenario template should list the human and equipment resources necessary to run the scenario. Any 'props' required should be detailed – high-quality images, test results, simulation equipment, training kits, manikins, telemedicine units. When the scenario stipulates five personnel are required, it should outline the role of each person including any consistent verbal script.

7. The time required for the scenario and debrief to occur should be clearly highlighted.

8. Identification of any specific location to conduct the simulation is important. For this particular scenario, it is necessary to use two separate areas – one to simulate the 'rural hospital' and one to simulate the location of the PHRM team clinical coordinator with access to the telemedicine system.

The simulation can be as simple or complex as required. The priority is to design a simulation that will assess the criteria against which the participant is to be assessed.

Simulation is an excellent modality to test the human-factor skills needed by a high-performing PHRM team.

Where specific skills are required for a clinical scenario, these may be better taught and assessed utilising a focused skill station. Skill stations encourage the development of muscle memory and 'drill' the skills necessary, particularly for low-frequency, high-consequence procedures. Frequent exposure to a focused skill station allows the skill to become 'second nature' to the operator, which, when put into the context of common PHRM challenges in a high cognitive load environment, allows the clinician the bandwidth to manage the overall situation, while avoiding task fixation. In this case, it would be ideal to set up a 'difficult airway' skill station to familiarise clinicians with the use of the fibre-optic scope to exchange the LMA for a TT. Affording all staff ample opportunity to 'drill this skill' prior to their participation in the simulation scenario, allows clinicians to refine their procedural skill set prior to application of the skill (or, in this case, guiding another clinician through the procedure) within the context of the scenario (see Cases 45 and 48).

Avoid any participant ambiguity by clearly stating in the instructions what the assessed criteria are and what is expected of them.

Discussion 55.2

Many PHRM services appoint a senior clinician to lead and oversee training and education. This person will be responsible for ensuring all staff members are adequately trained, and, ideally, they will form part of a multidisciplinary training and education team.

Ensuring that all staff are afforded the opportunity to participate in both the skill station, and then the simulation scenario, will require dedicated time. The timeframe will be roster dependent and needs to allow for part-time staff, roster patterns (week-on, week-off), leave and busy (mission) periods.

The skill station should be the priority, while the scenario is being developed. Once staff have had the opportunity to attend the skill station to 'drill the skill', the simulation should be set up and ready to be used on a daily basis. A method to track clinicians who have completed the skill station and the scenario should be developed prior to either being made available. A service-wide communique highlighting this opportunity should be sent, outlining the expectation of the education and training team that all clinicians undertake; firstly, the skill station, followed by the simulation scenario. It will be necessary to name the clinicians that are recognised assessors, so staff realise who they can approach to run the simulation scenario. The availability of the skill drill station and the simulation scenario should be reinforced at the PHRM service team brief (see Case 48).

Discussion 55.3

Assessment of competence is essential for patient safety but is also necessary to ensure the PHRM service can demonstrate good governance and accountability for its staff. A PHRM service needs to firstly determine what systems/procedures/equipment are to be measured and secondly, determine the timeframe of the competency expiry. Utilising an electronic system to enter assessment documents and dates of assessment and expiry allows the education and training team and the management team visibility of currency for all staff. The same system could be used/set up to track competency sign-off against the scope of clinical practice elements. This system can be used to guide the PHRM service's month-to-month, or bi-annual, teaching and training requirements.

Key points

- Educational frameworks in PHRM should follow standard adult education principles, e.g. acquisition of knowledge and skills, practice of skills ('drill the skill') and translation to clinician practice (scenario training).
- Assessment and recording of competence and audit of PHRM educational activities is core to good PHRM clinical governance.

Incident

A tropical storm (typhoon) has made landfall in the Pacific causing catastrophic damage, significant loss of life and making hundreds of thousands of people homeless. Members of the local PHRM team have been activated as part of the national disaster medical assistance response team.

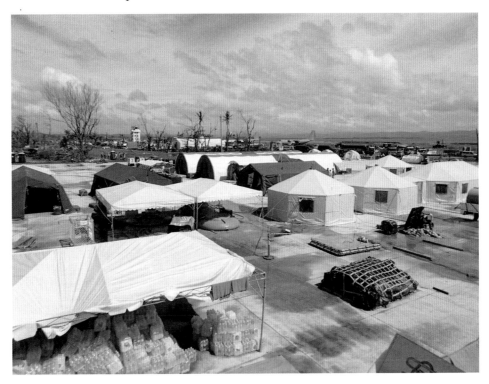

Question 56.1

What are the key strategic issues for consideration in such a deployment?

Question 56.2

What are the key principles of the humanitarian response in these circumstances?

Question 56.3

What are the priorities following arrival on-scene?

Question 56.4

What types of personnel are required?

Question 56.5

What types of pathology are to be expected?

Question 56.6

What are the main risks to personnel on deployment?

Discussion 56.1

Decompensated major incidents can occur globally and responses are almost invariably coordinated through national governments or major non-governmental organisations (NGO). In such circumstances, it is important that humanitarian aid is requested by the affected country and not simply assumed. Not all humanitarian aid requests require medical assistance teams. The necessary politics behind such decisions are beyond the scope of this question but the country or NGO sending humanitarian workers into such an environment will carry the responsibility for the welfare of those workers. This includes:

- Realistic appraisal of response capabilities (not all organisations will have the capacity for full surgical or critical care facilities)
- Selection of appropriate staff
- Safety of staff, including from ongoing natural hazards
- Healthcare and necessary vaccinations (require prior planning)
- Visas (if required), movement to the affected country and within that country
- Medico-legal immunity
- Travel to and from the scene of the incident.

The first step in such a deployment would be a formal 'needs assessment', which allows appraisal of the situation on the ground and formulation of the overall response.

Discussion 56.2

The core principles of the medical humanitarian response can be summarised as an avoidance of the Seven Sins of Humanitarian medicine (see box below).

Seven Sins of Humanitarian medicine
Sin #1: Leaving a mess behind
Sin #2: Failing to match technology to local needs and abilities
Sin #3: Failing of NGOs to cooperate and help each other, and to cooperate and accept help from military organisations
Sin #4: Failing to have a follow-up plan
Sin #5: Allowing politics, training or other distracting goals to trump service, while representing the mission as 'service'
Sin #6: Going where we are not wanted, or needed and/or being poor guests
Sin #7: Doing the right thing for the wrong reason

Source: Welling et al 2010

The Sphere handbook (Sphere 2018), first released in 2011, has attempted to deliver a common ground for governments and NGOs, and to help improve the quality and accountability of the humanitarian response. The handbook focuses on four technical chapters:

- Water supply, sanitation and hygiene promotion
- Food security and nutrition
- Shelter and settlement
- Health

The Sphere handbook also offers a humanitarian charter, which encapsulates the core beliefs of humanitarian organisations. Box 1 below highlights the common principles, rights and duties of the charter and box 2 demonstrates the four basic protection principles that inform all humanitarian actions.

Box 1: Common principles, rights and duties

- The right to life with dignity;
- The right to receive humanitarian assistance; and
- The right to protection and security.

Box 2: Four basic protection principles

1. Enhance the safety, dignity and rights of people, and avoid exposing them to harm.
2. Ensure people's access to assistance, according to need and without discrimination.
3. Assist people to recover from the physical and psychological effects of threatened or actual violence, coercion or deliberate deprivation.
4. Help people claim their rights.

Discussion 56.3

Humanitarian response teams need to be 100% self-sufficient (or have clear support arrangements between responding agencies) and must avoid worsening the situation on the ground by consuming local resources. Primary objectives on arrival of the team will involve securing a suitable location (as identified by the needs assessment team) and assembling the shelter that was brought in as part of their team response. Prior training by the individuals in the team will ensure that everyone understands the importance of working together in these early stages to allow a prompt deployment of the humanitarian response. Only when the team has established its own shelter, food and water arrangements can they focus on assembling the field hospital and commencing the delivery of aid. They should, however, be prepared for the possibility that casualties may arrive before the facility is completed and have plans for how these may be managed.

Discussion 56.4

Team composition will vary according to local need and patient demographics and this should have been identified during the needs assessment. Teams should endeavour to complement both local resources and other responding groups. As such, individual foreign medical teams may organise to support particular areas, such as public health/surgery/paediatrics, etc., or a larger team response may incorporate many or all of these.

Personnel can include the following:

- Logisticians – the key to any deployment. Personnel with knowledge and skills in setting up all necessary equipment brought by the response team. Responsible for shelter, food and water security and general welfare (for the team)
- Doctors
  - Depending on the situation and other responding agencies – emergency medicine, general surgeons, paediatricians, anaesthetists, general practitioners with augmented skill sets, e.g. obstetrics, paediatrics, etc.

- Nurses (and midwives)
- Radiographer(s)
- Pharmacist(s)
- Other Allied Health such as physiotherapists

Teams must be trained and prepared in advance. Many jurisdictions operate a system whereby suitable staff volunteer to become a member of the local Foreign Medical Team (e.g. AusMAT in Australia, UK-Med, NZMAT, etc.). Such teams should already be assessed and classified according to international standards (WHO 2013). These volunteers do orientation courses together, including time spent on training exercises, which allow the opportunity for team bonding as well as familiarisation with equipment. On top of the training exercise(s), volunteers may be deployed a few days prior to leaving to go overseas. This allows further refreshment of kit and acclimatisation prior to deployment.

Discussion 56.5

The pathology found on deployment is also very dependent on the nature of the disaster. In addition to all 'usual' presentations that might be expected in a primary or emergency healthcare clinic, a typhoon would lead to:

- Trauma
  - Initially: both major and minor injuries
  - Subsequently: wound infections, and sometimes the consequences of earlier wound management (such as inappropriate closure of highly contaminated wounds)
  - Delayed presentations of primary injuries
- Infectious diseases
  - Diarrhoeal illness, respiratory infections
  - Vector-borne diseases and other local/tropical diseases
- Pre-existing pathologies and chronic conditions
  - Worsening due to loss of medication/therapy, or lack of access to healthcare
  - Worsening due to disease progression
- Obstetrics and paediatrics

It is critically important to understand that resources will be limited and follow-up particularly challenging, so treatment plans and expectations must be realistic and match the local environment (pre-disaster). As an example, while a team may have the technical ability to insert complex orthopaedic metalwork, the local facilities may have no ability to manage or remove these, and the subsequent infection risk will be much higher, so some fractures may be more appropriately managed by non-operative means which are understood locally. The humanitarian response team will be present for a limited time and afterwards the local healthcare providers will be required to provide ongoing management to these cases using only local resources.

Discussion 56.6

The risks to the team can be divided as follows:

- Physical safety – despite government led security arrangements there are still risks associated with deployment. These risks include those related to the environment (e.g. weather, unstable structures) as well as those related to the local population (e.g. violence, theft).

- Trauma – a common array of minor injuries can be expected among the response team which can usually be managed 'in house', although consideration needs to be given to how more serious injuries may be managed or evacuated without impacting the wider response.
- Disease – preparation for disease prevention among the deployed teams is essential and will have been carried out prior to deployment. Awareness of local diseases is important, so that responders are prepared. Vaccinations and malaria prophylaxis form the backbone of medical prevention along with scrupulous attention to camp hygiene and water/food security.
- Psychological – while deployment is a unique and often uplifting experience, there are emotional challenges at many stages. The inability to deliver healthcare to the standards to which clinicians are accustomed can take a psychological toll, as can the stress of deployment in a foreign and often unstable environment. Isolation from regular support (such as family) may worsen this stress.

Key points

- PHRM team members have the requisite skills and training to be effective members of international disaster response teams.
- Disaster response teams should only deploy when requested by the host country and must be able to function independently of local resources.

References

Sphere. The Sphere Handbook 2018: humanitarian charter and minimum standards in humanitarian response. Sphere, 2018. Online. Available: https://spherestandards.org/handbook-2018/.

Welling DR, Ryan JM, Burris DG, Rich NM. Seven sins of humanitarian medicine. World J. Surg. 2010; 34(3):466–470.

World Health Organization (WHO). Classification and minimum standards for foreign medical teams in sudden onset disasters. WHO, 2013. Online. Available: https://www.who.int/docs/default-source/documents/publications/classification-and-minimum-standards-for-foreign-medical-teams-in-suddent-onset-disasters.pdf?sfvrsn=43a8b2f1_1.

Additional reading

Advanced Life Support Group. Major incident medical management and support (MIMMS), 3rd ed. Wiley, 2011.

Norton I, Trewin A (Eds). Australian medical assistance team training, version 3. AusMAT National Critical Care and Trauma Response Centre, 2011. Online. Available: https://www.nationaltraumacentre.nt.gov.au/sites/default/files/PDFs/AUSMAT_2011_web.pdf.

SECTION D

Paediatric and Neonatal Medicine

Foreword to the Paediatric and Neonatal Section

Success in treating the newborn, infant or child whose illness or injuries are beyond the hospital caring for them is a world-wide challenge. In recent decades much has been done to optimise high risk birth occurring in 'the right place' through improved ante-natal risk recognition and action. Where safe, injured patients may be taken directly from the scene to a hospital capable of offering definitive care; bypassing the nearest hospital.

However, these strategies are limited; particularly in countries with a widely dispersed population and/or steep gradient in health care infrastructure. Even basic hospital care can be distant for rural and remote communities. Consequently, a critical care consultation and retrieval service is required to effectively bridge the distance and time gap between local and definitive care.

This second edition brings alive some very real scenarios facing clinicians providing pre-hospital and retrieval medicine. It shows the challenges faced by these teams covering the gamut of patient age; from preterm infant to adult and the differing perspectives – namely from the pre-hospital setting to the hospital context. I would encourage readers to view these cases as a stimulus to discussion as much as set formulae for action. While these cases could occur in any health care context, regional variation is inevitable and the learnings for any context will benefit from a case-based discussion.

Andrew Berry
AM MB BS (Adel.) FRACP
State Director, NETS (NSW)

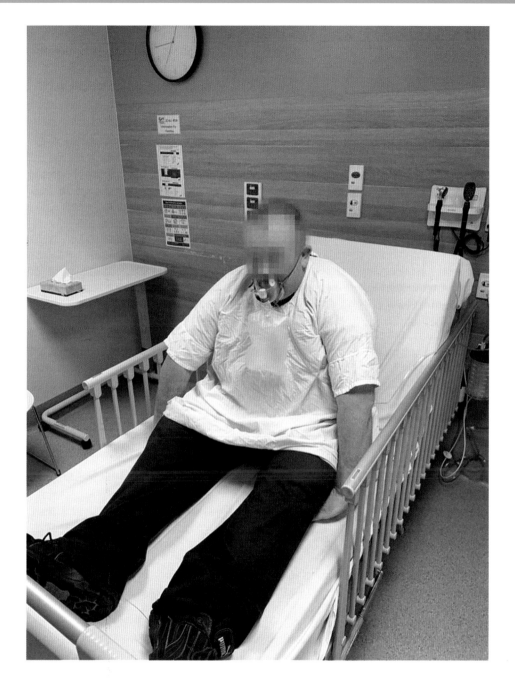

Incident

A 12-year-old boy with Trisomy 21 has been brought into a GP-run regional hospital after several days of shortness of breath, upper abdominal pain and fever.

Clinical information

- Obese (80 kg), blanching rash on torso.

- Airway: patent
- Breathing: Respiratory rate (RR): 28, moderately increased work of breathing, SpO_2 82% in air, improves to 94% on high-flow face mask oxygen at 15 L/min. Scattered coarse crackles in both lung bases.
- Circulation: Heart rate (HR) 170, blood pressure (BP) 75/30 (42), capillary refill time 1 second (flash).
- Disability: confused, agitated, taking off face mask, taking off monitoring equipment. GCS 13 (spontaneous eye opening, confused, localising to pain). Pupils equal and reactive.
- Exposure: temperature 39.1°C, blood glucose 8 mmol/L

The local General Practitioner has obtained intravenous access through which he has administered 2 g of ceftriaxone. Despite his best efforts, the patient's degree of agitation has prevented any further intervention.

Relevant information

- **PHRM team transport options**: Fixed-wing only, maximum one stretcher.
- **Additional resources:** On-call anaesthetist, hospital nurse (adult trained). Land ambulance (volunteer crew).
- **Retrieval options:** Paediatric hospital with intensive care capacity. Estimated flight time 2 hours.
- **Other:** Nil.

Question 57.1

What pre-retrieval advice to the local team would be appropriate?

While the retrieval team is en route, the patient has deteriorated.

On arrival: Grossly confused and agitated, not compliant with observations, pulling off monitoring and oxygen. IV access has been pulled out.

Question 57.2

Outline the arriving PHRM team's initial management.

Following your initial intervention, monitoring is established, oxygen by face mask is applied with improvement in saturations, and intravenous access is obtained. A venous gas show pH 7.08, pCO_2 32 mmHg (4.3 kPa), lactate 7.1 mmol/L. A bolus of 20 ml/kg of crystalloid is administered with some improvement in blood pressure. His respiratory distress is now more marked with saturations in the high 80s. Antibiotic cover is broadened according to local guidelines, in this case flucloxacillin 2 g IV.

Question 57.3

Outline your ongoing management.

Following the establishment of invasive ventilation, the patient's oxygen saturations deteriorate and he is noted to have poor bilateral chest rise and fall while lying flat. Ventilator settings are pressure support of 20 cmH₂O, PEEP of 5 cmH₂O, respiratory rate of 12 breaths per minute, inspiratory time 0.6 seconds. End-tidal CO_2 trace is visible on the patient monitor.

Question 57.4

How will you respond to this child's deterioration after invasive ventilation is established?

Just prior to departure, the patient's blood pressure starts to drop, and his heart rate trends upwards despite an increasing noradrenaline infusion rate.

Question 57.5

How will you use point-of-care ultrasound to guide your decision making and what are your priorities and considerations before departure?

Discussion 57.1

Clinical assessment is limited by telephone. If possible, telemedicine consultation may be helpful, particularly to gauge the degree of agitation of the patient and the extent to which this is compromising the local team's ability to care for him.

The working diagnosis in this case is pneumonia with septic shock and encephalopathy. Agitation may be caused by hypoxia, inadequate cerebral perfusion, metabolic disturbance or by CNS infection.

Generally speaking, interventions to address these reversible causes prior to arrival of the PHRM team might include face-mask oxygen, intravenous fluid bolus, a venous blood gas and correction of electrolyte/blood sugar abnormalities, and adequate antibiotic cover.

If agitation continues after these measures, the risks and benefits of gaining situational control through the administration of intravenous (0.25–0.5 mg/kg)/intramuscular (2–4 mg/kg) ketamine should be considered. In this case, upper airway obstruction, hypoventilation, and cardiovascular collapse should be anticipated and planned for.

Discussion 57.2

A key priority is to create a calm environment, with good 360-degree access to the patient and only key team members present, usually including the parents. It is often possible to de-escalate a critical situation by creating the correct environment. Children are often forced to lie down in a supine position which can hinder assessment and management. The child should be allowed to sit up in a position of comfort, or even be nursed in his mother's arms to facilitate O_2 delivery with 15 L/min via a non-rebreather. Poor O_2 delivery is a recurring theme during paediatric resuscitation. Oxygen delivery should be optimised during the initial remote assessment, e.g. poorly placed or kinked nasal specs, inadequate oxygen flow at the wall, inadvertent use of medical air, inappropriate use of a bag-valve-mask apparatus, etc.

If the child remains agitated despite optimising basic care, then situational control is the key initial treatment priority. It is uncommon to need to sedate children in this manner. The safety profile of ketamine makes it the ideal agent in this case. Midazolam has been used; however, it can be risky in the context of critical illness. Even a transient decrease in respiratory rate can decrease the physiological compensation for a metabolic acidosis and precipitate cardio-respiratory collapse.

Prior to ketamine administration, it is important for both the PHRM team and the local team to have a shared mental model for the anticipated clinical course. This would include intubation, ongoing difficulty with ventilation and anticipated cardio-vascular support.

Discussion 57.3

Once sedated, preparation for RSI can commence, including optimisation of pre-oxygenation and further attempts made to secure good IV or IO access.

Intubation should be planned using the same techniques as outlined in question 58. A focus on teamwork and human factors, including checklists, a pre-intubation brief as well as optimisation of sepsis physiology will add a layer of safety to a challenging and high-risk procedure. No assumptions should be made regarding the skill set of the local staff, equipment compatibility or serviceability, or access to necessary drugs or equipment. The transport ventilator and circuit must be thoroughly checked. PHRM teams are at risk of being overwhelmed by required critical tasks (task saturation). Prioritisation, delegation and clear communication are therefore key leadership and human-factor tools.

Pre-oxygenation must be optimised by providing 100% oxygen and PEEP. This can be provided using a t-piece, a ventilator in CPAP or BiPAP mode or a self-inflating bag with a PEEP valve. The self-inflating bag is potentially dangerous as the child in extremis may not be able to generate enough inspiratory flow to overcome the resistance of the duck-billed valve, and should only be used by an experienced operator who will provide assisted breaths. Efforts must be made to ensure that the mask is a good fit. If the patient is obtunded, ensure airway patency is maintained using airway-opening manoeuvres, oral or nasopharyngeal airways. A two-person BVM technique is strongly recommended. Decompressing the stomach with a gastric tube will reduce splinting of the diaphragm and can often dramatically improve respiratory distress. This would usually occur post intubation. In a smaller child a gastric tube may be placed prior to intubation; however, the benefits must be carefully balanced against the discomfort and distress caused by insertion.

Cardiovascular compromise is a predictable consequence after induction of anaesthesia in a septic child and a peripheral inotrope and/or vasopressor infusion should be commenced prior to intubation. A 'push dose' (e.g. 10 mcg) and a cardiac arrest dose (10 mcg/kg) of adrenaline should be pre-drawn and immediately available. A modified RSI using low-dose intravenous induction (e.g. ketamine 0.5 mg/kg) and high-dose intravenous muscle relaxant (rocuronium 1.6 mg/kg) should be considered.

It is vital to engage the parents prior to intubation to inform them of their child's progress and the subsequent risks involved. Ideally, informed consent should be obtained.

Discussion 57.4

The approach to sudden and significant clinical deterioration should be structured. In the case of hypoxia post intubation the acronym DOPE(S) is one example:

- Displacement
- Obstruction
- Pneumothorax (pulmonary embolus/oedema)
- Equipment
- Stacked breaths.

A more extensive assessment and response is detailed in the following flow chart. It is useful to follow the ventilation from the patient to the wall O_2 outlet.

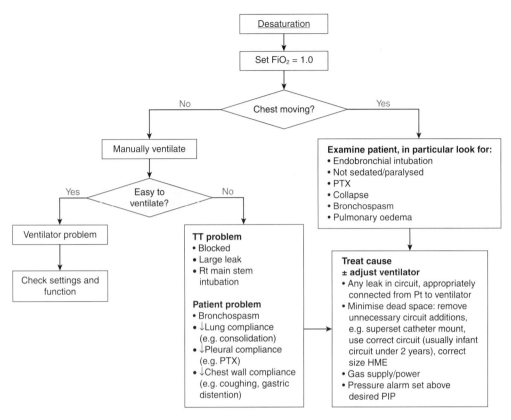

In this case, the patient should be placed in reverse trendelenberg 30°, disconnected from the ventilator, and bag ventilation commenced. Given the pathology and habitus, high airway pressures may be required due to poor lung and chest wall compliance. Oxygenation will likely be improved by increasing mean airway pressure, giving adequate tidal volumes not exceeding 6 ml/kg ideal body weight (high PEEP, low tidal volume strategy – see Case 30), with inverse I:E ratio (increased inspiratory time).

Discussion 57.5

Point of care ultrasound (POCUS – see Cases 39 and 44) may be used to further differentiate the shock state and to assess fluid responsiveness. In this case, US revealed no pericardial effusion but grossly impaired biventricular function. The inferior vena cava was dilated with no variation in diameter with ventilation. Lung ultrasound showed normal anterior lung sliding seen bilaterally (no evidence of pneumothorax). High PEEP in this case may contribute to impaired venous return and decreased cardiac output. Titrating PEEP to improve venous return while maintaining oxygenation should be considered. Ideally, a blood gas and CXR should also be performed prior to mobilising with this critically ill child.

The working diagnosis is of pneumonia with septic myocardial dysfunction which has been 'unmasked' by increasing systemic vascular resistance (afterload) with noradrenaline. Further administration of crystalloid is unlikely to improve perfusion; however, addition of an inotrope infusion (e.g. adrenaline) delete may do so. An arterial line is required, remembering that all taps should be visible at all times during the retrieval to prevent the risk of catastrophic bleeding. This is of critical importance in neonates and small children with low total blood volumes.

During this retrieval, the patient will need at least 4 transitions to move between various transport platforms. A vacuum mattress can facilitate easy transfers and has the advantage of providing limited protection against hypothermia, although some children will overheat in a 'vac mat'. Airway equipment, including drugs for re-intubation if required should be immediately available and a team member nominated to hold the TT for each episode of transfer.

A pre-departure checklist should be routinely used to minimise risk. This cognitive aid ensures that essential equipment accompanies the team on subsequent transport legs to definitive care.

This includes: patient identification, sedation, maintenance fluid, emergency equipment and drugs, patient adequately secured, all paperwork including radiology, consent obtained (see Appendix 4.2).

Prior to departure, it is essential to update the parents on their child's progress and give them the opportunity to spend some time together. Every effort is made to transport a parent with their child, although this is occasionally not possible. Many parents are understandably nervous pre-flight and time spent considering their comfort (bathroom, anti-emetic, phone charger and phone) is time well spent.

Key points

- Retrieval of children presents unique problems; thorough preparation and planning can reduce the risk of adverse events.
- Intubation of children with sepsis can lead to life-threatening circulatory collapse. Advanced planning, including adequate resuscitation, dose titration of induction agent, and peripheral inotrope infusion prior to intubation helps mitigate this risk.
- The DOPE(S) pneumonic is a helpful acronym for causes of post-intubation hypoxia and difficulty with ventilation.
- Sepsis resuscitation is dynamic and influenced by heart–lung interactions. Patient deterioration should prompt re-evaluation of the diagnosis and consideration of alternative therapies to support breathing and circulation.

Additional reading

Davis T. Ketamine dosing in obese adolescents. Don't Forget the Bubbles, 2014. Online. Available: https://dontforgetthebubbles.com/ketamine-dosing-obese-adolescents/. 7 September 2021. https://doi.org/10.31440/DFTB.6051.

Lanctôt J-F, Valois M. Echo guided life support: step by step ultrasound for resuscitation. Online. Available: https://www.echoguidedlifesupport.com/. 7 September 2021.

Long E, Barrett MJ, Peters C, et al. Emergency intubation of children outside of the operating room. Paediatr. Anaesth. 2020; 30(3):319–330.

Nickson C. Post-intubation hypoxia. Life in the Fastlane, 2020. Online. Available: https://litfl.com/post-intubation-hypoxia/. 7 September 2021.

Royal Children's Hospital Melbourne. Sepsis – assessment and management. Online. Available: https://www.rch.org.au/clinicalguide/guideline_index/SEPSIS_assessment_and_management/. 7 September 2021.

Weiss SL, Peters MJ, Alhazzani W, et al. Surviving sepsis campaign international guidelines for the management of septic shock and sepsis-associated organ dysfunction in children. Pediatr. Crit. Care Med. 2020; 21(2):e52–e106.

Incident

An 18-month-old male has been presented to a rural emergency department with noisy breathing that has progressed to increased work of breathing. He developed a fever and rhinorrhea 3 days ago and has had a progressive barky cough. He developed intercostal and subcostal indrawing over the past 12 hours. He has had a previous episode of croup 6 months ago that did not require intervention.

Relevant information

- **PHRM team transport options:** Fixed-wing aircraft.
- **Additional resources:** Regional GP-led hospital with on-call anaesthesia. Land ambulance and staff.
- **Retrieval options:** General hospital with paediatrician 40 minutes' flight time. Hospital with paediatric intensive care and anaesthetic capacity 90-minute flight time.
- **Other:** Nil.

Question 58.1

What is your differential diagnosis?

Question 58.2

What advice should be provided to the referring centre about managing this patient while the PHRM team is being mobilised?

Clinical information

On arrival, the following clinical information is available:
- Lethargic.
- P 165.
- RR 44.
- SaO_2 92% on room air.
- Biphasic stridor.
- Temperature 38°C (100.4°F).

Drugs administered:
- Intermittent nebulised adrenaline
- Oral dexamethasone 0.6 mg/kg.

Question 58.3

Discuss further management.

Discussion 58.1

Differential diagnosis includes epiglottitis, tonsillitis, laryngitis, aspiration of foreign body, tracheitis and anaphylaxis. Croup results from swelling of the mucosa in the subglottic area of the larynx. Viruses are the most common etiology, with parainfluenza virus types 1 and 3 being the most commonly identified. The disease has a gradual onset and usually develops after an upper respiratory tract infection. Patients with bacterial epiglottitis have a more acute and sudden onset of illness, characterised by high fever, drooling and muffled voice. Pain with breathing, swallowing, neck movement or laryngeal manipulation is characteristic of epiglottitis. Croup is much more common than epiglottitis in this post-immunisation era. The diagnosis of croup is a clinical one and obtaining an x-ray is generally not recommended as it is likely to cause significant distress leading to worsening obstruction. But if already done by the referring centre, anterioposterior radiographs of the neck may help confirm the diagnosis of acute epiglottitis or the possibility of a foreign body in the airway. The characteristic radiograph of croup includes a 'church steeple' or 'sharpened pencil' on anteroposterior films.

Discussion 58.2

There are two main priorities to be considered. Firstly, ensure optimal management of the child is undertaken. At this stage it is reasonable to consider croup as the diagnosis and start treatment accordingly. Secondly, consider and plan for the worst-case scenario, the need to intubate a potentially severely obstructed airway. If available, this child should be assessed remotely using telemedicine facilities.

The majority of cases of croup will resolve quickly with simple treatment and fewer than 10% will require hospitalisation. However, a small percentage of children will develop severe croup and require intensive care support including intubation and ventilation. Croup may present some management challenges to PHRM services as, despite a dramatic and severe presentation, a child with croup will often settle over several hours with good treatment and may not need retrieval.

Accurate assessment of severity, early management and settling the child are the keystones of a successful outcome (see table below).

Muscular laryngeal constriction that occurs with distress, crying or forceful breathing worsens the respiratory distress. A key priority is to keep the child calm and the following techniques may assist in this regard:

- Limit the noise and people in the room.
- Limit unnecessary interventions.

Table 58.1 Clinical assessment of croup

	Mild	Moderate	Severe
Behaviour	Normal	Intermittent mild agitation	Increasing agitation, drowsiness
Stridor*	No stridor, or only when active or upset	Intermittent stridor at rest	Persistent stridor at rest
Respiratory rate	Normal	Increased respiratory rate	Marked increase or decrease
Accessory muscle use	None or minimal	Moderate chest wall retraction	Marked chest wall retraction
Oxygen saturations			Hypoxia is a late sign which indicates life-threatening croup

*Loudness of stridor is not a good indicator of severity of obstruction. Soft stridor in the presence of a worsening clinical picture may be a sign of imminent airway obstruction.

- Allow the child to remain in the parent's arms (with monitoring on) if that is where they are more settled.
- Ask the parent what settles the child.
- Play nursery rhymes or cartoons on a phone.
- Ensure the child is nursed sitting up.
- Dim the lighting.
- For infants, consider wrapping or swaddling.

For severe croup, a single dose of dexamethasone (0.6 mg/kg orally) plus nebulised adrenaline (1 ml/kg of 1:1000) as needed is the cornerstone of management. Humidification of inspired gases is usually effective in improving respiratory distress and prevents drying of secretions. Cool air or cool mist therapies are not supported by evidence. Oxygen is usually not required and hypoxaemia suggests ventilation perfusion mismatching or copious secretions.

Nebulised adrenaline is the most effective initial drug therapy for children with croup. The duration of action is short and rebound oedema may occur. Treatments may be required every 1 to 2 hours and the child should be observed for at least 2 hours after treatment. Adrenaline may provide time to allow the steroids to take effect. Clinical improvement usually begins 2–3 hours after steroid administration and persists for 24–48 hours. Antibiotics are generally not indicated in the treatment of uncomplicated viral croup. However, antibiotics should be initiated if bacterial epiglottitis/tracheitis is suspected.

Failure of first-line treatment suggests ongoing oedema or obstruction caused by thick secretions or potentially a bacterial superinfection or a congenital airway malformation such as laryngomalacia. In these situations, or if the child appears exhausted from the work of breathing, relief of obstruction must be obtained through tracheal intubation followed by pulmonary suctioning. The clinical assessment of 'exhaustion' in children with croup may be difficult. Respiratory failure is characterised by rising pCO_2 level, hypoxia ($spO_2 < 92\%$ despite high-flow O_2 by mask > 5 L/min), moderate/marked recession and altered conscious level.

Importantly, securing the airway of a patient with severe obstruction is a high-risk procedure in limited resource settings. The risk of securing a difficult airway must be balanced with the risk of transporting a patient with a potentially unstable airway, and a thorough assessment of the clinical trajectory of the patient is an important consideration. For example, if the patient has had rapid deterioration over the past 12 to 24 hours, has required multiple adrenaline nebulisers and ongoing respiratory distress, then the safest approach would be to secure the airway prior to transport. Proper planning is essential for safe intubation prior to transport. Where possible, the most senior and experienced clinician should be included in the responding PHRM team, either in addition to or as a replacement for less experienced doctors.

Discussion 58.3

The child has deteriorated and will require intubation and ventilation prior to transport.

Ideally, intubations should be performed in the operating room (OR) under controlled anaesthetic conditions. The on-call anaesthetist can be called in to assist with stabilisation of the airway while the PHRM team is en route. While the presence of an ENT surgeon would be ideal, it is unlikely to be feasible in this case.

Different PHRM team members will possess different skill sets and may be comfortable with gaseous induction of anaesthesia. In such cases, the PHRM team should combine with the on-call anaesthetist to form a flash team.

Gaseous induction and intubation

General anaesthesia is induced with oxygen and sevoflurane with the child sitting up in a position of comfort. In epiglottitis, the large swollen epiglottis may flop down and obstruct the airway, particularly if the child is laid flat. Patients with epiglottitis often feel better if sitting fully upright or even leaning forward, for this reason. Spontaneous respirations are continued as the child is gently allowed to recline. When the child is deep under anesthesia, IV access can be established and secured.

Intravenous (IV) induction and intubation

For IV induction, careful planning and rigorous attention to detail is required to minimise the risk of this high-stakes procedure. This should include use of cognitive aids (checklist, standardised equipment, shadowboards), clear identification of roles and a pre-intubation brief to outline the plan for an unsuccessful intubation attempt and physiological deterioration. The most experienced airway operator should perform the procedure. A variety of tracheal tubes (TT) sizes, including croup tubes (see photo below) should be available, but it is reasonable to start with at least 0.5 mm internal diameter smaller than what would normally be used for a child of that age (formula: age + 3.5 for cuffed TT). Using videolaryngoscopy will allow optimal visualisation of the glottic opening. A stylet or bougie is essential because it provides rigidity and facilitates introduction of the TT through the obstructed airway. The choice of medications should focus on optimising intubating conditions and depend on the severity of illness of the child. In this example, since the child has deteriorated and there may be haemodynamic instability, ketamine 1 mg/kg followed by Rocuronium 1–2 mg/kg is appropriate. Optimising bag-mask ventilation (ie. two-handed technique) may be required to provide positive pressure ventilation through a severely obstructed subglottic trachea. Preparing for failure is essential and, although rarely required, having surgical back-up is ideal.

After intubation, the team should assess tracheal tube position and $ETCO_2$ waveform and insert a naso/orogastric tube. If a cuffed TT is used, then the cuff pressure should be checked with a manometer and should be < 20 mmHg. According to Boyle's law, gas expands with increasing altitude, so a TT cuff with air in it requires close monitoring/adjusting until cruise altitude is reached (see Case 27). Given the need for the

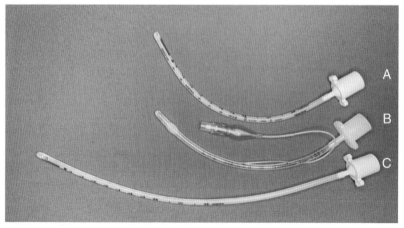

Figure 58.1 Examples of tracheal tubes that can be used in croup: A – uncuffed 4.5 mm diameter tube, B – cuffed 4.5 mm diameter tube, C – 4.5 mm diameter croup tube.

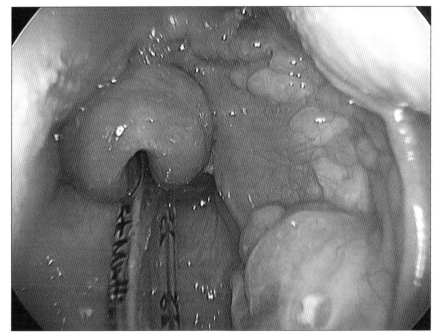

Figure 58.2 This child's difficult clinical course was explained by a diagnosis of bacterial epiglotittis. The swollen, cherry red epiglottis was seen at layngoscopy.

transferring of the patient to a stretcher and the vibration and general motion of ground and air transport, there is a risk of accidental extubation. All equipment for an emergency re-intubation should be ready and packed separately from all other equipment and kept in close proximity to the head of the patient. Some recommend the use of neuromuscular blockade in addition to IV sedation for all intubated patients with a difficult airway to decrease the risk of extubation en route. The TT should be very carefully secured by the PHRM team. One simple and effective method to ensure a well-secured TT is the Modified Melbourne strapping (see Appendix 1.1.7). All measures should be taken to avoid an accidental extubation and the need for re-intubation in the back of an aircraft or ground ambulance. Anticipate secretions that will require suctioning, particularly if the child has been deteriorating or tiring. Ensure intravenous access is adequate and secured. Maintenance fluids should be established and the patient should be prepared for transport.

For this case, there is a clear requirement for paediatric intensive care unit (PICU) support so the patient should be transported to the centre with PICU facilities, despite the longer travel time.

Key points

- Due to risk of catastrophic airway loss, planning in conjunction with the local team is essential prior to transport.
- Optimal management of presumed croup must be established prior to transport, including steroids and nebulised epinephrine.
- As with all low-frequency, high-consequence interventions, a risk–benefit analysis should occur regarding securing a potentially difficult airway prior to transport.

Additional reading

Long E, Barrett MJ, Peters C, et al. Emergency intubation of children outside of the operating room. Pediatr. Anesth. 2020; 30:319–330. https://doi.org/10.1111/pan.13784.

NHS Children's Acute Transport Service. Clinical guidelines: upper airway obstruction (UAO). January 2020. Online. Available: https://cats.nhs.uk/wp-content/uploads/cats_uao_2020-.pdf. 9 September 2021.

Royal Children's Hospital Melbourne. Croup (Laryngotracheobronchitis). Online. Available: https://www.rch.org.au/clinicalguide/guideline_index/Croup_Laryngotracheobronchitis/#assessment-of-severity. 8 September 2021.

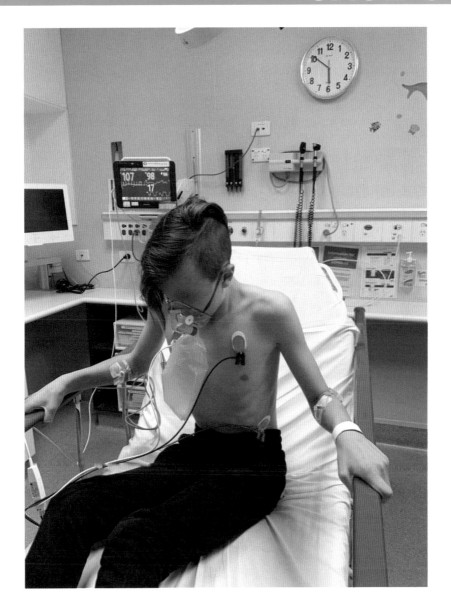

Incident

A 12-year-old boy has presented to a regional hospital with a 6-hour history of short-ness of breath, wheezing and decreased appetite. He has a history of severe asthma and poor compliance with his medications. He has had numerous previous admissions to hospital, with one previous PICU admission requiring intubation and ventilation at 6 years of age. His weight is 42 kg.

Clinical information

Clinical information on presentation to the regional hospital:
- Alert, anxious, speaking single words only.
- P 145.

- RR 34, accessory muscle use.
- SaO_2 91% on 15 L oxygen via nebuliser mask.
- Widespread expiratory wheeze.
- Temperature 37.5°C (99.5°F).
- The patient has had three back-to-back treatments of inhaled salbutamol (10 puffs) and atrovent (6 puffs) 20 minutes apart. He is now receiving intermittent nebulised salbutamol.

The above image is visible to you via telemedicine.

Relevant information

- **PHRM team transport options**: Fixed-wing.
- **Additional resources:** Regional GP-led hospital.
- **Retrieval options:** General hospital with paediatric intensive care capacity.
- **Other:** Estimated flight time 90 minutes.

Question 59.1

What advice should be provided to the referring centre about managing this patient while the PHRM team is being mobilised?

Unfortunately, the patient has deteriorated while the team was en route. Clinical assessment on arrival:

- Drowsy, unable to speak.
- P 159.
- RR 22, silent chest.
- BP 89/65 mmHg.
- SaO_2 88% on 15 LPM by non-rebreather face mask.

Ongoing management:

- An intravenous cannula has been placed and a 500 ml crystalloid fluid bolus given.
- Hydrocortisone 200 mg IV has been administered.
- Intermittent nebulised salbutamol every 20 minutes has been given.

Question 59.2

How would you stabilise and prepare this patient for transport?

Question 59.3

What are the complications that might arise on transport and what are your contingency plans for this patient?

Discussion 59.1

An acute asthma exacerbation in a poorly controlled asthmatic is a life-threatening situation. Clinical assessment is difficult by telephone/telemedicine, but it is important to determine the severity of illness and estimate the clinical trajectory (see Table 59.1). This patient is anxious, speaking words only and has low SpO_2 requiring supplemental oxygen. He has risk factors for ICU admission and death, including previous ICU admission and intubation.

Table 59.1 Rapid primary assessment of acute asthma in adults and children

Mild/Moderate	Severe	Life-threatening
Can walk, speak whole sentences in one breath (For young children: can move around, speak in phrases) Oxygen saturation > 94%	Any of these findings: • Use of accessory muscles of neck or intercostal muscles or 'tracheal tug' during inspiration or subcostal recession ('abdominal breathing') • Unable to complete sentences in one breath due to dyspnoea • Obvious respiratory distress • Oxygen saturation 90-94%	Any of these findings: • Reduced consciousness or collapse • Exhaustion • Cyanosis • Oxygen saturation <90% • Poor respiratory effort, soft/absent breath sounds

Notes

The severity category may change when more information is available (e.g. pulse oximetry, spirometry) or over time

The presence of pulsus paradoxus (systolic paradox) is not a reliable indicator of the severity of acute asthma.

If oxygen therapy has already been started, it is not necessary to cease oxygen to measure pulse oximetry.

Oxygen saturation levels are a guide only and are not definitive; clinical judgment should be applied.

Definitions of severity classes for acute asthma used in this handbook may differ from those used in published clinical trials and other guidelines that focus on, are or restricted to, the management of acute asthma within emergency departments or acute care facilities.

Australian Asthma Handbook v1.1

Differential diagnoses for wheeze also need to be considered, such as anaphylaxis, foreign-body aspiration, pneumonia and congestive heart failure. A focused history and a CXR can be helpful to rule in and out the differential diagnosis. For example, it can show lung hyperinflation consistent with asthma or a pneumothorax as a rare but potential complication. Furthermore, a CXR can assess the lung parenchyma for the presence of consolidation, atelectasis, foreign body or pulmonary oedema. If available, a peak flow meter can give valuable information when peak flows are compared with the child's normal values or 'personal best'. A peak expiratory flow of <60% of the patient's best value is another indicator of a severe exacerbation. Peak flow measurement adds little to the management of a patient with severe respiratory distress or those under 6 years of age.

The referring site should be instructed to escalate its current therapy since this patient is at high risk for respiratory failure.

Maximise oxygenation and ventilation

- Oxygen to keep SpO_2 levels above 92%. This is usually commenced at 15 L/min initially then titrated.
- Posture and positioning are important but often neglected considerations. A self-ventilating patient is best upright and leaning forward slightly in a 'tripod'

posture, which assists with the use of accessory inspiratory muscles, and increases lung volume. Supine and reclined posturing decreases lung volumes and flow rates. Lying flat should be avoided at all costs unless the patient arrests.

- NIV is controversial. In a self-ventilating asthmatic patient, PEEP should help splint airways, improve exhalation and reduce air trapping. However, NIV is generally poorly tolerated, impedes delivery of inhaled agents and may worsen fatigue.
- HFNC (high flow nasal cannula) may help to reduce the work of breathing and improve V/Q mismatch. Its role in asthma management is also controversial; however, it is favoured over NIV in the retrieval environment due to patient comfort and the ability to deliver warm, humidified oxygen.

Aggressive pharmacological treatment
- Salbutamol should be delivered by nebuliser if the child is on high flow rates of oxygen. On very high flow rates, the nebulised medication is mostly distributed around the room rather than inhaled, so oxygen flow rates need to be reduced. Salbutamol toxicity needs to be considered as extreme beta-adrenoceptor stimulation will increase whole-body cellular oxygen demands and, combined with the development of a lactic acidosis, this may worsen respiratory distress. However, in the acute salvage phase of critical asthma, salbutamol should be weaned as the patient settles. The effect of salbutamol can be monitored by looking for tachycardia, jitteriness and often a temporary dip in oxygen-saturation levels due to a short-term V/Q mismatch.
- Inhaled anticholinergics, such as ipratropium bromide, given with B2-agonists in the first hour have been shown to improve lung function and reduce hospital admission rates, but there is no evidence to support use beyond the first hour of therapy (National Asthma Council of Australia 2014).

Early corticosteroid administration is crucial as it will settle the inflammation triggering the clinical symptoms; however, it will take 4–6 hours to take effect. Giving parenteral corticosteroids (IV methylprednisolone 1 mg/kg, max 60 mg Q6H or Hydrocortisone 4 mg/kg, max 300 mg Q6H) will bypass the alimentary system (shortening time to effect by approximately 30 minutes) and will guarantee delivery of a dose.

Establishing IV access early is important and providing 10–20 ml/kg of fluid as a bolus is usually indicated as concomitant dehydration is common due to a combination of insensible losses and reduced intake.

Depending on the response to the above interventions, further treatment may be required.

- Magnesium sulphate infusion (25–50 mg/kg IV bolus, max 2 g) is an effective rescue medication in severe/critical asthma due to relaxation of both bronchial and vascular smooth muscle. The bronchodilator effect is relatively short lived (up to an hour or so) but can be very pronounced.
- Aminophylline was used extensively prior to the introduction of corticosteroid therapy but rapidly fell out of favour due to the low threshold for toxicity. However, it remains an effective therapy in serious/critical asthma in children. The usual recommendation is a loading dose (5 mg/kg over 20 minutes) then ongoing infusion if required, noting that the half-life is long (7–9 hours) and the clinical effects of the loading dose may be sustained.

- Administering salbutamol intravenously (loading dose 7.5 mcg/kg over 2–5 minutes, followed by an infusion of 1 mcg/kg/min, titrated up to a max of 5 mcg/kg/min) is often of little clinical advantage as, in a self-ventilating patient, nebulised/inhaled salbutamol is extremely well absorbed directly into the respiratory system and IV administration often leads to toxic side effects.
- Adrenaline is sometimes recommended in the management of asthma. Adrenaline has a much greater alpha and lesser β_2 adrenoceptor affinity than salbutamol. It is thought that the α_1 adrenoceptor effects may help to decrease airway oedema and increase venous return to the heart; however, there is little clinical evidence for this. Adrenaline is indicated in cardiac arrest due to asthma and should be used according to normal cardiac arrest protocols.
- Anaesthetic agents such as sevoflurane, ketamine and propofol all have bronchodilatory properties but should not be used in self-ventilating asthmatics as they may attenuate respiratory drive.

Other considerations

- Potassium levels often cause great concern in critical asthma as salbutamol drives potassium into cells causing a hypokalaemia. This is invariably asymptomatic, and giving potassium supplementation intravenously is unnecessary as it is transient, the total body potassium is unaffected, and it complicates management unnecessarily.
- Lactic acidosis unavoidably occurs in all intensively treated asthmatics. It should be observed, can sometimes be ameliorated with a small intravenous fluid load, but the main focus should continue to be on resolving the severe respiratory distress. It should, however, be an impetus to wean down salbutamol therapy as soon as clinically possible.
- Close observation is required to monitor for signs of impending respiratory failure, such as worsening mental status, inability to speak, a silent chest (absence of wheeze), and/or desaturation $<90\%$ SpO_2 despite supplemental oxygen. A normal or elevated CO_2 on blood gas should alert the clinician of impending respiratory failure.
- Intubation may be required and should be undertaken once other priorities are addressed. However, intubation should not distract from therapies aimed at reducing bronchospasm and the work of breathing, which may prevent the need for advanced airway management. While a cuffed tracheal tube protects the airway, it may not improve the underlying ventilation issue, which is due to hyperinflation and gas trapping. Care should be taken to focus on allowing exhalation, and resist the temptation to provide greater amounts of inspiratory pressure, which may lead to pneumothorax.

Discussion 59.2

The critical asthmatic is one of the most difficult patients to contend with in the retrieval environment. The patient has deteriorated significantly, showing evidence of impending respiratory failure. Simultaneous assessment and resuscitation, including aggressive bronchodilation, is required.

Given the clinical deterioration, and assuming all the advice given above has been implemented, this child is progressing towards the need for invasive ventilation.

Ensure the airway is patent and consider HFNC or NIV as a bridge to intubation. Consideration should be given to the possibility of a pneumothorax and rapid assessment should be done by clinical exam, urgent CXR and, potentially, bedside ultrasound. A second IV should be established and a 10–20 ml/kg bolus of crystalloid given. The majority of asthma exacerbations are triggered by respiratory infections that are from a viral source. Bacterial infections are uncommon; thus, empiric antibiotic treatment is generally not recommended.

If there is not a rapid improvement with this management, then emergency intubation is the next step.

Indications for intubation and ventilation

- Respiratory arrest is an absolute indication for ventilation.
- Exhaustion is commonly talked about but poorly defined. All patients tire, but it is the extreme loss of work of breathing that is the concerning sign, and will be occurring alongside decreasing air entry, increasing obtundation and rising pCO_2 rather than in isolation.

Induction, intubation and mechanical ventilation strategies

- Up to a quarter of children intubated for asthma experience significant adverse effects such as pneumothorax or cardiovascular collapse due to increased intrathoracic pressure from air trapping and hyperinflation. The procedure of tracheal intubation is high-risk and care in the post-intubation period with establishment of mechanical ventilation needs careful planning and rigorous attention to detail.
- It is important to have clear roles assigned to all team members and a shared mental model of the risks of tracheal intubation and emergency management of complications. If available and timing permits, the local anaesthetist should be called to assist the PHRM team. In particular, access to sevoflurane may help in the management of bronchospasm. Induction agents should be chosen to maximise bronchodilation and promote haemodynamic stability. Ketamine (1 mg/kg) and Rocuronium (1–2 mg/kg) are ideal agents. Ketamine has the added advantage of being a potent bronchodilator and provides relative preservation of cardiovascular stability, thus continuing a ketamine infusion for ongoing sedation following intubation is advantageous. Morphine and atracurium should be avoided due to histamine release. If an opioid is required, then fentanyl is a reasonable option. A cuffed tracheal tube with the largest diameter acceptable for age should be used, as high ventilatory pressures are often required (see picture below).

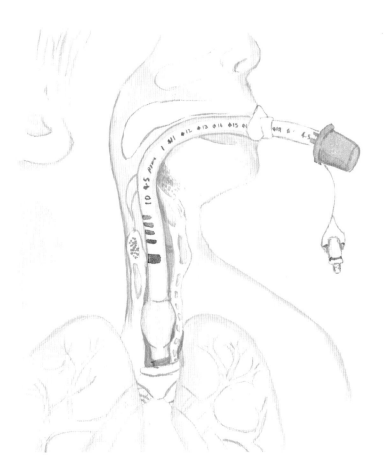

Cuffed vs uncuffed TT

Uncuffed tracheal tubes for children < 8 years were previously advocated to avoid exerting excessive pressure on the subglottic trachea. Cuffed TTs (especially micro-cuffed) for all ages have certain advantages and are now often preferred:

- Avoids need for re-intubation to eliminate leak, especially when high ventilatory pressures are required.
- High-volume/low-pressure cuff with shorter length and elimination of Murphy eye allows more distal position of the upper cuff border, reducing the risk of subglottic ischaemia and endobronchial intubation.
- Ultra-thin polyurethane cuff allows sealing at lower pressure and complete surface contact with minimal cuff folds.

Cardiorespiratory collapse during emergency intubation can occur for multiple reasons. Dynamic hyperinflation leading to pulmonary tamponade from air trapping commonly occurs, often due to overzealous use of BVM ventilation in the peri-intubation phase. Furthermore, profound bronchospasm and mucous plugging can lead to elevated pulmonary vascular resistance and right heart failure resulting in impending cardiac arrest. In addition, relative hypovolemia, coupled with the reduced preload from positive-pressure ventilation and the effects of anaesthetic agents on vascular tone, increase the risk of cardiovascular decompensation. Fluid status should be optimised in the preparation for intubation phase and further fluid boluses should be available. Consider initiating an adrenaline infusion at this stage (0.05 mcg/kg/min). Resuscitation drugs should be readily available as per the Paediatric Advanced Life Support (APLS) algorithms. All asthma therapy should be continued in the peri-intubation period, including all efforts to maintain continuous salbutamol admin-istration and 100% oxygen. Most modern ventilators have the capacity to deliver nebulised drugs. In-line metered dose inhaler devices may also be effective. Follow-ing intubation and maximal medical therapy, sevoflurane may need to be initiated and transport delayed until the patient is sufficiently stable. Paediatric Intensive Care consultation through the tasking agency may be required for ongoing management and situational awareness.

Intubated children with asthma are at increased risk of pulmonary tamponade, barotrauma, pulmonary oedema, cardiovascular dysfunction, and death (Krishnan 2021). Thus, ventilation strategy must be aimed at minimising air trapping and hyperinflation.

- A slow respiratory rate (1–10) and a prolonged expiratory time are key principles in ventilating an intubated asthmatic. Permissive hypercapnia (maintain arterial pH >7.2) may be required to allow adequate alveolar emptying.
- Utilising a pressure-regulated volume control mode allows for gas distribution to be optimised with a pre-set tidal volume while minimising the risk of baro-trauma. Peak pressures may be high (reaching upwards of 35 cmH$_2$O) due to profound bronchospasm, inflammation and mucous plugging. Calculating the driving pressure (plateau pressure – PEEP) may be more helpful in this setting. To minimise the risk of barotrauma, driving pressure should be 14–18 cmH$_2$O.
- Importantly, flow-time curves should be examined to determine whether expira-tory flow is complete at the end of each breath. For example, the expiratory flow curve must return to baseline prior to initiation of the next breath. If the curve does not return to baseline, adjustments can then be made with the inspiratory and expiratory time and PEEP as needed to ensure that there is full expiration with each breath.
- Ongoing bronchospasm can be identified by close examination of the shape of the end tidal CO$_2$ waveform which will demonstrate a 'shark fin' type appear-ance due to varying alveolar emptying on expiration (see Fig 59.1.)

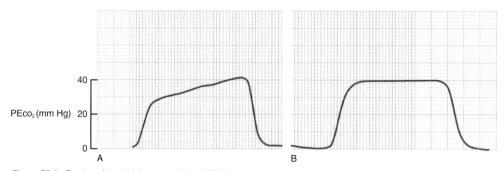

Figure 59.1 Tracing of end tidal carbon dioxide (ETCO$_2$) in a child with acute bronchospasm. Notice the slowly rising ETCO$_2$ value B, tracing from the same patient after administration of inhaled salbutamol. Note that the ETCO$_2$ waveform now has a flat plateau, indicating relief of the bronchospasm and efficient elimination of CO$_2$ from all areas of the lungs.

- Ensure that intrinsic ventilator pressure limits have been modified so that adequate tidal volumes will be delivered. The PHRM team should be alert to this issue and close attention paid to tidal volume, minute volume, peak inspiratory pressure and other ventilatory parameters.
- Tracheal suctioning is often required.
- PEEP in the invasively ventilated patient remains controversial; however, it can be used to stent open the small airways and facilitate full exhalation. Conversely it increases airway resistance, which may decrease passive exhalation. It is also known that an intubated, paralysed patient loses the normal physiological PEEP of 3–5 cm H_2O and PEEP may splint collapsing airways to improve passive exhalation.
- One recommendation is to periodically remove the patient from the BVM or ventilator tubing between breaths to reduce dead space and resistance during exhalation.

In an extreme clinical situation such as this, it is best to be aware of all the above concepts and be adaptable in moving from one to the other if the patient is deteriorating.

In the event of continuing deterioration despite maximal therapy, then triage to a centre with paediatric extracorporeal membrane oxygenation (ECMO) capabilities should be considered.

Discussion 59.3

The physiologic impact of acceleration and deceleration (e.g. take-off and landing) can be profound on patients with haemodynamic instability. Specifically, the force exerted by acceleration can cause a further decrease in venous return and cardiac output, worsening hypotension.

An arterial line should be placed prior to transport to assist in close monitoring.

This patient is also at risk of developing a pneumothorax; therefore, age-appropriate equipment for needle decompression and chest tube insertion should be available. In severe asthma, dead space can increase by ~50% and thus the $ETCO_2$ will underestimate the true arterial CO_2. Thus, point-of-care blood gas monitoring should be utilised to ensure adequate ventilation.

Mucus plugging is also common and attempts at chest physio and suction may be required on transport.

Key points

- Assessment and advice prior to retrieval should ensure early and appropriate escalation of therapy for presumed severe asthma.
- Emergency intubation of a severe asthmatic is a high-risk intervention. Vigorous use of BVM in the peri-intubation phase risks cardiovascular collapse.
- Once intubated, patients with severe, life-threatening asthma are at significant risk of barotrauma, air trapping, dynamic hyperinflation, pulmonary tamponade and haemodynamic instability.
- High pCO_2 may be tolerated until the bronchospasm resolves. Ventilation strategy should focus on preventing air trapping, ensuring adequate oxygenation and minimising barotrauma with low respiratory rate and long expiratory time.

References

Krishnan H. Acute severe asthma. In Krishnan K, Fine-Goulden MR, Raman S, Deep A. Challenging concepts in paediatric critical care: cases with expert commentary. Oxford University Press, 2021.

National Asthma Council Australia. Australian asthma handbook: quick reference guide, V1.0 2014. Online. Available: https://www.trmc.net.au/pdf/australian-asthma-handbook.pdf. 9 September 2021.

Additional reading

Cote CJ. A practice of anesthesia for infants and children, fifth edition. Elsevier Saunders, 2013.

Ortiz-Alvarez O, Mikrogianakis A. Canadian Paediatric Society, Acute Care Committee. Managing the paediatric patient with and acute asthma exacerbations. Paediatr Child Health 2012; 17(5):251–255.

Randle E. Clinical guidelines: Acute severe asthma. NHS Children's Acute Transport Service. January 2020. Online. Available: https://cats.nhs.uk/wp-content/uploads/guideline-asthma.pdf. 8 September 2021.

Royal Children's Hospital Melbourne. Acute asthma. Online. Available: https://www.rch.org.au/clinicalguide/guideline_index/Asthma_Acute/. 8 September 2021.

Incident

An 11-year-old girl presented to a GP-run regional hospital with a worsening history of profound lethargy and vomiting. Careful history by the local clinician elicited polyuria and weight loss, and a diagnosis of diabetic ketoacidosis (DKA) was made following a blood glucose reading of 'Hi'. Intravenous access was obtained, and IV fluids and insulin infusion have been commenced. The clinic is relatively close to the PHRM base and the team arrives within 15 minutes of the referral so treatment has only recently started. Weight of child is 32 kg.

Relevant information

- **PHRM team transport options:** Land ambulance.
- **Additional resources:** Nursing staff and GP.
- **Retrieval options:** Nearest centre with paediatrician 30 minutes by road. Nearest centre with paediatric intensive care and paediatric anesthesia 90 minutes by road.
- **Other:** Nil.

RADIOMETER ABL90 SERIES

ABL90 ABL 90 ED PATIENT REPORT	Syringe-S 65uL		08:31 Sample # 10572
Identifications			
Sample type	Venous		
Operator			
Patient ID			
Patient last name			
Date of birth			
T	37.0°C		
$PO_2(I)$	21.0 %		
Blood gas values			
↓ pH	6.787		(7.350 – 7.450)
↓ pCO_2	19.4	mmHg	(35.0 – 45.0)
↓ pO_2	51.5	mmHg	(80.0 – 105)
Electrolyte values			
cNa^+	144	mmol/L	(135 – 148)
cK^+	4.0	mmol/L	(3.5 – 5.3)
↑ cCl^+	114	mmol/L	(98 – 106)
↑ cCa^{2+}	1.79	mmol/L	(1.13 – 1.32)
Metabolite values			
cGlu	34	mmol/L	(–)
cLac	1.9	mmol/L	(0.5 – 2.0)
?↓ ctBl		mmol/L	(–)
Oximetry values			
ctHb	141	g/L	
↓ sO_2	81.1	%	(95.0 – 98.0)
PO_2Hb	82.2	%	
$PCOHb$	0.4	%	(–)
↓ $PMetHb$	−1.7	%	(0.0 – 15)
$PHHb$	19.1	%	
Calculated values			
Hct_c	43.3	%	
?↓ SBE_c	−31.8	mmol/L	(−2.4 – 2.3)
↓ $cHCO_2^-(P)_c$	2.9	mmol/L	(22.0 – 26.0)
Temperature-corrected values			
pH(T)	6.787		
$pO_2(T)$	51.5	mmHg	
$pCO_2(T)$	19.4	mmHg	

Question 60.1

What should the PHRM team be doing for preparation and stabilisation prior to transport?

Clinical information

On arrival, the following clinical information is available:
- Lethargic. Pale with cool peripheries
- P 137.
- RR 28. Deep Kussmaul breathing
- SaO_2 98% on room air.
- Temperature 36.3°C (97.3°F).
- Ketones (finger prick): 6 mmol/L
- Treatment administered: Normal Saline 1 L bolus just finishing. Insulin infusion at 3.2 units/hr (0.1 unit/kg/hr)

Question 60.2

Discuss ongoing management of this case and potential complications.

Discussion 60.1

It is important to establish the severity of the DKA, which will determine management priorities and will predict potential issues. A venous blood gas (see image), serum electrolytes and ketone levels are essential.

Management priorities
Assessment of dehydration and rehydration
An accurate clinical assessment of dehydration is notoriously difficult; however, many guidelines suggest that established DKA indicates at least 10% dehydration. In addition, chronic dehydration is subtly different from acute dehydration as the fluid loss has come from the intracellular space in addition to the intravascular and/or extracellular spaces. Rehydration should occur around two concepts: resuscitation to initially stabilise (if required) and then slow rehydration to allow equilibration across the fluid spaces. Large volumes of high chloride concentration fluids (such as normal saline 0.9%) will eventually lead to hyperchloraemic acidosis. Consideration should be made towards low chloride concentration iso-osmolar fluids as the resuscitation progresses.

This patient is profoundly dehydrated (estimated level of dehydration 10%) and shocked so the fluid bolus was appropriate. In this case the best approach would be to slowly re-establish iv fluids whilst the clinical situation is re-assessed and repeat blood gas analysis performed. Iso-osmolar should be used at 92 ml/hr (approximately 2/3 maintenance, assuming 10% dehydration corrected over 48 hours).

Insulin
Insulin is essential to switch off ketogenesis and should be continued even when euglycaemia is achieved as elevated ketone levels contribute to the vicious cycle of nausea, vomiting and anorexia. In this case, following a fluid bolus, the rate should be

reduced to 0.05 U/kg/hr (half the current rate). In severe cases, too rapid normalisation of glucose levels with high insulin doses may cause dramatic osmotic shifts risking cerebral oedema.

Sodium

One formula for calculating corrected sodium in hyperglycaemia is:

$$\frac{\left(\text{measured glucose} - \text{glucose upper limit of normal}\right)}{3} + \text{measured sodium} = \text{corrected sodium.}$$

In this case, the calculation is:

$$\frac{(34 - 7)}{3} + 144 = 153$$

Where glucose is 34, glucose upper limit of normal is 7 and measured sodium is 144.

Thus, this child has hypernatraemic dehydration. This has a lower association with cerebral oedema; however, may still cause neurological complications and dysfunction. After initial resuscitation, sodium levels should be reduced by no more than 0.5 mEq/L/h over 48–72 hours.

Hyponatraemic dehydration is associated with a higher risk of cerebral oedema and slow, careful rehydration and treatment is indicated to prevent this occurring.

Potassium

Most potassium (99%) is held in the intracellular space, and measured blood potassium level is usually falsely reassuring because acidosis causes potassium to move into the extracellular space. With the administration of insulin and correction of acidaemia, it is likely the blood potassium level will drop rapidly as it once again becomes intracellular. In addition, serum potassium is inversely related to serum pH and, as a rule of thumb, increases by 0.3 mEq/L for every 0.1 U decrease in pH below normal. In this case, the corrected potassium would be expected to be around 2.2.

Blood gas K^+ = 4.0 mmol/L

pH = 6.7

Decrease in pH = 0.6 × 0.3 = 1.8

Therefore potassium is 4.0 − 1.8 = 2.2 mmol/L

Cautious potassium replacement should commence once the patient's potassium is within normal range, and the patient is passing urine. The rate should not exceed 0.4 mmol/kg/hr. Adding 30 mmol potassium to a 1 L bag of plasmalyte would be normal replacement concentration in these situations.

Discussion 60.2

Monitoring

In a critically unwell patient with diabetic ketoacidosis in the retrieval environment, blood gases (including ketones, electrolytes and blood sugar level) should be performed hourly. It is likely that the acidosis will worsen as more acid (H+) comes out of the cellular space and into the vascular space in exchange for potassium. Clinical assessment of volume status must be regularly performed. Cardiorespiratory monitoring should be performed throughout and strict fluid balance documentation needs to be kept. Glasgow Coma Score should be recorded to monitor for early signs of cerebral oedema (see below).

Fluids

Once the patient is stabilised, maintenance and rehydration fluids should be commenced. Usually rehydration should occur over 48 hours and if there are concerns over cerebral oedema or hyper- or hyponatraemia, this can occur more slowly.

Once the blood glucose falls below 15 mmol, glucose should be added to the rehydration fluids, usually at 10% concentration.

Insulin

Insulin should be continued despite a falling blood glucose, as the end goal of treatment is to switch off the catabolic fat and protein gluconeogenesis processes that result in ketone production and switch energy production back to primarily carbohydrate metabolism. The success of this is measured by slow resolution of blood ketones which is ideally available during the retrieval phase of care.

Potassium

Ongoing potassium replacement should occur as it will take days to weeks to normalise whole body potassium levels. Consideration of phosphate replacement should also occur once the child is stabilised.

Cerebral oedema

Cerebral oedema is the most feared and life-threatening complication of DKA during the first 3–12 hours of resuscitation. Fluid shifts from the hypo-osmolar extracellular space to the osmotically active, dehydrated intracellular space within the brain result in swelling. Slow correction of glucose and electrolyte abnormalities are the key to prevention of cerebral oedema. Excess administration of IV fluids and any hypo-osmolar fluids must be avoided. Patients with DKA who remain obtunded, despite appropriate initial management, are assumed to have cerebral oedema and should be managed with appropriate medical therapy, including hypertonic saline or mannitol. Rapid sequence induction and intubation should be seen as a last resort as it can precipitate decompensation due to a rapid increase in pCO_2 with corresponding worsening acidaemia. To minimise this risk, a modified approach to RSI should be utilised. After administration of general anaesthesia and subsequent apnoea, the patient should be gently hand ventilated to maintain a low $paCO_2$.

Bicarbonate

Bicarbonate is rarely indicated in DKA as it is associated with an increased risk of cerebral oedema. However, it should be administered in patients with life-threatening hyperkalaemia.

Sepsis

DKA is uncommonly precipitated by systemic infection; however, broad spectrum antibiotics should be considered on a case-by-case basis.

Gastric stasis

Gastric stasis is common in DKA and consideration should be given to an enteric tube especially if aeromedical transport is planned.

Key points

- The prime issues in DKA are dehydration, acidosis, electrolyte disturbance and cerebral oedema.
- The retrieval phase of care presents the opportunity for therapeutic intervention in addition to the prevention of iatrogenic harm. Therefore careful management during this phase will significantly improve the patient's recovery and avoid complications such as cerebral oedema.

Additional reading

Paediatric BASIC: Basic assessment and support in paediatric intensive care, third edition. Online. Available: https://www.aic.cuhk.edu.hk/pae_basic/courses_ad.php?country= Australia.

Royal Children's Hospital Melbourne. Diabetic ketoacidosis. Online. Available: https://www.rch.org.au/clinicalguide/guideline_index/Diabetic_Ketoacidosis/. 10 September 2021.

Wolfsdorf J I, Glaser N, Agus M, et al. ISPAD clinical practice consensus guidelines: diabetic ketoacidosis and the hyperglycemic hyperosmolar state. Pediatr. Diabetes. 2018; 19(27):155–177. doi:10.1111/pedi.12701.

Incident

A 33-week gestation mother attends a rural emergency department with contractions and per vaginum (PV) loss of clear fluid. She is examined and found to be 6 cm dilated. The local obstetric team feels comfortable delivering the baby.

Relevant information

- **PHRM team transport options:** Fixed-wing aircraft.
- **Additional resources:** Local GP on-call to attend to emergencies. Land ambulance and crew.
- **Retrieval options:** Hospital with neonatal intensive care capacity 5 hours by road, 40 minutes' flight time.
- **Other:** Nearest centre with paediatrician 1 hour by road.

Question 61.1

What should be considered in preparation for a retrieval response?

The baby is delivered vaginally and weighs 1.75 kg at birth. Apgars are quoted as 7 at 1 minute and 8 at five minutes.

Clinical information

On arrival of the PHRM team, the following clinical information is available:
- Pale pink; 'flat' with some spontaneous movement.
- Subcostal and intercostal recession with nasal flaring.
- HR 120.
- RR 45.
- SaO_2 90% on room air.
- Temperature 36°C.

Question 61.2

What is your differential diagnosis?

Question 61.3

Discuss further management.

Discussion 61.1

The aim in the PHRM environment with regard to premature newborns should be to get the correct specialised team to the correct patient with the right equipment in a timely manner. In this case, the support of efficient ventilation and maintaining thermoregulation are the key priorities. While many peripheral units may request a specialist team to be present for the delivery, it should be noted that the duration of labour is unpredictable and a team may be tied up in a distant location for significant amounts of time if this path is followed. It is usually better to wait for the baby to be delivered or a definite delivery time to be decided (e.g. a caesarean section is started) before mobilisation of any resources (see Case 42).

It is always useful to raise the option of retrieving the mother with foetus in-utero. Depending on local resources, utilising a multidisciplinary perinatal advice line may be useful for decision making. Outcomes for premature and extremely premature newborns are improved by delivery in a tertiary neonatal/perinatal centre. Delivery in a larger centre may also present fewer risks for the mother in relation to management of pre-, peri- and postnatal complications. If the pregnant mother is moved with the baby in-utero, a single team (usually an adult team) can be tasked, limiting the logistical planning otherwise needed to transfer both baby and mother postpartum. If in-utero transfer is not possible, then it is important to try and keep mother and baby together as this will assist in establishing breastfeeding and other neurodevelopmental benefits of maternal contact. It should be remembered that recently delivered mothers will, in all likelihood, be in-patients, and the local team will need to arrange admission to the maternity service of the same hospital as her baby. It should be clear where responsibilities lie; the retrieval team is there for the baby and should not compromise their cognitive bandwidth by also assuming responsibility for the mother.

Once it is clear that the baby will be delivered in a peripheral unit, advice and support can be given while the PHRM team is mobilised.

- The most senior/experienced clinician should be identified and called in if they are not at the hospital.
- The delivery room should be kept as warm as possible, drafts minimised and the temperature raised.
- Adjuncts for thermoregulation should be identified: dry/warmed towels, blankets, plastic bags/wrap (for extremely premature infants).
- If a resuscitaire, or heated workspace, is available, it should be prepared.
- It may be useful to discuss airway management plans with the referring unit. If positive pressure ventilation and/or PEEP can be effectively delivered via face mask (ideally NeoPuff device) then it may be advisable to hold intubation until the PHRM team is present, particularly if the local team is not confident with this procedure.
- Neonatal resuscitative procedures are a niche skill set which many practitioners may not have performed recently, if at all. Following the principle that the first attempt should be the best attempt, it may be necessary for the tasking agency to reassure the referring team that certain procedures should be postponed until the arrival of the PHRM team.

Discussion 61.2

'Prematurity' as a diagnosis describes a range of delayed physiological adaptations on the journey from fetus to newborn. Birth at different gestational ages can be expected to present with particular challenges – for example, earlier gestations have significantly more fragile skin. However, there are a few broad groupings that may present challenges for the PHRM team:

- Airway – premature infants have small airways. Practitioners may be unfamiliar or inexperienced in the instrumentation of smaller airways. It is important to remember alternatives such as supraglottic airways or, in the case of extremely small neonates, good-quality bag-mask ventilation and avoiding fixation on advanced airway management.
- Breathing – premature infants have proportionally low muscle mass and will tire easily. Intubation/ventilation may be necessary for this factor alone. Abdominal

distension secondary to bagging can splint the diaphragm and cause compromise, a frequently aspirated gastric tube is essential, particularly if prolonged mask IPPV or CPAP is delivered.

- Ventilation/gas exchange – all premature babies will have some degree of lung immaturity. Alveolar development should be presumed to be delayed in any premature baby or small baby of uncertain gestation. This will impact on ventilation strategies and accepted blood gas parameters. It should be noted that premature babies tolerate hypercapnoea well, while even relatively mild hypocapnoea may be associated with increased risk of intraventricular haemorrhage. Particularly in the case of premature babies, discussion with a neonatal intensivist may be helpful in determining ventilation strategy.
- Circulation – in contrast to adults, most acute neonatal compromise is primarily respiratory. In an uncomplicated neonatal resuscitation, adequate ventilatory support will usually reverse a falling heart rate. However, volume replacement should be considered. Premature babies are more susceptible to fluid loss given their large surface area to volume ratio and their thin skin. Feto-maternal haemorrhage is difficult to diagnose acutely and in the case of a large peri-delivery maternal bleed, a blood transfusion for the baby may be indicated. Many neonatal retrieval services carry blood for this purpose.
- Temperature – newborns are extremely sensitive to changes in temperature. Babies who become cold have poor neurodevelopmental outcomes. This is a key capability of a neonatal transport cot. Continuous temperature monitoring (rectal, oesophageal or skin) is used as standard.
- Sugar control – regular BSLs should be taken and babies commenced on a 10% dextrose infusion if unable to be fed enterally.

Discussion 61.3

The management of premature newborns often causes significant stress for referring teams. While the incidence of premature delivery is around 10%, the majority of these take place in larger centres with dedicated teams and clinicians; therefore, many local teams will have managed this type of patient infrequently, if at all.

Premature delivery often places strain on local resources as both mother and baby will likely need management and treatment.

In addition to the unfamiliarity of the clinical scenario there is often a significant emotional burden associated with premature delivery and the possible long-term implications of resuscitation. It is important that teams have the opportunity to debrief, even if the resuscitation and retrieval are successful. Debriefing visits to the local unit may also be helpful both for them and the PHRM specialists.

Logistics

In this complex scenario the retrieval team may be required to serve as much logistically as clinically. Open communication is necessary between the clinical team and the coordination centre:

- Are there more experienced or specialist clinicians who could be tasked?
- Are additional teams required to manage mother and baby?
- Is coordination able to provide clinical support and advice while the team is en route?

● Are there other resources which could be leveraged (videoconferencing or neo-natal expertise at the receiving unit)?

PHRM teams specialising in neonatal retrievals are essential, particularly in cases of premature delivery as specialised equipment will be needed. Neonatal ventilation requires infant-specific ventilators or infant-specific software and circuits to deliver appropriate ventilation and humidification. Neonatal transport cots are needed to safely secure a small baby for transport and maintain their temperature.

A PHRM team will bring appropriately sized equipment to deal with the full range of neonatal patients from 500 g to 5 kg, or the maximum-size baby that will fit safely in a transport cot (see Appendix 2.2 and Figure 61.1 below).

Calculations

Neonatal dosing is based on patient weights. Calculating doses can be difficult in the heat of the moment. Doses should be double checked, but it is good practice to use a reputable drug/dose calculator. There is a range of online or app-based calculators that can provide dosing based on weight or gestation.

Intubation and ventilation

Intubation of premature infants is usually achieved using an uncuffed TT and a straight Miller blade. Increasingly, videolaryngoscopy is used in neonatal intubation.

The tubes should be inserted to: weight (in kg) + 6 cm.

This sizing is for an orally inserted tube. Neonates are much more susceptible to TT misplacement then adults, due to their proportionally shorter trachea; when the total tracheal length is less than 5 cm, 1 cm too deep or shallow is a significant length that

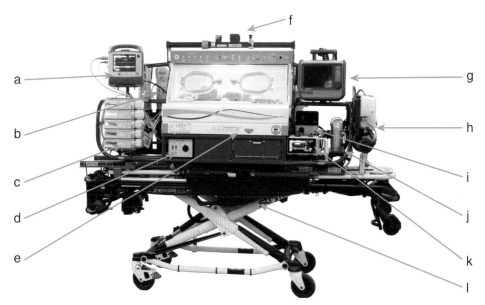

Figure 61.1 Key capabilities of a neonatal transport cot: a. advanced monitoring (arterial, central, temperature, ETCO$_2$, pre and post ductal SaO$_2$), b. gas mixing c. additional infusion pump d. Powered transport cot (temperature regulation, sound / vibration protection, storage of essential emergency equipment, radiant heat, lighting and a solid platform for procedural use) e. Stretcher base f. Bilitron (transport phototherapy), g. ventilator, h. inhaled nitric oxide (iNO), i. Humidification, j. Portable suction unit, k. Additional monitor." (With permission from Neocot.)

may lead to accidental extubation or ventilation of only the right lung, with a risk of pneumothorax. Tube depth should be calculated from a bony structure (the midline of the upper lip/maxilla) and secured there. Newborn facial structures are very mobile, TTs secured in the corner of the mouth are dangerous as they are prone to significant motion. As a rule, the tip of the tracheal tube will follow the tip of the nose. For example, flexing the patient's neck will result in advancement of the TT.

Some neonatologists will use a nasal intubation but this should only be performed by an experienced and confident operator. The TT should be secured in a way that the team is comfortable with. Newborn TTs are usually taped in place with some variation of a double trouser leg/Melbourne strapping (see Appendix 1.1.7). Unless the baby is in extremis, a CXR should be performed to assess for lung pathology and importantly to check TT position particularly if surfactant administration is required.

Premature newborns are by definition, surfactant deficient. Provision of appropriately stored surfactant via a TT is a key capability of a neonatal PHRM service. The advised dose is 200 mg/kg and it is recommended to round up the dose to the nearest whole vial. There are dedicated surfactant administration kits; however, in an emergency retrieval setting, surfactant can be drawn up and administered down the TT in two aliquots through a pre-measured size 5 Fr gastric tube or a blunt needle. After each aliquot, the baby should be hand ventilated or the ventilator re-connected. Surfactant can produce a rapid response and care should be taken to wean both PIP and FiO_2 to avoid iatrogenic injury.

Due to lung immaturity, surfactant deficiency and pathology, premature lungs are extremely susceptible to shearing trauma from ventilation. This baro/volu-trauma has significant implications for long term pathology of Chronic Lung Disease (CLD), also referred to as Bronchopulmonary Dysplasia (BPD). Volume-targeted ventilation with a tidal volume starting at 4 mL/kg aims to reduce the risk of this shearing force.

Provision of IV medications and central monitoring

Peripheral IV insertion can be challenging for local teams to achieve. An appropriately trained PHRM team can gain peripheral and central IV and arterial access for the purposes of administering medication and fluids and for monitoring. Point-of-care testing is another key capability of the PHRM team.

Sepsis/Infection

While spontaneous premature delivery does occur, there is usually a pathophysiological trigger to account for the initiation of labour.

Bacterial infection is a common cause of premature birth and subsequent pathology. The most common causative agent is Group B Streptococcus (GBS) which is exquisitely sensitive to penicillins. Generally, GBS is managed with penicillin and gentamicin for putative synergistic effect. Maternal vaginal swabbing is not necessarily reassuring in the context of GBS.

Given the potential benefit of antibiotic therapy in the reduction of morbidity and mortality, and the low risk of any adverse effect, any premature baby should be started on antibiotics.

As with the majority of cases, premature neonates have the best outcomes when basic care is done extremely well. Maintaining adequate temperature and supporting ventilation with minimal airway instrumentation may be of greater benefit than embarking upon more complex interventions with unproven benefits.

Key points

- The threatened pre-term labour presents significant logistical challenges for the clinical coordination team.
- The out-born premature neonate presents significant clinical challenges.
- Out-born premature neonates are at risk of poor outcomes but this can be mitigated by high-level neonatal response.
- Neonatal retrieval medicine encapsulates the core principles of PHRM, whereby delivering the right team, with the right equipment in the right timeframe will maximise positive clinical outcome

Additional reading

Cheo Ed Outreach. Neonatal Resuscitation Drug Calculator. Online. Available: https://outreach.cheo.on.ca/emergency-drug-calculator/14. 10 September 2021.

Newborn and paediatric Emergency Transport Service (NETS). NETS clinical calculator. Online. Available: https://www.nets.org.au/NETS-Clinical-Calculator.aspx. 10 September 2021.

Royal College of Paediatrics and Child Health (RCPCH). Neonatal electronic dose calculator. https://qicentral.rcpch.ac.uk/medsiq/safe-prescribing/neonatal-electronic-dose-calculator-acute-neonatal-transport-service/. 10 September 2021.

Incident

A 9-year-old boy has been mountain biking in the local foothills with his friends. He slipped and fell, hitting the right side of his head against a rock. He was wearing a helmet. He was witnessed to have a brief (10-second) period of loss of consciousness and appeared to stop breathing. This resolved spontaneously and he was taken to the local healthcare facility. Having initially been confused and agitated, he is reported to be improving and is now (at 2 hours post injury) GCS 14 (M6, V5, E3). He has post-event amnesia and has vomited once.

Relevant information

- **PHRM team transport options:** Rotary-wing aircraft; land ambulance and crew.
- **Additional resources:** Regional hospital with GP cover and no CT scanner.
- **Retrieval options:** Nearest hospital with general surgery capability and CT scanner is 30 minutes by road. Nearest major trauma centre with paediatric intensive care and paediatric surgery 90-minute's flight time.
- **Other:** 21:00 hours. Rain forecast for the night.

Question 62.1

What advice could be offered to the local GP attending the patient?

Question 62.2

Should a PHRM team be tasked to this case?

Clinical information

After further examination, 3 hours post-injury, the GP re-engages the PHRM clinical coordinators:

- GCS 13 (M6, V4, E3). Lethargic and erratic with responses. Boggy, tender swelling to right fronto-temporal region, not previously appreciated. Pupils 3 mm and reactive bilaterally. No neck pain but cervical spine not formally cleared. Tender left wrist.
- P 98.
- RR 15.
- SaO_2 98% on room air.
- BP 110/80.

Drugs administered:
Fluid bolus 10 mL/kg 0.9% NaCl
Paracetamol IV 15 mg/kg
Ondansetron 4 mg IV

Question 62.3

How does this additional information influence your decision making?

Due to weather delays, the GP has sent the patient to the nearby hospital with access to a CT scanner. The patient remains clinically unchanged. The CT scan is shown below.

Question 62.4

How does this alter your management plan?

Discussion 62.1

This patient appears to have suffered at least a mild traumatic brain injury (TBI). Mild TBI may present with altered cognition and/or consciousness, headache and vomiting. A deterioration in condition is usually predictive of other injuries, particularly intracranial haemorrhage causing raised intracranial pressure.

Signs of skull fracture should be sought, such as bruising around eyes and behind the ears, otorrhea or rhinorrhea or any boggy swelling on the scalp. Any evidence of a skull fracture is suggestive of a corresponding intracranial bleed. The patient should be examined for neurological deficit with an emphasis on repeated GCS and pupil assessment.

Impact brain apnoea

Traumatic brain injury often results in a period of apnoea. From animal studies, it has been demonstrated that the period of apnoea is proportional to the degree of force. Impact brain apnoea is underappreciated in humans because healthcare workers do not usually witness the apnoeic period, and the hypoxic brain damage that may result can mistakenly be attributed to diffuse axonal injury. Impact brain apnoea may also be associated with cardiovascular instability. Although it is often stated that hypotension cannot be caused by an isolated head injury (implying you should look for other causes of hypovolaemia), a small proportion of hypotensive trauma patients (SBP <90 mmHg) may have an isolated head injury and this hypotension can be attributed to impact brain apnoea.

Other injuries

It is assumed that this patient has suffered an isolated head injury; however, given the mechanism and ongoing symptoms, there is a high probability of other injuries. Occult injuries to the abdomen, chest and perineum (particularly due to handlebar impact) are often initially missed in these situations. Therefore, a full secondary survey needs to be performed while maintaining C-spine protection.

If he continues to vomit, a non-sedating anti-emetic should be administered, along with simple analgesia.

Discussion 62.2

The need for transfer is questionable at this point. The patient's sole identified injury is a mild TBI with evidence of moderate concussion, and observation in an appropriate sensible environment would be the mainstay of management.

The main indications for transferring the patient include:
- Access to a CT scanner
- Observations in a neurosurgical centre.

Those against transfer include:
- Patient is easily managed locally
- Night helicopter transfer in bad weather carries aviation risks.

Discussion 62.3

This update changes the clinical situation dramatically. The boggy swelling and the fact that the patient has an ongoing altered GCS more than two hours after the injury is highly suggestive of a skull fracture with associated intracranial pathology (Osmond et al 2010).

An urgent retrieval to a neurosurgical centre is now indicated and a PHRM team should be dispatched by helicopter.

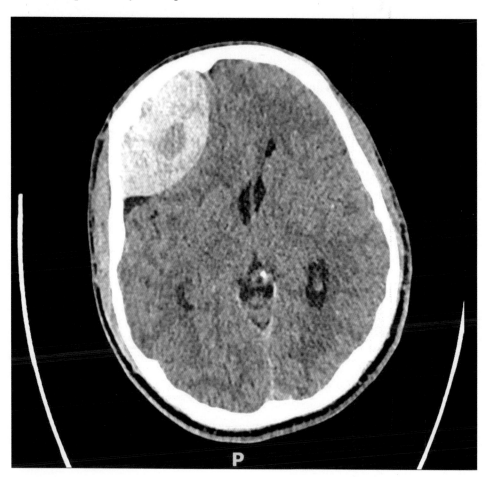

Discussion 62.4

The CT scan demonstrates an acute extradural haemorrhage with mass effect.

The primary active treatment of an enlarging extradural haemorrhage is operative drainage – everything else is temporising. Many clinicians advocate intubation and ventilation in anticipation of the predictable sequelae of this condition. There is an alternative school of thought that leaving the patient conscious at this point in time is advantageous for several reasons: it allows easier assessment for deterioration; the act of intubation is not without risk and may cause a spike in ICP if not managed properly. Indeed, a number of extradural haematomas are managed conservatively.

However, this patient has ongoing neurological signs >3 hours post injury and is at risk of complications, including seizures and rapid decompensation due to raised intracranial pressure. These would be extremely difficult to manage should they occur acutely during transport in a helicopter at night. For this reason, intubation and ventilation of this patient would be appropriate.

Discussion with the receiving neurosurgical team and PICU team needs to occur through the clinical coordination centre. Consideration may be made to transfer an appropriately skilled neurosurgical team to the patient to allow drainage and stabilisation at the referring hospital. While this is an option, the time taken to arrange personnel and necessary additional equipment on an ad hoc basis often makes this option impractical.

Post intubation, the child needs to be closely observed for signs of raised intracranial pressure, and preparations should be made for emergency treatment should he deteriorate (see also Case 10):

- Raise the head of the bed to 30 degrees.
- Suppress cough with adequate sedation.
- Have gastric tube on free drainage.
- Maintain euvolaemia (preferably at 2/3 maintenance IV fluids).
- Consider osmotic agent (either mannitol or hypertonic saline 3%) after discussion with neurosurgical centre.
- Ventilate to a low–normal pCO_2 (e.g. 30–35 mmHg [4–4.5 kPa]).
- Consider seizure prophylaxis.
- Take care with cerebral venous drainage – TT ties/c-spine collar.

Key points

- Key features in the history and examination of a child following head injury may significantly change the management plan and need to be actively sought during the initial consultation.
- The following risk factors in a head-injured child suggest significant intracranial pathology that may require urgent neurosurgical intervention:
  - GCS <15 two hours post injury
  - Clinical evidence of a skull fracture
  - Worsening headache (or irritability in a baby).
- The decision to perform paediatric emergency anaesthesia requires a careful risk–benefit analysis.

References

Osmond MH, Klassen TP, Wells GA, et al, for the Pediatric Emergency Research Canada (PERC) Head Injury Study Group. CATCH: a clinical decision rule for the use of computed tomography in children with minor head injury. CMAJ, 2010; 182(4):341–348. doi:https://doi.org/10.1503/cmaj.091421.

Additional reading

Babl FE, Tavender E, Ballard DW, et al, for the Paediatric Research in Emergency Departments International Collaborative (PREDICT). Australian and New Zealand guideline for mild to moderate head injuries in children. Emerg. Med. Australas. 2021; 33(2):214–231. doi:10.1111/1742-6723.13722.

Royal Children's Hospital Melbourne. Head injury. Online. Available: https://www.rch.org.au/clinicalguide/guideline_index/Head_injury/. 14 September 2021.

Samuels M, Wieteska S (Eds). Advanced paediatric life support: a practical approach to emergencies (Advanced Life Support Group), 6th edn. BMJ Books, Wiley Blackwell, 2017.

Incident

A 2-year-old boy has presented to a regional emergency department with a short history of fever, cough and coryza. During a prolonged period in the waiting room, he has further deteriorated and his mother has approached the triage nurse with concerns about his increasing agitation and an evolving rash to his trunk. After rapid assessment, he is rushed into the resus bay and the PHRM service is contacted. The following image is sent to the PHRM service.

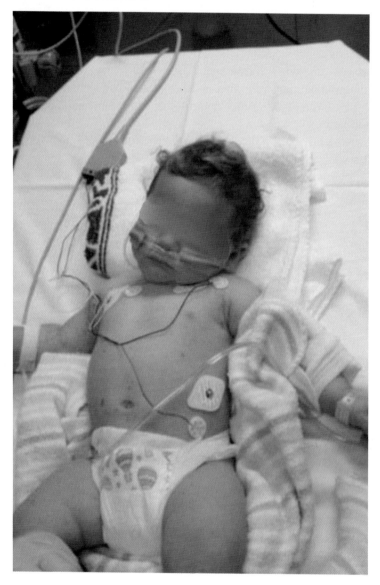

Clinical information

During the initial consult, the following clinical information is provided:
- Weight: 12 kg.
- Hot to touch centrally, non-blanching rash to trunk and limbs.

- Airway patent, child remains agitated on mum's lap.
- RR 80, O_2 delivered via NRBM (15 L/min), SaO_2 – poor trace.
- HR 180 (sinus tachycardia), CRT 6 seconds, peripheral pulses not able to be palpated, automated BP unrecordable.
- Unable to obtain IV-access.
- Drugs/Fluid administered: nil.

Relevant information

- **PHRM team resources:** Rotary-wing.
- **Additional resources:** Regional ED with emergency physicians. Land ambulance and crew.
- **Retrieval options:** Nearest centre with on-site PICU is 30 minutes' flight time. Nearest centre with on-site PICU and ECMO is 120 minutes' flight time.
- **Other:** Nil.

Question 63.1

What are the treatment priorities for the local team?

Question 63.2

Outline key considerations in the retrieval response.

On arrival of the PHRM team, the above interventions have been initiated; however, the child's conscious level has deteriorated, and he is now unresponsive. He remains tachypnoeic with a tightly fitted NRBM with 15 L/min O_2, HR 220 (sinus tachycardia), central pulse palpable only, SaO_2 and BP remain undetectable. Widespread purpura fulminans.

Question 63.3

What should the PHRM team be doing for preparation and stabilisation prior to transport?

Discussion 63.1

Commencement of treatment cannot be delayed till arrival of the PHRM team, no matter their proximity.

As soon as a clinical diagnosis of suspected septic shock (inadequate tissue perfusion, signs of SIRS and suspected infection) has been made by the local team, the patient should be moved to the highest acuity area in the hospital. In most cases this will be the allocated resuscitation area within the emergency department. Full (age-appropriate) cardiorespiratory monitoring should be applied and the most senior clinicians (preferably with advanced airway skills) should be informed and attend. This patient will require significant nursing care, and allowances within the department should be made to achieve this. Timely recognition and resuscitation of septic shock is vital to ensure optimal outcomes as associated mortality with treatment delay is significant.

Treatment priorities in chronological order are:

- Assessment of airway and breathing
- Simultaneous application of supplemental O_2 to help prevent tissue hypoxemia
- Rapid establishment of vascular access.

Intravenous access is often difficult to achieve. Larger veins such as the cubital, long saphenous and external jugular should all be considered, and ultrasound guidance used as required. If not established within 5 minutes, attempts should be abandoned, and intraosseous access should be obtained. Blood samples should be collected on insertion and the following investigations organised.

- Blood cultures and a venous blood gas (glucose/ionised calcium/lactate) take priority over all other tests; however, ideally, a complete set of laboratory tests should be obtained
- FBC, UEC, LFTs, Calcium, Magnesium, Phosphate
- CRP/Procalcitonin/Viral and bacterial PCRs
- Coagulation studies
- Group and hold.

Further diagnostic tests such as urinalysis, CXR and lumbar puncture should be delayed until stabilisation is achieved. Hypoglycaemia and hypocalcaemia should be anticipated and treated promptly.

Ideally, two points of IV/IO access should be established as required for ongoing resuscitation. Empiric broad-spectrum antibiotics as an IV/IO push should be administered immediately as per local antimicrobial guidelines. In the rare situation where IV/IO access has not been established after 15 minutes, intramuscular ceftriaxone 100 mg/kg should be given in all age groups. In addition, acyclovir (20 mg/kg IV) for potential herpes simplex virus infection and/or Clindamycin (15 mg/kg IV) for suspected toxin-related disease should be given. Special antimicrobial considerations for immunocompromised patients should be made, and local guidelines followed.

The first fluid bolus should be given as soon as practically possible (via 'push-pull' or rapid infuser over 5–10 minutes) in the form of 10–20 mL/kg of either a balanced crystalloid or normal saline, and patient fluid responsiveness should be assessed. If the patient still appears fluid-responsive and no signs of fluid overload are present, the bolus can be repeated as required to a maximum of 40 mL/kg. If there is no improvement in perfusion and/or there is ongoing circulatory failure, start vasoactive support early. In the majority of cases, initiation of a peripheral adrenaline infusion would be appropriate (see Case 29). An easy method for drawing up and administering an adrenaline infusion rapidly would be 6 mg adrenaline in a 1 L bag of NaCl 0.9% dose range 0.5–5 mL/h (0.05–0.5 mcg/kg/h). Concurrent fluid resuscitation can take place if patient remains fluid-responsive.

If considered, HFNC/NIV instead of supplemental O_2 can be used as long as consciousness is maintained, and it does not delay plans to establish tracheal intubation.

Discussion 63.2

PHRM team composition

This is a critically ill child at serious risk of long-term morbidity and death. The most experienced and skilled PHRM team should respond to this case. This may be achieved by augmenting the PHRM team with a paediatric intensive care specialist. A standardised process and fixed communication pathways should be in place to facilitate this rare requirement, and this should not unnecessarily delay the PHRM team response.

Ongoing resuscitation

It is important for the patient to avoid the therapeutic vacuum while the retrieval response is coordinated. During this 'golden hour' of resuscitation, ongoing clinical assessment and updates to the PHRM service are vital, so goals of treatment can be tailored to the individual patient and ongoing care can be arranged as indicated. This would include advice from paediatric critical care experts through the coordination centre.

Retrieval options

Note there are two paediatric critical care units available; however, only one of these has ECMO capability. It is currently too early to definitely decide on the need for ECMO. Any child with fluid refractory septic shock and vasoactive treatment will require PICU-level care, and thought should be given to the availability of extracorporeal organ support availability of ECMO within the receiving paediatric intensive care unit prior to transfer. This potentially definitive option should be considered early using multiparty discussions facilitated by the coordination centre.

Discussion 63.3

It is well recognised that early resolution of septic shock has a significant positive impact on subsequent end organ perfusion and overall survival. On balance, the PHRM team should be prepared to spend some time on the ground optimising the patient's haemodynamic status prior to transport, to minimise the time spent in septic shock. This constitutes definitive care and is independent of location. Ongoing resuscitation during transfer is required, especially when initial treatment has not adequately restored the circulation, and judicious fluid resuscitation, appropriate respiratory support and titration of vasoactive drugs should all continue.

Induction of anaesthesia and tracheal intubation for fluid- and catecholamine-resistant septic shock prior to transfer is indicated due to altered level of consciousness (agitation, lethargy or reduced GCS) and worsening respiratory status. Intubation provides a protected airway, reducing the risk of aspiration, improved oxygenation and ventilation, significant reduced metabolic demand and left ventricular afterload reduction.

Hypoxia, myocardial depression and afterload reduction are associated with induction of anaesthesia and intubation and can lead to respiratory and circulatory collapse. Optimisation of the patient as recommended above should take place prior to induction. Careful planning of a modified rapid sequence induction is required (see Cases 57–59). Prior to induction the patient should have received:

- Volume resuscitation
- Ongoing vasoactive support
- Pre-oxygenation
- NGT insertion
- Anaesthetic drugs drawn up as per local weight-based resuscitation guidelines:
  - Ketamine (0.5–1 mg/kg) and rocuronium (1.6 mg/kg) would be suggested for patients >3 months of age. Ketamine should be replaced by fentanyl (1–2 mcg/kg) in the <3 months of age patient population. Both ketamine and fentanyl should be given slowly to prevent side effects.
  - Push-dose and resus-dose adrenaline drawn up and ready (see Appendix 7).
- A gaseous induction is contraindicated due to the cardiovascular side effects, unless superseded by a (suspected) difficult airway.
- Propofol, thiopentone and benzodiazepines all have an unfavourable cardiovascular side-effect profile and should be avoided.

Use of a paediatric intubation checklist and 'time-out' is recommended and careful role allocation should make optimal use of each individual's skill set during this anticipated high-risk procedure. It can be useful to allocate a team member to palpate the femoral pulse and alert the team to PEA arrest early. Tracheal tube placement should be confirmed with continuous $ETCO_2$ monitoring and CXR. Ongoing sedation with an opioid infusion $+/-$ low-dose midazolam and non-depolarising muscle relaxant use can be considered.

A protective lung-ventilation strategy should be implemented.

Optimisation of cardiovascular status and frequent reassessment should take place prior and during transfer. Addition of vasopressin as a third agent with adrenaline and noradrenaline is reasonable and can be considered in consultation with the receiving PICU. The establishment of central venous access should be assessed on a case-by-case basis and is not automatically required when adequate IV/IO access is already in place. Invasive arterial blood pressure monitoring is preferred. Evaluation of cardio-vascular state includes repeated blood gas monitoring with specific attention to the change in lactate, and, if central venous access via the internal jugular has been estab-lished, can include a central venous saturation. Urine output is also a good marker of cardiovascular state and POCUS can be helpful (see Case 57).

Routine neurological assessment should include assessment and management of any signs of raised intracranial pressure, especially if meningitis is suspected (see Cases 10 and 62).

Electrolyte abnormalities should be corrected, especially hypocalcaemia and hyper-kalaemia. Regular blood glucose levels are required, especially if there is a previous episode of hypoglycaemia, and an ongoing infusion of dextrose saline will be required to maintain adequate blood glucose levels. The patient should remain fasted during transfer.

Septic shock is often associated with disseminated intravascular coagulopathy, and, if clinically significant bleeding is present, platelets, FFP and/or cryoprecipitate can be administered. Abnormal coagulation studies in isolation are not an indication for blood product transfusion. A pragmatic approach to red blood cell transfusion would be to aim for an Hb 90–100 g/L in a patient with fluid and catecholamine refractory septic shock with ongoing signs of inadequate tissue oxygenation. Otherwise, a transfusion threshold of 70 g/L is sufficient.

For fluid and catecholamine refractory shock, a stress dose of hydrocortisone should be considered, although definitive paediatric evidence is lacking.

Prior to transfer, antimicrobial treatment should be re-evaluated to ensure appropriate cover has been achieved. Source control should be identified and addressed if possible.

On occasion, a window of stability to transfer the patient may not be achieved and this should prompt renewed discussion with the PICU and the ECMO centre.

Although challenging, it is important that during the initial assessment, ongoing resuscitation and transfer process, the PHRM team builds rapport with the accompany-ing family members/carers. Empathetic, thoughtful and honest communication is vital to ensure shared decision making in the care of this critically unwell patient.

Key points

- Sepsis remains a rare but important cause of morbidity and mortality in the paediatric age group.
- Early aggressive intervention improves outcomes.
- A comprehensive PHRM response provides the best opportunity to improve outcomes for children presenting outside of tertiary centres.

Additional reading

Martin K, Weiss SL. Initial resuscitation and management of pediatric septic shock. Minerva Pediatr. 2015; 67(2):141–158.

Royal Children's Hospital Melbourne. Sepsis – assessment and management. Online. Available: https://www.rch.org.au/clinicalguide/guideline_index/SEPSIS_assessment_and_management/. 14 September 2021.

Southampton Paediatric Retrieval Service. Guidelines for the retrieval and management of severe sepsis and septic shock in infants and children. Online. Available: https://www.uhs.nhs.uk/Media/SUHTInternet/Services/IntensiveCare/PICU/SevereSepsisandSepticShockGuidelines.pdf. 14 September 2021.

Weiss SL, Peters MJ, Alhazzani W. Surviving Sepsis Campaign international guidelines for the management of septic shock and sepsis-associated organ dysfunction in children. Pediatr. Crit. Care Med. 2020; 21(2):e52–e106.

Weiss SL, Pomerantz WJ. Septic shock in children: ongoing management after resuscitation. Online. Available: https://www.uptodate.com/contents/septic-shock-in-children-ongoing-management-after-resuscitation?search=ongoing%20management%20after%20resuscitation&source=search_result&selectedTitle=1~150&usage_type=default&display_rank=1. 14 September 2021.

Weiss SL, Pomerantz WJ. Septic shock in children: rapid recognition and initial resuscitation (first hour). Online. Available: https://www.uptodate.com/contents/septic-shock-in-children-rapid-recognition-and-initial-resuscitation-first-hour?topicRef=86881&source=see_link#H19450291. 14 September 2021.

CASE 64

Incident

A 6-day-old neonate has presented to a regional hospital with a 12-hour history of poor feeding, lethargy and increased work of breathing. During a feed he was noted to be cyanosed and cool to his hands and feet. He was brought into hospital by ambulance. He was born at 39 weeks, following an uncomplicated pregnancy.

Clinical information

On arrival to the regional hospital, the following clinical information is available:
- Lethargic with low tone.
- P 175.
- RR 60.
- Capillary refill time 6–7 seconds, femoral pulses not palpable.
- SpO_2 90% (right arm) on room air with poor trace.
- Temperature 35.5°C (95.9°F).
- Blood glucose 0.9 mmol/L

Interventions done:
- Placed under warmer.
- 2 mL/kg of 10% Dextrose solution (D10W) administered.
- Hi-flow nasal cannula (HFNC) 2 L/kg/min FiO_2 40%.

Relevant information

- **PHRM team transport options:** Fixed-wing aircraft.
- **Additional resources:** General paediatrician in a regional hospital. Land ambulance.
- **Retrieval options:** Tertiary hospital with paediatric intensive care capacity and paediatric cardiac intensive care is an estimated 90-minute flight away.

Question 64.1

What is your differential diagnosis?

Question 64.2

On arrival, discuss how you will stabilise the neonate and prepare for transport?

Question 64.3

In the event of cardiac arrest at the referring centre or during transport, what are the key considerations if CPR is to continue throughout the retrieval?

Discussion 64.1

The differential diagnosis for a previously healthy newborn who presents in profound shock is broad. The most common causes are cardiac disease, sepsis and metabolic disorders. There can be considerable overlap in the presenting signs and symptoms, making it difficult to delineate a clear aetiology in the acute resuscitation phase. Less common, but important, differential diagnoses include respiratory, endocrine neurologic and gastrointestinal disorders. It is equally important to consider the possibility of non-accidental injury (NAI) or trauma.

Discussion 64.2

Given the emergent nature of the presentation it is important to simultaneously resuscitate the neonate while attempting to ascertain a diagnosis. An initial approach assessing the patient's airway, breathing and circulation (ABC) is important. The neonate in shock may have respiratory distress for many reasons, including primarily a respiratory or cardiac aetiology, or secondarily as compensation for metabolic acidosis or anaemia. A plan should be made to transfer the patient to a centre with broad paediatric critical care capacity, including neonatal extracorporeal membrane oxygenation (ECMO) if available.

The first step in providing resuscitative care is to ensure airway patency and to apply supplemental oxygen. Giving early positive end expiratory pressure (PEEP) via anaesthetic T-piece or CPAP/BiPAP mask is beneficial. Neonates in profound shock often require intubation. The indications for intubation include apnoeas, respiratory failure and shock. Intubating a sick neonate is a high-risk procedure, especially in a small regional centre that does not have the support of paediatric critical care or anaesthesia. It is important to have clear roles assigned to all team members and a shared understanding of the risks of tracheal intubation. Neonates have high oxygen consumption and a closing capacity that exceeds their functional residual capacity, putting them at increased risk of desaturation. In addition, there is a high risk of cardiovascular compromise. The anticipation of cardiovascular collapse is important.

Vascular access is required urgently, either peripherally if possible or via the intraosseous route. Umbilical venous access can be considered if the stump remains attached. An arterial line and/or central line is often indicated and should be inserted as soon as possible if within the scope of practice of the PHRM team. Bloods should be drawn for POC analysis including: blood gas, glucose, electrolytes and renal and liver function. Additional blood will be required for blood cultures. It is likely these blood cultures (plus other microbiology) will need to accompany the neonate to the tertiary facility. Repeat blood sampling will be required at the tertiary facility and this will include coagulation profile and ammonia level. Two separate points of vascular access should be established prior to transport. A patient like this should be resuscitated with a balanced crystalloid fluid in 10 mL/kg aliquots, with close assessment of response to each bolus, with prompt cessation of fluid administration if signs of cardiac compromise are noted (increased work of breathing, hepatomegaly, worsening perfusion). In addition, given the risk of cardiovascular collapse with the provision of anaesthetic agents, an inotrope infusion, such as adrenaline at a dose 0.05–1 mcg/kg/min should be established prior to induction. All resuscitation drugs should be readily available and administered as required as per the Advanced Paediatric Life Support (APLS) algorithms. The goal of providing induction agents in this setting is to optimise intubating conditions and could include fentanyl 1 mcg/kg or ketamine 0.5 mg/kg and rocuronium 1–2 mg/kg. Atropine (20 mcg/kg) should be drawn up and available should the neonate develop bradycardia. A term neonate whose size is appropriate for gestational age should be intubated with a size 3.5 internal diameter uncuffed tracheal tube (TT).

A preliminary assessment for the presence of congenital heart disease (CHD) is important in the initial management of a sick neonate, especially in the first week of life as this is when the ductus arteriosus typically closes, which can cause cardiovascular collapse in a neonate with a duct-dependent heart lesion. This patient was noted to have absent femoral pulses. This clinical finding raises the suspicion for a heart lesion in which the systemic circulation is duct dependent, such as coarctation of the aorta. Additional tests that may be useful in assessing for CHD are: checking preductal and postductal SpO_2 (right arm = preductal, lower limb = postductal), checking blood pressure in all four limbs, and conducting a hyperoxia test:

- Place the infant on 100% oxygen for 10 minutes.
- A lack of improvement in SpO_2 is suggestive of duct-dependent CHD.

A CXR and ECG should be readily available in most centres. Paediatric echocardiography is the gold standard but is unlikely to be available locally. When there is suspicion of duct-dependent CHD, a prostaglandin infusion (10-50 nanograms/kg/min) should be urgently initiated. High doses may be required to open a closed duct; this should be done in consultation with a paediatric intensivist/cardiologist. Close monitoring for the side effects (apnoeas, hypothermia, hypoglycemia and hypotension) of prostaglandin is required. A mean blood pressure of 40 is a reasonable target blood pressure for a term neonate. As described above, fluid boluses of 10 mL/kg should be administered with close re-assessment after each one. In cases of congenital heart disease, fluid resuscitation may precipitate heart failure, whereas a neonate in septic shock will potentially require significant intravascular volume resuscitation and the diagnosis is rarely clear at the outset.

The signs of sepsis in a neonate are often non-specific. Neonates with sepsis typically present without fever and they may have hypothermia. Other clinical findings include tachycardia or bradycardia, tachypnea, hypoglycaemia and increased or decreased leucocyte count. All neonates who present in shock require blood cultures and expeditious administration of broad-spectrum antibiotic and anti-viral coverage (as per local guidelines; e.g. Ampicillin + Gentamicin OR Cefotaxime + Acyclovir). The most common organisms include: Group B strep, E.coli and Listeria. At presentation, sepsis cannot be ruled out, even if an alternative diagnosis is present; thus, it is imperative to treat for presumed sepsis until culture results are available.

The presentation of a neonate in shock from an underlying metabolic disease can be variable. Presenting features may include metabolic acidosis, metabolic alkalosis, hypo- or hyperglycaemia, elevated lactate, hyperammonaemia, apnoea and seizures. The cornerstones of treatment include: stopping feeds, providing IV fluid with adequate dextrose and electrolytes, supportive care with inotropes, intubation and fluid resuscitation. Urgent transfer to PICU is required for definitive management, which includes further supportive care and, potentially, initiation of intensive medical therapies, such as dialysis.

A neonate in shock may also present with lethargy, encephalopathy or seizures. Seizures should be aggressively treated as per local guidelines (see Case 65). Initial treatment typically includes the use of a benzodiazepine such as lorazepam or midazolam, followed by a second agent such as phenobarbital or levetiracetam if needed. Biochemical causes (including hypoglycaemia, hyponatraemia and, hypocalcaemia) need early consideration. A neonate with an abnormal neurological exam should undergo an urgent CT head. Consider if this can be done locally without delaying transfer to definitive care.

Neonates have low glycogen stores putting them at significant risk of hypoglycaemia. The profound hypoglycaemia seen in some neonates with shock may be a result of critical systemic illness or could be indicative of an underlying metabolic disorder. The glucose needs to be closely monitored and adequate glucose must be provided. If the glucose is below 2.9 mmol/L then a bolus of 2–5 mL/kg of D10W should be administered and the glucose rechecked shortly thereafter. Maintenance of intravenous fluids with an adequate dextrose concentration, such as 10% Dextrose in saline (D10NS), should be administered during the transport. An adequate glucose infusion rate (5–8 mg/kg/min in neonates) must be provided, and blood glucose should be checked during transport, using a point-of-care device. The administration of hydrocortisone is indicated when adrenal insufficiency is suspected. This typically manifests as refractory shock with hypoglycaemia in sepsis or hyponatraemia, hyperkalaemia and hypoglycaemia if the diagnosis is congenital adrenal hyperplasia (CAH).

The neonate should be placed under a radiant warmer on presentation, and close monitoring of the temperature is essential. Hypothermia can lead to negative physiologic consequences, such as bradycardia and clotting problems. If the neonate is anaemic with an Hb <70 g/dL or there is evidence of bleeding and shock, a packed red blood cell (PRBC) transfusion should be given. If the bleeding is significant, then other blood products should be administered in addition to the PRBCs, such as fresh frozen plasma, cryoprecipitate and platelets, although these may not be available in the retrieval setting (see Case 33). An intracranial haemorrhage due to trauma or haematological disease (e.g. vitamin K deficiency) should be considered in the patient who is anaemic with neurological findings or evidence of trauma (bruising, etc.). In the absence of an urgent CT scan, any evidence of increased intracranial pressure, such as a bulging fontanelle, bradycardia and hypertension, pupillary dilatation or asymmetry needs to be treated aggressively with either mannitol or hypertonic saline.

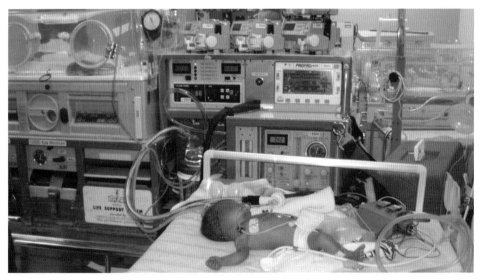

A critically unwell neonate post stabilisation and ready to move into the adjacent transport cot

Discussion 64.3

The neonate in shock is at significant risk of cardiopulmonary arrest. Resuscitation should follow the appropriate APLS algorithms. Reversible causes should be sought out and treated aggressively. Early discussion through the tasking agency with the accepting PICU is critical, both to help support the team and to help determine whether a transport during CPR should be considered.

The following criteria for transport to an ECMO centre during CPR have been proposed (Noje et al 2017):

- Witnessed arrest at local hospital.
- Patient is thought to have a reversible condition (such as congenital heart disease amenable to surgery, myocarditis, sepsis, toxic ingestion, ice-water-drowning).
- High-quality CPR is initiated immediately and maintained throughout.
- Total transport time is estimated to be <60 minutes.
- Parents agree to transport and the decision is supported by the receiving centre following a multiparty discussion.

In addition to the above, the safety of the transport team is the priority and needs to be considered throughout. All precautions should be taken to ensure the safety of the crew while providing CPR in transit, and regional guidelines should be followed. This applies to both aviation and land-based transport platforms. Notwithstanding regional variation, the following should be considered:

- Seat belts should be worn whenever possible.
- Mechanical compressors should be used when available.
- 'Lights & sirens' driving should be avoided when staff are not able to wear seat belts.
- In the aviation context, cabin and occupant safety takes absolute priority, and the pilot has authority in this regard.
- With pilot approval, restraint devices may be removed during flight; however, aviation safety standards mandate the wearing of restraint harnesses for all occupants during take-off and landing.
- In this case, as per the above criteria, transport under CPR would not be indicated (transport time over 60 minutes).

Key points

- The differential diagnosis for a neonate in shock is broad. Resuscitative interventions by the PHRM team need to be provided prior to a definitive diagnosis being made.
- Given the broad differential, the PHRM team should consider simultaneous treatment with antibiotics, prostaglandin infusion and dextrose titrated to response.
- Neonates in shock should ideally be transferred to a centre capable of providing neonatal ECMO. Transport of a patient actively undergoing cardiopulmonary resuscitation should be considered in certain circumstances.

References

Noje C, Fishe JN, Costabile PM, et al. Interhospital transport of children undergoing cardiopulmonary resuscitation: a practical and ethical dilemma. Pediatr. Crit. Care Med. 2017; 18(10):e477–e481.

Additional reading

NHS Children's Acute Transport Service (CATS). Clinical guidelines: Duct dependent congenital heart disease. January 2020. Online. Available: https://cats.nhs.uk/wp-content/uploads/guideline-congenitalheartdisease.pdf. 14 September 2021.

Randle E. Clinical guidcline: CATS metabolic referrals. NHS Children's Acute Transport Service (CATS). January 2020. Online. Available: https://cats.nhs.uk/wp-content/uploads/guideline-metabolic.pdf. 14 September 2021.

Randle E. Clinical guidelines: neonatal collapse. NHS Children's Acute Transport Service (CATS). January 2020. Online. Available: https://cats.nhs.uk/wp-content/uploads/guideline-neonatalcollapse.pdf. 14 September 2021.

Samuels M, Wieteska S (Eds). Advanced paediatric life support: a practical approach to emergencies (Advanced Life Support Group), 6th edn. BMJ Books, Wiley Blackwell, 2017.

CASE 65

Incident

A 7-year-old girl has been brought into a regional hospital in a rural town, post-ictal following a 12-minute focal seizure.

Clinical information

- 23 kg child.
- Airway: No obstructive noises with child in the lateral position.
- Breathing: Respiratory rate: 26, no additional work of breathing, SpO_2 100% on 10 L via NRBM.
- Circulation: Heart rate 124, blood pressure 105/68, capillary refill time 1–2 s.
- Disability: rouses and localises to painful stimulus, no response to verbal prompts, pupils equal and reactive.
- Exposure: temperature 37.1°C (98.8°F), blood glucose 6.1 mmol/L.

Management

Patient has been placed in the recovery position with oxygen delivered via a non-rebreather mask. No medication has been given and IV access has not been obtained.

Relevant information

- **PHRM team transport options:** The PHRM team is 30 minutes' rotary-wing flight from the regional facility.
- **Additional resources:** GP registrar and 2 x nursing staff in attendance. GP anaesthetist on-call within 30 minutes. No other acutely unwell patients currently in the facility. Ground paramedic crew available immediately.
- **Retrieval options:** Regional hospital with paediatrics, CT and MRI 30 minutes by air, 100 minutes by road. Tertiary children's hospital with PICU and neurosurgery approximately 2 hours by air.
- **Other:** Time of day 19:45; ambient temperature 25°C (77°F).

Question 65.1

What initial advice should be provided by the clinical coordination team?

After an assessment and 10 minutes of further observation, it is established that she is an otherwise entirely well girl with no developmental concerns and without syndromic features, rash, neurocutaneous stigmata or signs of trauma. She is fully immunised with no known drug allergies. She had a febrile, coryzal illness one week previously, but this seems to have resolved and she was afebrile at the time of seizure onset. There is no relevant birth or family history.

During the assessment, she starts to have a generalised tonic-clonic seizure.

Question 65.2

What further advice should now be given?

At 25 minutes into the initial resuscitation, oxygen is being provided via a non-rebreather mask and two points of IV access have been established. The patient has received one dose of intra-nasal midazolam at 0.3 mg/kg and one dose of intravenous midazolam at 0.15 mg/kg. She has also received 40 mg/kg of Levetiracetam and 20 mg/kg of

Phenytoin. POC bloods show a glucose of 6.1 mmol/L, Na of 139 and ionised Ca of 1.13. She is continuing to seize. The GP anaesthetist has arrived at the facility and a PHRM team has been dispatched.

Question 65.3

Outline the considerations regarding airway management.

Question 65.4

On arrival of the PHRM team, outline the approach to intubation.

In addition to continuous 3 lead ECG monitoring, the non-invasive blood pressure cuff is set to cycle every 2 minutes. The patient has been intubated with 2 mg/kg Ketamine and 1.5 mg/kg Rocuronium and a nasogastric tube has been inserted. A chest x-ray confirms appropriate tracheal and nasogastric tube positions, and a normal appearance of the lungs. Ventilation is commenced using synchronised intermittent mandatory ventilation (SIMV) with a tidal volume of 140 mL (6mL/kg), a rate of 25 breaths per minute and PEEP of 5 cmH$_2$O. Further blood is taken for a venous blood gas.

Question 65.5

Describe your approach to sedation and ongoing seizure management.

Question 65.6

The patient is still seizing after 60 minutes. Outline your approach to further treatment and monitoring.

Discussion 65.1

The focal nature of the seizure would suggest that, at a minimum, neuroimaging and paediatric involvement would be appropriate. While the patient is not fully recovered, she is not currently actively seizing, is protecting her own airway and is haemodynamically stable. There are three main reasons that she remains obtunded following her seizure, none of which mandate urgent escalation of therapy (e.g. intubation) or retrieval.

1. Degree of hypercarbia
2. Post-ictal, generally with a mild degree of cerebral oedema that will resolve spontaneously
3. Effects of bendiazepines

In general, patients in this condition will improve with airway and breathing support (best delivered with a T-piece) and close monitoring.

Retrieval or transport at this time of day will require either a road or air journey in the dark, which increases risk. The resources of the local hospital are not currently overwhelmed, and the child is receiving adequate care. Fever with a seizure in this age group would be concerning for an infective cause as she is too old for a simple febrile convulsion. Any signs of trauma with a focal seizure would mandate urgent neuroimaging. The patient currently has neither of these and the trajectory of her recovery will determine both whether immediate transport is required and the appropriate destination for that transport. If she fully recovers from this episode within a short timeframe, then urgent outpatient follow-up at the regional hospital would be sufficient. It would therefore be reasonable to observe for a further 30 minutes before making a decision about patient movement, though the potential need to attend this patient should be considered when arranging other patient movements using the same assets.

Discussion 65.2

If their airway appears partially obstructed, careful suction may be possible. Trismus often precludes both effective suction or use of an oropharyngeal airway and nothing should be forced into the mouth. Note also that the patients gag reflex may well be intact. Nasopharyngeal airways are well tolerated and ideal in this circumstance. Oxygen should be applied via non-rebreather mask regardless of saturations. Ideally IV access is obtained, and blood withdrawn for point of care blood gas analysis. Significant abnormalities in glucose, sodium and calcium should be excluded. Midazolam IV or IO (0.15 mg/kg) or IM, IN or buccal (0.3 mg/kg) should be given 5 minutes into the seizure and should not be delayed in the event of difficulty with IV access. A second midazolam dose is given after a further five minutes. If IV access has not been established in time for this second midazolam dose it would be appropriate to insert an intraosseous needle. Current guidelines suggest after 2 doses of midazolam and 15 minutes of seizure time, levetiracetam (bolus) should be given, immediately followed by phenytoin (infused over 20 minutes with cardiac monitoring) if the patient is still seizing. Ensure that the GP anaesthetist has been called and is on the way. The consultation should continue via telemedicine if available. The image below can be seen on the clinical coordination centre telemedicine link.

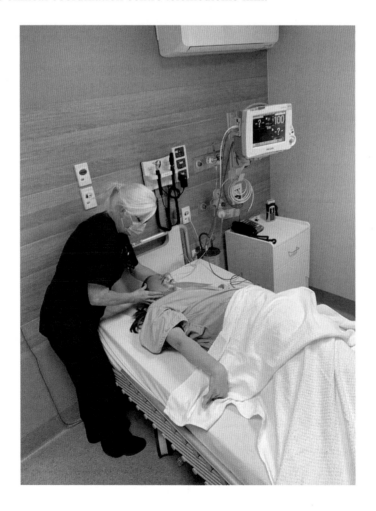

Discussion 65.3

This child is now considered to be in refractory status epilepticus, having had ongoing seizures despite adequate doses of benzodiazepines followed by a second (and subsequently third) antiepileptic drug. The goal of therapy is to terminate seizure activity as soon as possible. A detailed discussion with the GP anaesthetist should occur regarding their level of comfort in managing the child's airway. Unless they have recent and ongoing experience in this area, they should be encouraged to provide basic airway and ventilatory support only until the PHRM team arrives.

Discussion 65.4

Prior to intubation, specific consideration should be given to oxygenation and haemodynamic support. The GP anaesthetist is present and should become a part of the team (a flash team). Positive-end expiratory pressure should be delivered via a T-piece with the patient in a reverse Trendelenburg position. A dose of 10 mL/kg of normal saline is given as a bolus through the second IV while the phenytoin is running through the first. Ketamine is the preferred induction drug. Rocuronium is used as the paralytic agent, despite making assessment of ongoing seizure activity more difficult. Tracheal intubation should be completed as previously outlined (see Case 58).

Discussion 65.5

The ketamine dose used for induction may terminate the seizures. However, if she remains in convulsive status epilepticus, it may take some time to be able to detect the signs of ongoing seizure activity, owing to the effects of the rocuronium. Non-convulsive status epilepticus is very common and signs of this include:
- Autonomic changes (hypertension and sinus tachycardia)
- Eye signs (deviation, dysconjugate gaze, hippus, twitching)
- Lacrimation
- Subtle motor signs (muscle twitching, myoclonus).

Given the uncertainties in being able to adequately assess her neurological status following intubation and muscle relaxation, continuous infusions of sedation and analgesia should be commenced soon after intubation. Morphine or fentanyl is ideal to assist with comfort and tube tolerance. Midazolam or propofol can be used for ongoing sedation as they also possess anti-epileptic properties. A plan should be made to manage ongoing seizures with bolus doses of midazolam and increasing the rate of sedative infusion.

Discussion 65.6

In order to gain control of this child's seizures, the goals of sedation have shifted. Initially, the aim is to keep her comfortable and safe during invasive ventilation and transport. However, her sedation must be deepened in order to aim for pharmacological coma and seizure termination. This is done by giving the child an additional bolus of midazolam 0.15 mg/kg and increasing her background infusion rate. On arrival at the tertiary centre, this child will need continuous EEG monitoring in order to guide the dose titration. The higher doses of midazolam infusion required to achieve these new goals may compromise the patient's haemodynamics and require invasive blood-pressure monitoring and vasopressor support.

Key points
• Paediatric status epilepticus should be managed using standardised algorithms.
• Hypoglycaemia, hyponatraemia and hypocalcaemia represent reversible causes and should be excluded early in the course of seizure management.
• Seizures are a common source of referral to retrieval services and most will resolve spontaneously or with minimal intervention. High-level clinical advice, appropriate treatment and understanding of an anticipated clinical course may obviate the need for unnecessary intervention and retrieval.

Additional reading

Archibald J, Murphy C. Febrile infection-related epilepsy syndrome (FIRES). Don't Forget the Bubbles, 2021. Online. Available: https://dontforgetthebubbles.com/febrile-infection-related-epilepsy-syndrome-fires/. 22 September 2021.

Children's Health Queensland Hospital and Health Service. Status epilepticus – emergency management in children. 2021. Online. Available: https://www.childrens.health.qld.gov.au/wp-content/uploads/PDF/guidelines/CHQ-GDL-60014-status-epilepticus.pdf. 22 September 2021.

Samuels M, Wieteska S. (Eds) Advanced paediatric life support: a practical approach to emergencies, 6th edn. Advanced Life Support Group, BMJ Books, Wiley Blackwell, 2016.

Incident

A 40+12-week (12 days post term) gestation baby is delivered at home. A paediatric PHRM team with neonatal expertise is requested by the paramedics on-scene. The baby's mother has not engaged with maternity services and little is known of the antenatal history. The baby was 'free-birthed' (delivered by the father/friends with no medical input) and the ambulance called at approximately 10 minutes of age because of maternal bleeding.

The location is a short 5-minute rapid-response drive from the PHRM base.

The paramedics on-scene report the following:

- Significant meconium-stained liquor
- Reduced effort of breathing currently requiring assisted ventilation with a bag and mask
- Weight uncertain but appears 'well grown'.

Relevant information

- **PHRM team transport options:** Dedicated paediatric/neonatal ambulance with transport cot.
- **Additional resources:** 2 ambulance paramedics. Land ambulance.
- **Retrieval options:** Tertiary hospital with neonatal intensive care capacity is 60 minutes away by road. Regional hospital with emergency department is 15 minutes by road.

Question 66.1

What considerations are relevant when clinically coordinating and responding to this scenario?

Clinical information

On arrival, the following clinical information is noted:

- The infant is covered in thick meconium.
- Subcostal and intercostal recession with nasal flaring.
- Grunting.
- 'Starfish' posture with little movement.
- HR 120.
- RR: ventilated via bag and mask 45 bpm.
- SaO_2 81% on room air.
- CRT 7 seconds.
- Temperature 35°C (95°F).

Question 66.2

What differential diagnoses would explain the infant's current clinical condition?

Question 66.3

Discuss management of these conditions in the PHRM environment.

Discussion 66.1

Attending a home-birth scenario with both a mother and baby can be logistically complicated. It is important to ensure that the right number and type of resources are mobilised to the scene. The following should be considered:

- Rendezvous options: Can the paramedic team mobilise with the baby and meet the PHRM team at the local emergency department? This may allow for earlier assessment, resuscitation and warming in a better resourced environment.
- Are additional resources (e.g. extra teams or advanced neonatal expertise) required and/or available? Is an additional adult PHRM team required for the mother? How many paramedics are present currently and are others en route?
- Conference-calling (either video or voice only) to connect the PHRM team with the clinical coordination centre to bring in additional expertise if required (e.g. a tertiary neonatologist).

Most of the equipment required to manage a home birth will be included in a paediatric/neonatal PHRM team kit; however, many services will have an additional 'home birth' pack containing further equipment (see Appendix 2.2).

A home birth represents a unique environmental challenge and, following initial resuscitation, it is important to safely transport the baby in a neonatal transport cot, which will usually have been left in the back of the ambulance. This environment is essential for thermoregulation and provides a safe and stable platform to perform life-saving procedures such as intubation and IV access insertion (see Case 61). The baby can be safely restrained and transported to the tertiary hospital. (See image below)

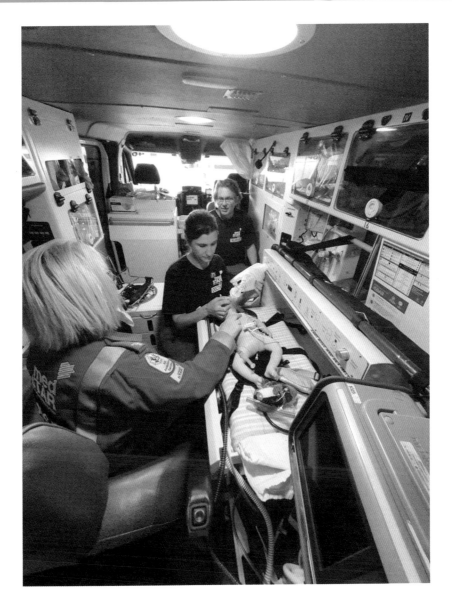

Discussion 66.2

The presence of significant amounts of meconium in a term or post-term newborn with respiratory distress should raise concerns of the possibility of **meconium aspiration syndrome (MAS)**. MAS is a complex constellation of physiological and anatomical insults, and their attendant responses.

Persistent Pulmonary Hypertension of the Newborn (PPHN) is associated with MAS but should be considered when there is any difficulty in oxygenation of term babies.

Hypoxic Ischaemic Encephalopathy (HIE) occurs in term babies and is associated with post-term delivery, meconium aspiration, prolonged or difficult labour, antepartum haemorrhage, but may also occur idiopathically.

Discussion 66.3

Hickam's Dictum states 'Patients can have as many diseases as they damn well please' and this may be true within intensive care medicine, particularly NICU, more so than other specialties (Blaser et al 2021). It is likely that a newborn with the described history would have a combination of HIE, PPHN and MAS. Successful management involves minimising the clinical impact from all three of these conditions.

HIE

HIE should be suspected in all term babies requiring prolonged resuscitation following a perinatal event, such as a placental abruption or prolonged second stage of labour.

HIE is diagnosed on the following criteria:

- Gestation of 36 weeks or more *and at least one of:*
  - Apgar score ≤5 at 10 minutes of age (see Appendix 7.4)
  - Continued resuscitation at 10 minutes of age
  - pH <7 within 60 minutes of birth on ANY gas (arterial, venous, cord or capillary)
  - Base excess ≥ –16 within 60 minutes of birth on ANY gas

and

- Seizures or all three of:
  - Reduced consciousness
  - Abnormal reflexes
  - Hypotonia/flaccidity (general or focal).

Whole-body hypothermia has been shown to be effective in treating HIE. There is a six-hour window from birth for the initiation of cooling, though there may still be some effect if started later.

In the PHRM environment, cooling can be initiated on-scene; however, local practice may vary and, if in doubt, the case should be discussed with the receiving neonatologist through the clinical coordination centre. Cooling, and discussions around it, should not get in the way of active resuscitation

This is a procedure that can be performed on retrieval using 'transport cooling packs' (see figure 66.1).

Uncontrolled hypothermia is associated with poor outcomes in newborns including coagulopathies and worsening PPHN; therefore, central temperature monitoring is essential.

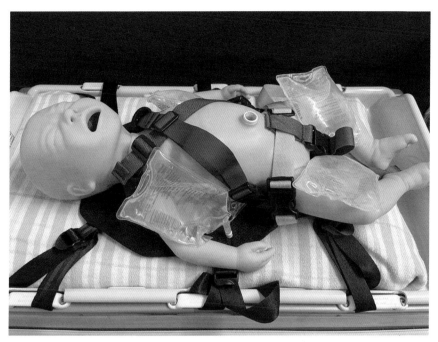

Figure 66.1 Example of a simple, low-tech transport cooling, using four cooled (4-10 degree C) bags of 0.9% NaCL. Saline bags are shown in position without cotton covers for illustration purposes. Servo-controlled cooling systems are available (eg tecotherm, criticool) however their use is limited by the transport environment.

MAS

Meconium is passed by infants in distress so its presence is a suggestion of a difficult delivery in itself.

Aspirated meconium causes multiple problems and should be considered in unresponsive babies who have thick or significant meconium visible on their skin.

Although initially sterile, meconium is an extreme irritant and causes a chemical pneumonitis. This compromises oxygenation, makes mechanical ventilation more difficult, and may worsen or cause PPHN.

Once aspirated, meconium is difficult to remove. Suctioning down a tracheal tube may be helpful in dislodging large clumps but will do little to reverse the effects of aspirated meconium. Surfactant lavage has been trialled but there is little evidence for this and it would not be recommended in a PHRM setting.

Meconium is also very sticky. When in smaller airways it produces a 'ball valve' effect where gas passes through to the alveoli but cannot escape them. The ball-valve effect can lead to patches of over-distension and the risk of pneumothorax. A prolonged expiratory time can help to lessen the negative effects of this phenomenon. If the ventilator is capable of delivering high-frequency oscillatory ventilation (HFOV), then this should be considered in the field.

PPHN

As mentioned above, PPHN can be caused or worsened by either MAS or HIE, but may also exist in isolation.

In utero the lungs are not in use and in order to maximise blood flow through the placenta, the pulmonary vascular pressure is extremely high. The pulmonary pressure normally drops in response to oxygen in the lungs and the changing intrathoracic pressure of the first breaths; in the absence of these changes and the presence of pathology, such as MAS, the pulmonary pressure remains high and deoxygenated blood is shunted across the ductus arteriosus. The presence of the ductus lends to a simple diagnostic test for PPHN. The arterial circulation for the right upper limb branches from the aorta prior to the insertion point of the ductus arteriosus. By placing saturation probes on the right wrist (pre-ductal) and any other limb (post-ductal), a difference between pre- and post-ductal saturations can be measured. A difference of more than 10 percentage points strongly suggests the presence of significant shunting and, therefore, PPHN.

Management of PPHN can be achieved by either reducing pulmonary vascular resistance (PVR) and/or increasing systemic blood pressure above pulmonary pressure. Given the risks of significantly elevating systemic pressure, the former, or at most a combination of the two, is to be preferred. In a PHRM setting with limited resources, inotropic support to increase mean systemic pressure is a good initial option. Ideally, these should be used in conjunction with arterial pressure monitoring (via an umbilical arterial catheter UAC), although in this particular case the UAC could be deferred until arrival at the tertiary centre. Adrenaline or noradrenaline are readily available and other options include milrinone which, if available, can be considered following discussion with the receiving neonatal unit via the clinical coordination centre.

Oxygen is a potent vasodilator and high inhaled oxygen fractions should be used to reduce PVR. If available, inhaled nitric oxide (iNO) can also be used to reduce PVR significantly. iNO is usually delivered via dedicated equipment (see Figure 66.2) and started at 20 ppm. This dose is usually sufficient to cause noticeable reduction in PVR and improvement of physiology. iNO is generally safe, but teams should be aware that airframes need to be specifically certified for flight with iNO, and detection equipment is mandatory. With adequate equipment, service infrastructure and clinical governance, iNO can be initiated within a few minutes in the PHRM environment.

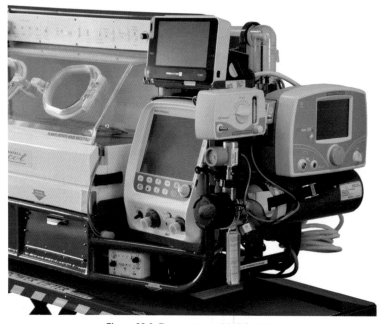

Figure 66.2 Transport cot with iNO delivery system.

Key points

- A critically unwell newborn, born at home or in a peripheral hospital represents a unique challenge for the PHRM team, both medically and logistically.
- An emphasis on preparation, planning and early communication is key.
- In the case of a home birth, the PHRM team should be capable of delivering the full suite of complex neonatal critical care interventions in a neonatal transport cot in the back of the ambulance or aircraft.

References

Blaser S, Schaye V, Hwang J, et al. Hickam's dictum, Occam's razor, and Crabtree's bludgeon: a case of renal failure and a clavicular mass. Diagnosis (Berl). 2021 Aug 5. doi:10.1515/dx-2020-0149. Epub ahead of print. PMID: 34355545.

Additional reading

State of Victoria: Victorian Agency for Health Information and Safer Care Victoria. Neonatal ehandbook. Online. Available: https://www.bettersafercare.vic.gov.au/clinical-guidance/neonatal. 23 September 2021.

Sydney Local Health District. Royal Prince Alfred Hospital newborn care clinical guidelines, 2021. Online. Available: https://www.slhd.nsw.gov.au/rpa/neonatal/protocols.html. 23 September 2021.

Incident

Following a domestic disturbance, a parent has accidentally reversed their 4 x 4 over their 11-year-old child in the driveway of the family home. He has sustained a compound tibia-fibula fracture. The parent is on-scene with the child. Both are visibly distressed. You are part of a PHRM team that has been tasked and has just arrived on what is an emotionally highly charged scene.

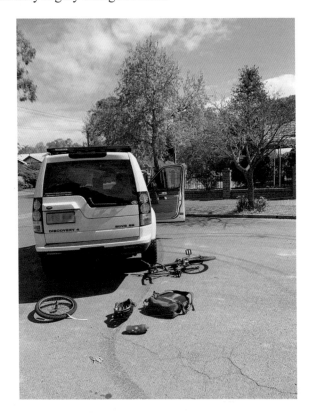

Question 67.1

What communication techniques could be utilised on-scene?

Question 67.2

Outline and discuss potential immediate debrief strategies for the PHRM team.

Discussion 67.1

During a medical or traumatic experience, patients and their families are highly open to suggestion (suggestible), and it is important to be aware of how we communicate with them. As trained healthcare professionals, we are well versed in what we need to do to help clinically in an emergency situation. In addition, what we say and how we say it can also have a profound physical and emotional effect. There is almost always an opportunity to say something that promotes a better outcome.

How we communicate within and between the PHRM and other emergency services teams in front of the patient is equally as important.

What to say and how to say it

Techniques for the patient and their family

Calm is contagious. During an emergency situation, approach the patient with the intention of instilling a sense of calmness and control. Speak as slowly and softly as possible. The effects on children (and adults) who have undergone a traumatic event can be very profound. To date, there is little specific evidence regarding communication techniques in the acute setting. However, evidence exists around the beneficial use of relaxation techniques to lower the 'stress' response as measured by serum cortisol and adrenaline.

The following phrases can be used to assist in rapidly gaining rapport and trust, and may work towards positively engaging suggestible patients. These opening phrases are good examples of techniques to reduce feelings of helplessness and vulnerability that the patients may have.

- 'My name is Dr Smith, but my friends call me John'…
- 'I've got you … you are safe now … I will stay with you for as long as you need …'
- 'I am sure you will want to listen to what I say and do as much as you can to help me help you.'

Try to follow with statements designed to convey the following ideas, adapted to fit the situation at hand. They should include constant emphasis on the idea that the patient is safe and in control.

- 'The worst is over, you are safe now.'
- 'Everyone is here to help you keep safe and comfortable.'
- 'They are getting everything ready at the hospital to make you safe and keep you comfortable while we take you there as quickly and as safely as possible.'
- 'Tell me what you need right now.'
- 'Tell me what you are feeling.'
- 'I can see {your leg} needs my attention … is there anything else I need to pay attention to that will make you feel more safe or comfortable?'

Often, asking about an uninjured part will direct attention away from the injured area to a part that does not hurt. This is an effective distraction therapy, e.g.

- 'Wow, you must be very strong because most of your body is healthy now.'

At this point, the focus can turn to relaxation and removing the stress of the situation. Try to avoid using words such as 'pain' or 'pain score' or 'pain killer'.

- 'Because I am a doctor (nurse, paramedic, trained first aider) you can start to relax a little now and let your body do what needs to be done.'
- 'Is there somewhere you would rather be right now … where would that be? While I am here looking after you, your mind can go there and you can begin to relax even more and start feeling more comfortable.'
- 'Wherever you go, whoever is with you, know you can continue feeling more and more comfortable.'

While these techniques can be used for all age groups, some phrases can be specific for children. For example, children can be encouraged to become an active part of the PHRM team by asking them if they want to be a partner like Batman and Robin or any other superhero pair.

- 'Now that we are partners, we can work together to make you feel more comfortable.'

Techniques for use within the PHRM team and other emergency services personnel

The tendency for the crew/staff to move towards a highly aroused 'Fight or Flight' response invoked by external environmental stimuli is common. As such, management of 'personal state' has a powerful effect on your own comfort and resourcefulness on-scene.

Once the crew arrive, given their authority status, people at the scene will mirror the state of the crew, which explains why calm and panic can be extremely contagious. Therefore, the crew needs to be aware that perceptions of their personal state can be manifested by other people on-scene. So, if the PHRM team arrives out of breath, sweaty and anxious, this can alter the entire mood of the scene. Accessing a calm, focused, controlled state in the face of confronting and potentially overwhelming situations can be difficult. Four distinct, evidence-based, performance-enhancing psychological skills (PEPS) are listed below (Lauria et al 2017):

- **Breathe:** e.g. 'box breathing'
- **Talk:** positive self-talk
- **See:** visualising the successful outcome of the situation
- **Focus:** using a familiar word or gesture that reminds you of a time when you felt calm, confident and totally focused and in control.

PHRM teams should be familiar and practised with these techniques to control their personal state to ensure they are able to remain focused, calm and in control. Stress inoculation, through repetitive drills and simulation, allows teams to practise these various techniques and to ultimately utilise them in a crisis situation.

Discussion 67.2

Team debriefs can either be clinical (systems/medical management and performance aspects that could be improved) or psychological (to de-escalate sympathetic activation and minimise potential psychological trauma in team members).

Immediate debrief after traumatic events requires an individualised approach as there are many elements involved. Immediate counselling of people following trauma has not been shown to be helpful unless asked for. When utilised, techniques that may be helpful should focus on reducing the stress associated with increased adrenaline and cortisol to achieve a more relaxed personal state and promote a healthy psychophysiological response. This can potentially reduce the likelihood of developing negative psychological outcomes. Any PEPS (or 'anti-anxiety technique') that reduces sympathetic activation and promotes parasympathetic dominance is beneficial.

Immediate debriefing is best accomplished using a script to cover the following points (Eppich & Cheng 2015):

- Setting the scene and objectives
- Reaction: 'how are you feeling?'
- Description: 'can someone please summarise the case so that we're on the same page'
- Analysis: Advocacy-inquiry (i.e. explore frames with genuine curiosity) can be useful
  - 'I observed…'
  - 'I think…'
  - 'What was going through your mind at the time?'
- Clinician self-assessment and reflection

- Opportunity for question: 'any outstanding issues before we wrap up?'
- Application/summary:
  - Two learning points to take away
  - Summarise key learning types

A more detailed dissection is best left until some time has elapsed since the event and a trained facilitator and/or a clinical psychologist should lead the session.

Key points
• Communication in a crisis is critical and if done expertly can have therapeutic value.
• Performance-enhancing psychological skills need to be considered and practised for career longevity and well-being.
• Immediate debrief should focus on clinical issues and de-escalation of psychophysiological response.
• Team well-being needs to be incorporated into the PHRM service culture and not only considered on an ad hoc basis.

References

Eppich W, Cheng A. Promoting excellence and reflective learning in simulation (PEARLS): development and rationale for a blended approach to health care simulation debriefing. Simul. Healthc. 2015; 10(2):106–115.

Lauria MJ, Gallo IA, Rush S, et al. Psychological skills to improve emergency care providers' performance under stress. Ann. Emerg. Med. 2017; 70(6):884–890.

Additional reading

Benson H. Timeless healing: the power and biology of belief. Fireside, 1997.

Glo Clinical Hypnosis, Adelaide. Online. Available: https://www.glohypnosis.com.au. 23 September 2021.

Hearns S. Peak performance under pressure: lessons from a helicopter rescue doctor. Core Cognition, 2019.

International Critical Incident Stress Foundation (ICISF). Critical incident stress information sheets. Online. Available: https://icisf.org/wp-content/uploads/2020/06/CRITICAL-INCIDENT-STRESS-INFORMATION-SHEETS.pdf. 23 September 2021.

Jacobs DJ. Patient communication for first responders and EMS personnel: the first hour of trauma. Brady, 1997.

Tolgou T, Rohrmann S, Stockhausen C, et al. Physiological and psychological effects of imagery techniques on health anxiety. Psychophysiology 2018; 55(2). doi:10.1111/psyp.12984.

van der Kolk B. The body keeps the score: brain, mind and body in the healing of trauma. Penguin, 2014.

CASE 68

Incident

A 72-hour-old male neonate presented to a regional hospital with a 12-hour history of poor feeding and 3-hour history of green, bile-stained vomiting.

The neonate was born at 39+1 by normal vaginal delivery, following an uneventful antenatal course. At birth, the Apgar scores were 9 and 9, and the child roomed in with his mother. The neonate was established on breastfeeds and stooling normally prior to discharge home at just over 24 hours of life.

Clinical information

Following the child's arrival to the regional hospital, the following clinical information is available:

- Appears alert, warm and pink.
- P 131 beats/min.
- Capillary refill time is brisk (<2 seconds), and the femoral pulses are easily palpable.
- RR 35 breaths/min, no grunting or other signs of respiratory distress.
- SpO$_2$ 100% on room air with good trace (right arm).
- Temperature 36.6°C (98°F).
- Blood glucose 4.3 mmol/L
- Abdominal examination: not distended, soft, with no tenderness, masses or inguinal herniae. The anus is patent and orthotopic in its position.

Interventions performed:
- Placed under warmer.
- Remains on room air, with no respiratory supports.
- IV bolus of 10 mL/kg of 0.9% NaCl administered.
- IV maintenance fluids commenced to follow above bolus.

Relevant information

- **PHRM team transport options:** Fixed-wing aircraft.
- **Additional resources:** Local paediatrician based in regional hospital with limited neonatal intensive care capacity and adult general surgery service. Land ambulance.
- **Retrieval options:** Nearest centre with neonatal ICU and paediatric surgeon 5 hours by road, 1.5 hours' flight time.
- **Other:** Nil.

Question 68.1

What is your differential diagnosis?

Question 68.2

What other clinical features impact the differential diagnosis?

Question 68.3

How will you stabilise this neonate and prepare for transport?

Question 68.4

How would the management differ if the child was born prematurely (30 weeks)?

Discussion 68.1

The differential diagnosis for a previously healthy neonate who presents with bile-stained vomiting is broad (see Table 68.1 below) (Hutson et al 2015). However, the seriousness and time-critical nature of midgut malrotation *with* volvulus makes this the primary diagnosis until proven otherwise.

Large national and single centre audit series show approximately 1 in 4 bile-stained vomiting neonates referred for retrieval have a surgical cause. Further, almost 1 in 10 of these have a surgical cause in which delayed treatment may result in bowel loss, including the catastrophic bowel loss associated with untreated midgut volvulus (Malhotra et al 2010, Ojha et al 2017).

Any neonate with bilious vomiting should still be managed as a time-critical emergency, even if they look systemically well.

The absolute importance of avoiding delay in this process demands an urgency of response and action at every step in the neonate's care, be that in referral, preparation, retrieval, reception, investigation or definitive surgical management. This approach aims to reduce the morbidity and mortality associated with delayed treatment.

Discussion 68.2

When making or taking a referral for retrieval of a neonate with bile-stained vomiting, the colour of the vomit, systemic status and examination of the abdomen are key considerations.

a. What color is the vomit?

The presence of bile in vomit can manifest in many shades of green, varying from lightly stained with bile (near yellow) to heavily stained with bile (near black). Neonatal vomitus should be milk or curdled milk and any yellow, green or black in the vomit should prompt an urgent review. Bespoke colour-matching charts are available to assist in determining whether an observed vomit is bile-stained, or not (Walker at al 2006).

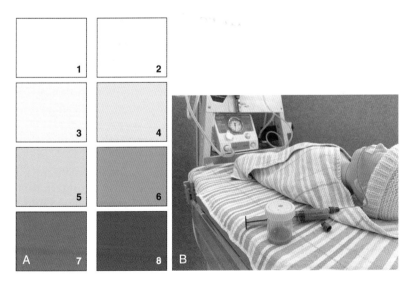

Table 68.1 Causes of neonatal bile-stained vomiting: *surgical vs medical*

Surgical	Medical
Midgut malrotation +/– volvulus*	Systemic sepsis +/– ileus
Duodenal atresia and stenosis	Gastroesophageal reflux
Jejunoileal atresia	Feed intolerance
Meconium disease‡	
Hirschsprung disease ± enterocolitis	
Anorectal malformation	
Small left colon	
Colonic atresia	
Inguinal hernia	
NEC§	

*The presence or absence of a volvulus in addition to midgut malrotation may not be constant, but a safety-first approach insists that volvulus be presumed present and established, as indeed it may well dangerously be.
‡ Meconium disease includes meconium ileus, meconium plug.
§NEC, Necrotising enterocolitis, in the appropriate clinical setting, which can include term delivery with superadded congenital heart disease and/or perinatal sepsis.
Source: Hutson et al. 2015

A child with bile-stained vomit should be referred and retrieved for urgent paediatric surgical care. If there is any doubt, expert specialist advice should be sought without delay from the receiving neonatal and paediatric surgical services via the clinical coordination centre.

In this early and undifferentiated stage, blood in the vomit and/or nasogastric aspirates (fresh or altered) should increase the level of clinical concern. Blood may be a sinister finding, indicative of gut ischaemia and injury as a complication of untreated causes, including midgut malrotation *with* volvulus.

b. Is the neonate systemically unwell or well?

It is well recognised that a neonate with midgut malrotation and volvulus can be systemically *entirely well* at presentation. Without due attention to this possibility, the referring team and PHRM service may be falsely reassured. This can lead to injurious delay in this neonate accessing necessary care.

It is also well recognised that if untreated, a neonate with midgut malrotation can become progressively, rapidly and dangerously unwell.

Therefore, the bile-stained vomit in a neonate presenting systemically unwell implies established disease requiring emergent surgical intervention. In this situation, the neonate will need a full paediatric / neonatal PHRM team to assist with resuscitation with the understanding that the child's life is threatened.

In both scenarios, there is importance and benefit in appraising the relevant neonatal and paediatric surgical teams of this neonate and their expected needs on arrival at the receiving centre. Early communication with these specialist teams is a key part of the retrieval process but the time-critical retrieval should not be delayed while awaiting acceptance from a surgical team that may be difficult to contact.

c. Is there accompanying abdominal distension?

In broad terms, the presence of abdominal distension in a neonate presenting with bile-stained vomiting may be indicative of the level of obstruction: more proximal levels of obstruction, e.g. midgut pathology vs more distal levels of obstruction. Distal bowel obstruction results in multiple bowel loops being distended by air and fluid, which manifests as distension of the abdomen.

Other factors may contribute to abdominal distension which are independent of the level of obstruction. These include systemic and/or intra-abdominal sepsis, gut ischaemia, ascites and bowel perforation.

A systemically unwell neonate presenting with established midgut malrotation with abdominal tenderness and distension, and possibly passing blood per rectum is considered to be in immediate life-threat. In the tertiary centre, exploratory laparotomy on the basis of clinical assessment alone, avoiding even the delay of a confirmatory upper gastrointestinal contrast study may be indicated.

Thus, whether well or unwell, non-distended or distended midgut malrotation *with* volvulus remains possible, and cannot be safely discounted prior to specialist assessment in the receiving centre.

For the PHRM service, this information should be incorporated into decision making regarding team configuration. Physiologically normal neonates may be suitable for nurse-led transfers, whereas even early and mild physiological compromise may suggest the need for a full PHRM team. In all cases, the infant should be transferred as early as possible. This information is summarised in Figure 68.1 below.

Discussion 68.3

Once the time-critical nature of this case is established, the management of the neonate in preparation for and during transport follows expected and relatively standard protocols for the surgical neonate:

- ABC
  - Respiratory, cardiac and other intensive supports as required
- Nasogastric tube
  - In a term neonate, use 8 Fr gauge to ensure adequate decompression
  - Free drainage and regular aspirates to ensure position of gastric tube or if any signs of increased distension or respiratory distress develop.
  - Replace significant nasogastric losses using 0.9% NaCl
- IV fluids
  - IV fluid resuscitation as required (bearing in mind, third space losses in intra-abdominal sepsis)
  - IV fluid maintenance in accordance with standard local rates/fluid choices
- Nil enteral
- Ensure blood sugar is monitored (e.g. every 4–6 hours)
- Sepsis considerations
  - Blood cultures

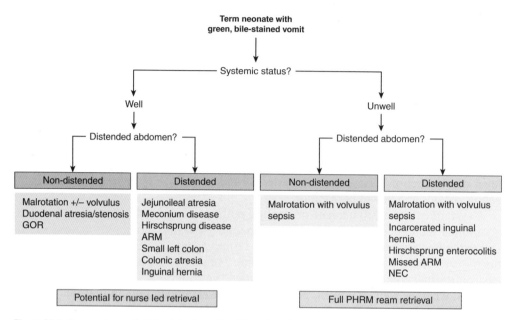

Figure 68.1 Causes of neonatal bile stained vomiting. Meconium disease includes meconium ileus, meconium plug. ARM = anorectal malformation.

- Broad spectrum antibiotic cover suitable for systemic and abdominal sepsis in the neonate, e.g. benzylpenicillin + gentamicin + metronidazole

Electronic (or hard copy if electronic transfer not available) copies of any plain x-rays, contrast studies or abdominal ultrasound imaging should accompany the neonate to the receiving centre. However, these investigations may contribute little to immediate care priorities of the neonate, and so should not delay departure of the neonate.

This neonate may need consent given for emergency surgical procedures soon after arrival in the receiving centre. Under normal circumstances, one or other of the parents would be expected to accompany the neonate during the transfer. If this is not possible, contact details for the parent(s) should be obtained. While there are typically clinical governance allowances for emergency life-saving interventions to proceed in the absence of parental consent, it is ideal and compassionate to rapidly update and advise the parent(s) of the emergency care their newborn requires.

If in *this* case weather conditions were to preclude air ambulance transfer for 6 or more hours, the retrieval service would need to consider alternative strategies to facilitate access to suitable surgical and neonatal services. This may include multi-leg road ambulance transfers.

In the rare and desperate scenario that even these alternative transport options are unavailable, and with the present-day capabilities of telemedicine, it is possible for a paediatric surgeon to assist a suitably trained adult general surgeon to perform an exploratory laparotomy and treat the volvulus.

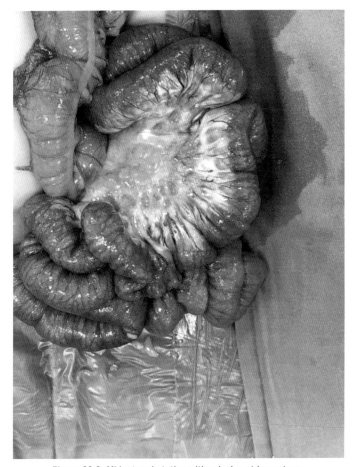

Figure 68.2 Midgut malrotation with volvulus at laparotomy.

Discussion 68.4

The above case, discussion and recommendations relate specifically to the differential diagnosis and priorities of a *previously well* term neonate with bile-stained vomiting. This neonatal population is distinct from the medically complex, premature population.

Such neonates are more likely to have complex conditions arising from their prematurity such as NEC and its obstructing sequelae, and medical causes including 'prem gut' and sepsis. The need for early transport and assessment of these neonates in a tertiary facility remains; however, the provision of definitive care may not include time-critical surgical intervention.

Key points

- The previously well neonate with bilious vomiting should be considered seriously unwell and managed accordingly.
- While the differential diagnosis for the neonate with bile-stained vomits is broad, best care is served by presuming the cause is midgut malrotation *with* volvulus, until proven otherwise.

References

Hutson JM, O'Brien M, Beasley SW, et al (Eds). Bowel obstruction. In 'Jones' Clinical Paediatric Surgery, 7th edn. John Wiley & Sons, 2015.

Malhotra A, Lakkundi A, Carse E. Bilious vomiting in the newborn: 6 years data from a Level III Centre. J. Paediatr. Child Health 2010; 46(5):259–261.

Ojha S, Sand L, Ratnavel N, et al. Newborn infants with bilious vomiting: a national audit of neonatal transport services. Arch. Dis. Child. Fetal Neonatal Ed. 2017; 102(6):F515–F518.

Walker GM, Nielson A, Young D, Raine PAM. Colour of bile vomiting in intestinal obstruction in the newborn: questionnaire study. BMJ, 2006; 332(7554):1363. doi:10.1136/bmj.38859.614352.55.

Additional reading

Neonatal Transfer Service (NTS) London. Bowel obstruction. Online. Available: https://london-nts.nhs.uk/wp-content/uploads/2015/01/Bowel-Obstruction-NTS-Guideline.pdf. 13 July 2015.

NHS Thames Valley & Wessex Operational Delivery Networks. Wessex care pathway for term infants referred with bilious vomiting for exclusion of malrotation. Online. Available: https://www.sort.nhs.uk/Media/SONeT/Guidelines/NetworkClinical/Wessex%20Bilious%20Vomiting%20Pathway%20-%20Malrotation%20guideline%20final%20version%201.3%20(1).pdf. 24 September 2021.

Sydney Local Health District. Royal Prince Alfred Hospital Guideline: Bilious vomiting in the term neonate. Online. Available: https://www.slhd.nsw.gov.au/RPA/neonatal%5Ccontent/pdf/guidelines/Bilious_Vomiting_SLHD_Guideline.pdf. 24 September 2021.

Victorian Agency for Health Information and Safer Care Victoria. Vomiting in neonates. Online. Available: https://www.bettersafercare.vic.gov.au/clinical-guidance/neonatal/vomiting-in-neonates. 24 September 2021.

Incident

A 20-month-old male has been taken by ambulance to his regional hospital emergency department following an immersion incident at home. The child was found outside, submerged in a pool during winter. He had been 'missing' for approximately 10 minutes. Local ambulance officers performed cardiopulmonary resuscitation (CPR) at the scene and during the 10-minute transfer to the ED. The child has been intubated and is being hand ventilated. Two doses of intravenous adrenaline have been given for asystole and the patient has had a return of spontaneous circulation (ROSC) with a heart rate of 70.

Relevant information

- **PHRM team transport options:** Rotary-wing aircraft.
- **Additional resources:** Adult emergency medicine physicians in attendance. Full nursing staff complement. Land ambulance available.
- **Retrieval options:** Tertiary-level paediatric hospital with pediatric intensive care capacity 40 minutes by road, 10 minutes' rotary flight time.
- **Other:** Local temperature 2°C (36°F).

Question 69.1

Outline the PHRM team's preparations while en-route to the emergency department.

On arrival of the PHRM team in the ED, there are two emergency physicians providing manual ventilation, three nurses and the two ambulance officers who attended the drowning scene and provided pre-hospital CPR. The parents are waiting outside the resuscitation room.

Clinical information

The following clinical information is available:
- Intubated and manually ventilated at 24 breaths per minutes in 100% oxygen; no spontaneous ventilation; SaO_2 unrecordable.
- HR 70, sinus, occasional ventricular ectopics; BP unrecordable; capillary refill 7 seconds.
- GCS 3; pupils fixed and dilated.
- Temperature (tympanic) 34°C (93.2°F).
- Drugs administered:
  - Adrenaline 1:10,000 1.3 mL x 2 doses IV
- Estimated 'down' time approximately 30 minutes prior to ROSC

The patient becomes asystolic as the PHRM team is taking verbal handover. The single IV cannula is now not functioning.

Question 69.2

What is your immediate management of this evolving clinical situation?

Question 69.3

Discuss ongoing management.

Discussion 69.1

In Australia, accidental drownings cause an average of 281 deaths per year with 24% of these in children under the age of 5 years (Peden et al 2018). In addition, for every fatal drowning there are 2.7 non-fatal drownings with 58% of these in children under 5 years of age. While the vast majority of drownings occur in swimming pools or natural bodies of water (80%), a significant amount occur in smaller bodies of water like bathtubs (8%).

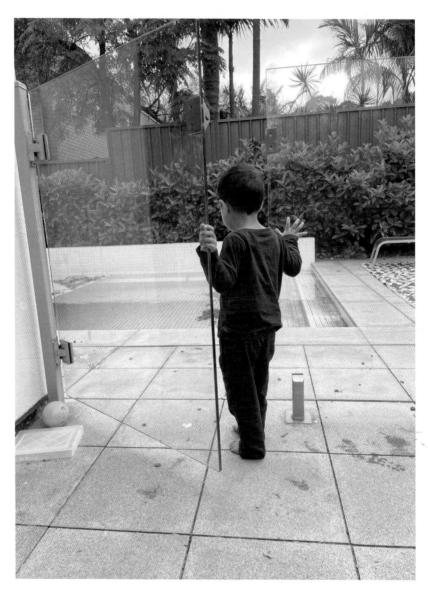

Team preparation prior to arrival at the case will involve practical planning for patient stabilisation and transport as well as preparing for the psychological impact of the case.

Practical preparation should proceed in a structured manner (A, B, C) with discussion around approach to assessment and management of the current clinical situation and likely clinical progression. The adequacy and security of the intubated airway (A) will need to be assessed. A cuffed 4.0 TT should be in situ and taped securely at 13.5 cm at teeth. If an uncuffed TT has been used, it should be left in situ unless there are problems with leakage, airway pressures or ventilation. If re-intubation is required, appropriate laryngoscope and blades with a backup LMA (size 2.0) will be required. Despite the degree of obtundation, intubation may be possible without medications, but appropriate muscle relaxants and induction agents are still recommended with dosing for an estimated 13 kg child. Breathing (B) adequacy should be assessed and $ETCO_2$ monitoring is mandatory. Circulation (C) preparation includes ensuring two functioning and well-secured vascular access points (IV or IO). Crystalloid fluid boluses of 10 mL/kg aliquots may be required but persistent hypotension unresponsive to fluids will require inotropic support, and the dilution and dosing for an adrenaline infusion should be calculated prior to arrival. Planned packaging of the patient will require age-appropriate restraints and active warming strategies including heat packs and space blankets, with central temperature monitoring as part of targeted temperature management. It should be recognised that this phase of care runs a reduced risk of 'afterdrop' (see Case 17) and active re-warming up to 32°C (89.6°F) is appropriate. The PHRM team needs to prepare for further deterioration, including the possibility of TT dislodgement or failure and the need to suction or re-intubate en route, as well as possible further cardiac arrests requiring CPR and adrenaline.

The psychological impact of this case is significant. The distressed parents will need clear and calm communication regarding the status of their child and the plan moving forward. Wherever possible, parental presence in the resuscitation room is encouraged, reducing their distress and anxiety, and, in anticipated poor outcomes, allowing them to start the grieving process (Phillips 2020). The local healthcare team is also likely to be highly invested in the outcome, having successfully obtained ROSC, and their expectation and hope for a positive result will be significant. The local team should be actively included in discussions around ongoing management. The impact of the case on the PHRM team members must also be recognised with planned debriefing immediately after the case and access to peer support in the days to come.

Discussion 69.2

Working with the local health team, CPR must immediately recommence. Team roles will be rapidly assigned, utilising available staff resources. Cycling CPR roles between team members every 2 minutes will assist in ensuring good-quality resuscitation. Urgent vascular access is required with an intraosseous insertion the fastest option. The asystole advanced paediatric life support algorithm should be followed with a dose of intravenous adrenaline (10 mcg/kg), followed by a flush and then 2 minutes of CPR. The 4 Hs (hypoxia, hypovolaemia, hypothermia, hypokalaemia/calcaemia) and 4 Ts (toxins, thrombus, tension pneumothorax, tamponade) should be actively sought and corrected. Urgent review of the adequacy of ventilation should occur to identify hypoxia from possible TT dislodgement or blockage or tension pneumothorax. An urgent core temperature will assist in excluding hypothermia as a contributing cause.

Hypothermia with core temperatures <30°C (86°F) can be neuro-protective in the context of cardiac arrest (Corneli 2012). The old adage 'no one is dead until they're warm and dead' is still applicable in situations of arrest with significant hypothermia. In these cases, it is recommended to withhold declaration of death and continue resuscitative efforts until core temperatures reach 32°C (89.6°F) or greater for 30 minutes or more

(Corneli 2012). In this clinical case, if the core temperature is actually 34°C (93.2°F), it is appropriate to follow standard resuscitation protocols and durations.

Defibrillation below 30°C (86°F) is unlikely to be successful and should be avoided. As per adults (see Case 17) adrenaline should also be withheld at this temperature.

Discussion 69.3

The ongoing management of this patient is complex and sensitive. Resuscitative efforts were in progress for 30 minutes prior to ROSC, and prior to the recurrence of asystole, there were no spontaneous respirations, no recordable BP and fixed and dilated pupils. Termination of resuscitative efforts requires consideration of both medical and non-medical factors (Campwala et al 2020). Medical factors include:

- Duration and adequacy of resuscitation
- Response to treatment
- Underlying cause of arrest
- Likelihood of intact survival.

Failure to restore spontaneous circulation after 20 minutes of advanced resuscitation, in the absence of refractory VF/VT, toxins or hypothermia, is an appropriate time to consider cessation of resuscitative efforts. Non-medical factors, however, play a significant role in this decision-making process. In this case, consideration of local team expectations and parental involvement and their acceptance will be important before any decision to terminate resuscitation. If the decision is made to cease resuscitation, bringing the parents in to the resuscitation room prior to ceasing CPR can be helpful for both the family and the staff involved (Campwala et al 2020).

If only intermittent ROSC is achieved during the resuscitative efforts, but the child remains profoundly unstable despite maximal therapy including inotropic support and ventilation, consideration of the need to transfer the patient should occur. Patient long-term survival is unlikely and ceasing resuscitation and providing comfort care locally may be an option. The risks and benefits associated with or without transfer should be considered. Allowing the patient to die locally has the potential to enable local support for the family and may reduce the stress associated with unfamiliar places and unknown people. Road and aeromedical transfer of a highly unstable patient places the PHRM team at increased risks as they may be required to provide CPR while unsecured. Conversely, transferring the patient to the paediatric hospital may reassure the parents and local team that everything that could have been done was done and allow time for absent friends and family to gather for grieving. In some cases, transferring a terminal patient to a tertiary centre may allow organ donation to be considered, although this is unlikely to be an option in this case due to severe hypoxic insult.

Key points

- Drowning is a common cause of death and children under the age of 5 are over-represented.
- The decision to cease resuscitative efforts requires careful consideration of both medical and non-medical factors.
- The possibility of not transferring a pre-terminal patient and providing focused end-of-life care may be appropriate in some cases.

References

Campwala RT, Schmidt AR, Chang TP, Nager AL. Factors influencing termination of resuscitation in children: a qualitative analysis. Int. J. Emerg. Med. 2020; 13(12). https://doi.org/10.1186/s12245-020-0263-6.

Corneli HM. Accidental hypothermia. Pediatr. Emerg. Care. 2012; 28(5):475–480.

Peden AE, Mahony AJ, Barnsley PD, Scarr J. Understanding the full burden of drowning: a retrospective, cross-sectional analysis of fatal and non-fatal drowning in Australia. BMJ Open 2018; 8:e024868.

Phillips B. Towards evidence-based medicine for paediatricians. Should family members be present at resuscitation? Arch. Dis. Child. 2020; 105(5):506. doi:10.1136/archdischild-2020-319198.

Additional reading

Government of Western Australia Child and Adolescent Health Service. Hypothermia. Online. Available: https://pch.health.wa.gov.au/For-health-professionals/Emergency-Department-Guidelines/Hypothermia. 24 September 2021.

Samuels M, Wieteska S. (Eds) Advanced paediatric life support: a practical approach to emergencies, 6th edn. Advanced Life Support Group, BMJ Books, Wiley Blackwell, 2016.

APPENDIX 1: PROCEDURES

1.1 Airway
1.1.1 RSI flowchart

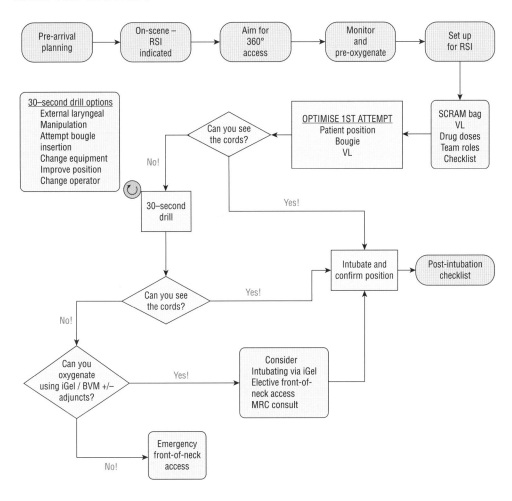

1.1.2 RSI checklists

RSI preparation	Equipment check	Team brief	Post RSI
✓ Optimise patient position & access	✓ BVM with O_2	✓ Airway assistant	✓ Waveform $ETCO_2$ confirmed
✓ O_2 cylinder > half full & back-up	✓ ETT mount & HME	✓ M.I.L.S	✓ Check obs
✓ Nasal prongs ApOx	✓ Laryngoscopes x 2 tested	✓ Drug giver	✓ Tube secured & position noted
✓ Pre-oxygenation	✓ Blade size	✓ RSI drug doses	✓ Ventilation
✓ OPA & NPA	✓ Suction tested	✓ Consider cricoid pressure	✓ Analgesia/Sedation
✓ Vascular access	✓ Bougie or stylet		✓ Paralysis
✓ Fluids run easily	✓ ETT & cuff tested		✓ Consider oro/nasogastric tube
✓ BP set at 2-minute cycles	✓ Syringe		✓ Temperature probe
✓ Baseline obs	✓ Tube tie		✓ Cuff pressure
✓ $ETCO_2$ connected to monitor & on	✓ LMA (inc iLMA)		
	✓ Surgical airway kit		

30-second drill options:
1. Release cricoid pressure
2. External laryngeal manipulation
3. Adjust patient position
4. Adjust operator position
5. Change equipment
6. Change operator

JAWS:
- Jaw thrust
- Airways – OPA/NPA
- Work together – 2-person
- Small volumes, easy squeeze

CHALLENGE & RESPONSE

CO_2.B.O.L.T.S

IMMEDIATE/ PERI-ARREST INTUBATION CHECKLIST

CO_2 – $ETCO_2$ connected to monitor and on

B – Bougie/BVM

O – Oxygen

L – Laryngoscope

T – Endotracheal tube

S – Suction/syringe

CHALLENGE & RESPONSE

Confirm ETT placement

1.1.3 RSI pandemic checklist

CLEAN ZONE | ADULT Preparation for COVID-19 modified RSI

Equipment

Intubation kit dump (as per equipment check)
- Plan A on trolley
- Rescue airway bag = (Plan B, C & D) – double ziplock bag immediately available
- BVM set-up (as per BVM below)
- Gauze swabs

Ventilator set-up (as per Ventilator circuit below)
- Pre-set Vt 6mL/kg/PBW, FiO_2 1.0, RR 16–20/min, PEEP 5–10 cmH_2O, I:E 1:2
- Set High PAW hard alarm to 50 cmH_2O

Drugs
- Rocuronium ≥ 1.5 mg/kg pre & post induction
- Ketamine 1–2 mg/kg (consider dose reduction if CVS unstable)
- Metaraminol **drawn up & present during RSI**
- Post-intubation sedation loaded on T34L

Rescue airway bag

PLAN BCD
- iGel
- Laryngoscope
- Mac Blade
- VL angled blade and introducer
- Bougie/stylet

FONA
- 6.0 ETT
- 20 Scalpel
- Maxi-swab

RSI considerations

- Adequate IV / IO access
- Consider Fluid load (250–500 mL)
- 3-minute pre-Ox with well-sealed BVM (2-person technique advised), 25° head-up
- Avoid apnoeic oxygenation
- Avoid BVM ventilation in apnoeic period unless critical desaturation
- If BVM used for IPPV, ensure full exhalation before mask seal released
- Clamp ETT for ALL circuit disconnections
- Start sedation promptly
- Paralysis post-intubation
- Adjust ventilation as per ARDSnet strategy

Other considerations

- Invasive line insertion (IA / CVC)
- Vasoactive infusion commencement

Team & personnel

- Sitrep to MRC
- **Don full PPE as standard – Contact, Droplet & Aerosol precautions**
  - **PPE buddy checks**
- Brief 'clean runner' on their role
- **Have we forgotten anything?**
- **Confirm any equipment deficits**
- Enter patient care area

BVM
- BVM
- PEEP valve
- $ETCO_2$
- HME filter
- Catheter mount
- Mask

Ventilator
- Circuit
- $ETCO_2$
- HME filter
- Catheter mount
- In-line suction

Set up both circuits. Clamp tube to swap between them.

379

HOT ZONE   ADULT COVID-19 modified RSI Checklist: COVID-19

RSI preparation

✓ Optimise patient position & access

✓ Intubation and ongoing sedation drugs

✓ O_2 supply identified

✓ Vascular access x 2

✓ Fluids run easily

✓ BP set at 2-minute cycles

✓ Baseline vital signs

✓ Ventilator pre-set with circuit attached

✓ $ETCO_2$ functioning

✓ Pre-ox sealed BVM 3 mins

Equipment check

✓ BVM set-up

✓ Laryngoscope + blade tested (VL preferred)

✓ Bougie or stylet

✓ ETT x 2 with cuffs tested

✓ ETT clamp

✓ Syringe & tube tie

✓ Rescue airway bag

✓ OGT / NGT & temperature probe

✓ Cuff manometer

✓ Suction tested & on

30-second drill options:
1. External laryngeal manip
2. Adjust patient position
3. Adjust operator position
4. Change equipment
5. Change operator

Team brief

✓ Intubator

✓ Airway assistant

✓ Drug giver

✓ RSI drug doses

✓ Prompt ETT cuff inflation

✓ Vocalised plan A and rescue plan

Ventilator connection:
1. ETT cuff inflated
2. Waveform $ETCO_2$ on BV
3. TIME OUT
4. Change $ETCO_2$ from BV to vent at zoll monitor
5. Clamp ETT
6. Connect to vent circuit
7. Unclamp ETT
8. Start ventilation

Post RSI

✓ Waveform $ETCO_2$ confirmed

✓ Tube position confirmed, secured & noted

✓ Check vital signs

✓ Sedation started

✓ Consider maintaining paralysis

✓ OGT / NGT

✓ Temperature probe

✓ ETT cuff pressure

✓ Patient ready for departure

✓ Outer PPE doffed

V 1.3 March 2020

Government of South Australia
SA Health

SA Ambulance Service

CHALLENGE & RESPONSE

med STAR

1.1.4 RSI paediatric pandemic checklist

CLEAN ZONE | PAEDIATRIC MODIFIED RSI Checklist: COVID-19 / < 12 years preparation

Equipment

Intubation kit dump (as per equipment check)
- Plan A on trolley
- Rescue airway bag = (Plan B, C & D) - double ziplock bag immediately available
- BVM set-up (as per BVM below)
- Gauze swabs

Ventilator set-up (as per Ventilator circuit below)
- Pre-set Vt 7 mL/kg/PBW, FiO$_2$ 1.0, RR & IT age appropriate, PEEP 5–10 cmH$_2$O, I:E 1:2
- Set High PAW hard alarm to 50 cmH$_2$O

Drugs
- Rocuronium ≥ 1 mg/kg pre & post induction
- Ketamine 2 mg/kg (consider dose reduction if CVS unstable)
- Post-intubation sedation loaded on T34L

Rescue airway bag

PLAN B&C
iGel
Consider Video laryngoscopy
Needle Cricothyroidotomy >1y
Surgical airway >8Y

BVM
- BVM
- PEEP Valve
- ETCO$_2$
- HME filter
- Mask

Ventilator
- Circuit
- ETCO$_2$
- HME filter
- In-line suction

Set up both circuits. Clamp ETT to swap between them.

RSI considerations

- Adequate IV / IO access
- Consider Fluid load 10 mL/kg
- Pre-ox with well-sealed BVM (2-person technique advised), 25° head-up
- Avoid BVM ventilation in apnoeic period unless critical desaturation
- If BVM used for IPPV, ensure full exhalation before mask seal released
- Clamp ETT for ALL circuit disconnections
- Start sedation promptly
- Maintain paralysis post-intubation
- Adjust ventilation as per ARDS strategy

Other considerations

- Invasive line insertion (IA / CVC)
- Vasoactive infusion preparation
- Maintenance fluids + T34L pump
- Other medications

Team & personnel

- Sitrep to MRC
- Don full PPE as standard – Contact, Droplet & Aerosol precautions
  - PPE buddy checks
- Brief 'clean runner' on their role
- **Have we forgotten anything?**
- **Confirm any equipment deficits**
- Enter patient care area

HOT ZONE | PAEDIATRIC MODIFIED RSI Checklist: COVID-19 / <12 Years

RSI preparation

- ✓ Optimise patient position & access
- ✓ Intubation and ongoing sedation drugs
- ✓ O$_2$ supply identified
- ✓ Vascular access x 2
- ✓ Fluids run easily
- ✓ BP set at 2-minute cycles
- ✓ Baseline vital signs
- ✓ Ventilator pre-set with circuit attached
- ✓ ETCO$_2$ functioning
- ✓ Pre-ox BVM sealed

Equipment check

- ✓ BVM set up
- ✓ Laryngoscope + blade tested (VL preferred)
- ✓ Stylet or bougie
- ✓ ETT x 2 with cuffs tested
- ✓ ETT clamp
- ✓ Syringe & tube tapes
- ✓ OGT / NGT & temperature probe
- ✓ Cuff manometer
- ✓ Rescue airway bag
- ✓ Suction tested & on

30-second drill options:
1. External laryngeal manip
2. Adjust patient position
3. Adjust operator position
4. Change equipment
5. Change operator

Team brief

- ✓ Intubator
- ✓ Airway assistant
- ✓ Drug giver
- ✓ RSI drug doses
- ✓ Prompt ETT cuff inflation
- ✓ Vocalised plan A and rescue plan

Ventilator connection:
1. ETT cuff inflated
2. Waveform ETCO$_2$ on BV
3. TIME OUT
4. Change ETCO$_2$ from BV to vent at zoll monitor
5. Clamp ETT
6. Connect to vent circuit
7. Unclamp ETT
8. Start ventilation

Post RSI

- ✓ Waveform ETCO$_2$ confirmed
- ✓ Tube position confirmed, secured & noted
- ✓ Check vital signs
- ✓ Sedation started
- ✓ Maintain paralysis
- ✓ OGT / NGT
- ✓ Temperature probe
- ✓ ETT cuff pressure
- ✓ Patient ready for departure
- ✓ Outer PPE doffed

CHALLENGE & RESPONSE

medSTAR

Government of South Australia
SA Health

SA Ambulance Service

V 1.3 March 2020

1.1.5 Surgical cricothyrotomy

Surgical airway equipment should be immediately to hand for the anticipated difficult airway. If possible, the cricothyroid membrane should be palpated and marked prior to induction. Possible difficulties may be expected in:

- Airway trauma
- Difficult anatomy
- Burns to face and/or neck
- Presumed airway burns.

There are many emergency surgical airway techniques (not all described here). The technique of adult surgical cricothyroidotomy described here is rapid, reliable and relatively easy. The key is not to lose anatomical landmarks following the initial incision and to minimise local haemorrhage.

Surgical cricothyroidotomy technique	
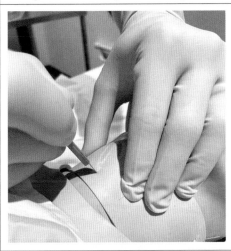	1. Palpate the larynx and identify the cricothyroid membrane. Stabilise the thyroid cartilage with the non–dominant hand and perform a horizontal stab incision at 90 degrees with a large broad–blade scalpel to a depth of approximately 1.5 cm.
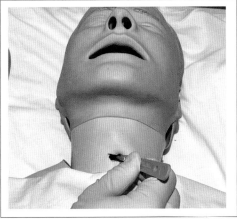	2. Lean the scalpel handle in a lateral direction to open the formed incision through into the laryngeal lumen.

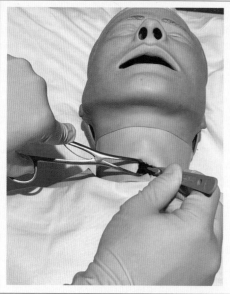

3. Some services use tracheal dilators and others do not. If using dilators, place the tips of the tracheal dilators along the blade of the scalpel until they 'fall off' the end of the scalpel blade. Do not remove the scalpel until the dilators are deployed. This ensures minimal haemorrhage and maintenance of landmarks.

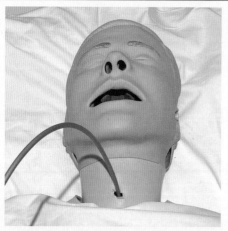

4. Place a bougie through the cricothyroidotomy incision into the trachea. Remove the tracheal dilators.

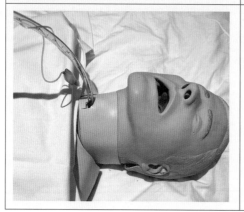

5. Place a size 6 tracheal tube over the bougie. The tracheal tube must only be inserted to a minimal distance (for example up to the vocal cord black marker on the tube). Inflate the tube cuff to minimal occlusive volume ideally using a cuff manometer. Assess for adequate ventilation.

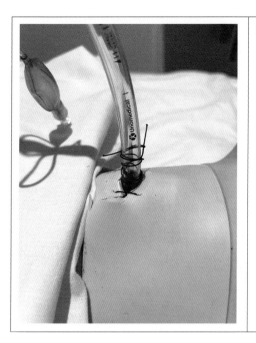

6. Secure with either a suture, ribbon tape or a tracheal tube tie. The method shown in the picture uses a suturing technique.

1.1.6 Paediatric needle cricothyrotomy and jet oxygenation

Needle cricothyroidotomy should be considered in a CICO scenario where a surgical airway is not possible (i.e. child <8 years). Ensure continuous attempts at apnoeic oxygenation are in progress via supraglottic airway (e.g. iGel) connected to O_2.

Equipment required:
- 14G cannula over 8 years (18G under 8 years)
- 5 mL luer-slip syringe
- Saline ampoule
- Custom-designed oxygen-delivery device (e.g. Rapid O_2™)
- Oxygen cylinder or wall oxygen outlet.

Needle cricothyroidotomy technique

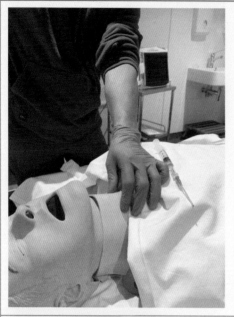

1. Draw up 2 mL of normal saline into the 5 mL syringe and attach syringe to cannula. Stand to left of patient if right-hand dominant or vice versa. Extend head fully on neck (unless c-spine immobilisation required). Palpate the larynx and identify the cricothyroid membrane. Stabilise the thyroid cartilage with the non-dominant hand.

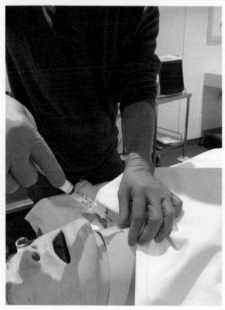

2. Hold 5 mL syringe in dominant hand using an 'aspirate as you go' technique. Insert cannula through skin at 45 degrees to the trachea, aiming caudally. Confirm successful airway cannulation with free aspiration of air up the full length of the barrel of the syringe.

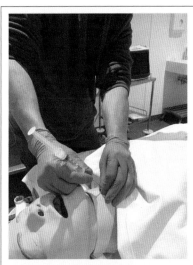

3. Stabilise catheter hub with non-dominant hand. Move dominant hand under syringe to rest against patient's neck and stabilise trochar. Advance catheter over trochar and into trachea with non-dominant hand. Remove trochar while stabilising catheter.

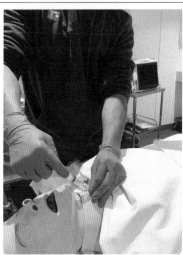

4. Detach trochar from syringe, expel air and re-check position, by attaching syringe to catheter and freely aspirating air. Attach Rapid O$_2$™ to catheter.

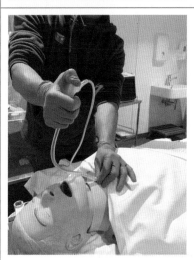

5. Jet oxygenation:
Attach oxygen tubing to Rapid O$_2$™.
  Connect oxygen tubing to oxygen supply at 15 L/min (or 1 L/min per year of age, if child).
Screw luer-lock end of Rapid O$_2$™ gently to catheter in airway.
Cover open limb of Rapid O$_2$™ with thumb to deliver first jet of 4 seconds duration.

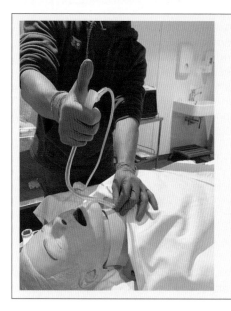

6. Jet oxygenation (cont.):
Wait for SpO_2 to rise to a peak.
Once SpO_2 has dropped by 5% points from peak, deliver second jet of 2 seconds.
Repeat cycle of jetting once SpO_2 has dropped by 5% points from peak.
If no SpO_2 reading, deliver 2-second jet every 30 seconds.
Consider conversion to cuffed tube using available equipment (e.g. Melker cuffed cricothyrotomy catheter) or by conventional intubation (jet insufflation may open up the glottis, improving original view).

Source: Heard A. Percutaneous emergency oxygenation strategies in the 'can't intubate, can't oxygenate' scenario. Smashwords, 2013.

1.1.7 Options for securing tracheal tubes

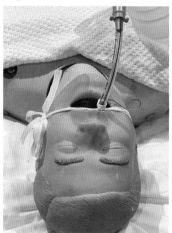

Tracheal tube cloth option

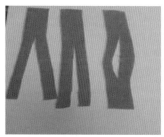 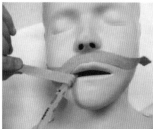 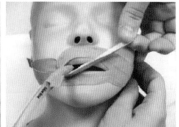

Modified Melbourne strapping used by the Children's Acute Transport Service (CATS), London. Source: Sarfatti A, Ramnarayan P. Transport of the critically ill child. Intensive Care 2017; 27(5):P222–228.

1.2 Vascular access

1.2.1 Central access: common femoral vein

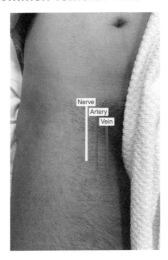

The femoral vein is located medial to the common femoral artery, which is found at the mid–inguinal point (halfway between the anterior superior iliac spine and the symphysis pubis). Ideally, an ultrasound should be used to identify and aid insertion of the catheter. The vein can be cannulated rapidly using a catheter over needle or Seldinger technique. Standard multi–lumen central access catheters can be used; however, large bore catheters (e.g. 9 Fr) may be preferable in trauma patients. The femoral artery lies immediately lateral to the vein and can be accessed for invasive arterial pressure monitoring or an introducer sheath for REBOA, if indicated.

1.2.2 Central access: subclavian and internal jugular vein

Subclavian vein cannulation allows resuscitation of a patient who has had significant pelvic trauma. The subclavian vein is a continuation of the axillary vein and arches cephalad behind the medial clavicle before joining the internal jugular vein. The infra-clavicular approach is most commonly used. This can either be performed using anatomical landmarks or with ultrasound. If the patient has a chest drain or thoracostomy, it is preferential to use that side first. The right subclavian vein cannulation is preferred as it avoids the thoracic duct, and the right pleural apex is lower than the left.

Anatomical landmarks (subclavian):

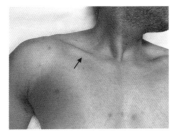

Skin insertion sites include 1 to 2 cm inferior to the clavicle at the junction of its medial and middle thirds or just inferior to the clavicle. The needle is then advanced medially under the clavicle towards the sternal notch until the vein is accessed.

Ultrasound guidance (subclavian):

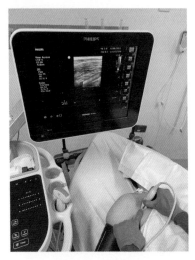

With the patient supine, the probe is placed in the infraclavicular fossa both in the long and short axis view to identify the subclavian vein, artery and axillary vein. Cannulation occurs more laterally than in the landmark approach, hence the axillary vein is usually cannulated using this method.

The internal jugular vein remains the most common site for central access, and internal jugular catheters should always be sited under ultrasound guidance. In trauma patients, access to the neck for catheter placement can be challenging in view of concurrent airway management and spinal immobilisation.

1.2.3. Intraosseous (IO) access

The following pictures show the ideal locations for intraosseous access using mechanised placement devices (e.g. EZ–IO).

Intraosseous access: proximal humerus

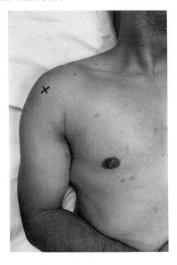

The patient should be positioned supine with their arm adducted and the elbow positioned posteriorly. The humerus should be palpated until the greater tubercle is felt.

This position is also two finger widths inferior to the coracoid process and the acromion. The IO needle is inserted into the greater tubercle.

Intraosseous access: proximal tibia

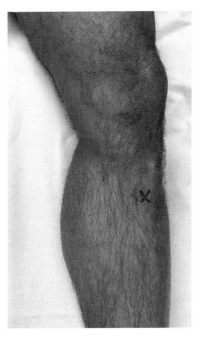

The IO needle is inserted one finger width medial to the tibial tuberosity.

Intraosseous access: distal tibia

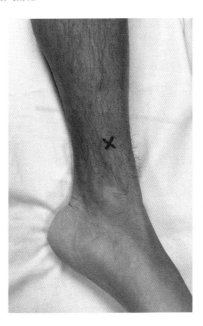

The IO needle is inserted two finger widths proximal to the medial malleolus, midline on the medial tibial shaft.

1.2.4 Umbilical vein and umbilical artery catheters

Introduction

UVC insertion provides a rapid, safe means to achieve central venous access in the unwell infant. Umbilical arterial catheterisation should be considered when continuous blood pressure monitoring (e.g. for titrating inotropes) or frequent blood gas sampling is required.

Umbilical catheterisation can be performed as a formal sterile procedure in premature infants or in those requiring central access or as part of emergency resuscitation. It is usually possible to use the umbilical vein for access until around 72 hours of age and this route can be considered in infants presenting from home in this time period.

If the expertise and confidence of the operator is sufficient, a formal, sterile UVC/UAC may be considered. However, this is a slow process and requires imaging to determine position.

In the case of an infant under active CPR it is impractical to insert a sterile UVC to a calculated depth. A rapid, non-sterile line may be necessary to administer adrenaline. This is not a sterile procedure and so eliminates use of the umbilical vein in the longer term. For this reason, rapid UVC access should not be undertaken routinely except in the context of active CPR.

Catheter size

A size 4 or 5 Fr. line is usually sufficient for any UVC/UAC insertion. Smaller sizes may be available for extremely premature babies, but these gauge lines are frequently used for these babies in tertiary units.

Depth of insertion

There are multiple online tools to calculate the depth of insertion, and these have been validated.

The following formula may also be used:

$$\text{UAC: } (3 \times \text{birthweight \{kg\}}) + 9$$
$$\text{UVC: UAC/2}$$

- The length of any umbilical stump should also be included in addition to the calculated length.
- The tip of both the UAC and UVC should be seen on XR.

UVC: should either traverse the ductus venosus to sit in the inferior vena cava close to the right atrium at T8–10 (at the level of the diaphragm) or be 'low' and short of the portal vein in the umbilical vein.

UAC: has two potential positions – 'high' or 'low'.

- The high position is at the level of thoracic vertebral bodies T6–T10. This position is above the coeliac axis (T12–L1), the superior mesenteric artery (T12–L1), and the renal arteries (L1–L2). This position is 'above the diaphragm'.
- The low position is at the level of lumbar vertebral bodies L3–L4. This position is below the structures above and is above the aortic bifurcation (L4–L5). The inferior mesenteric artery arises from L3–L4.
- Intermediate positions should be corrected to the 'low' position.

Equipment required:

- Fabric tape (umbilical tape is ideal but intubation tape or any fabric tape is usable)

- Umbilical clamp
- Umbilical catheter, primed with 0.9% NaCl
- Three-way tap and bungs
- Scalpel, size 11
- Umbilical vessel dilator (curved non-toothed forceps)
- Sterile plastic drapes, gloves and gown
- Cleaning solution, e.g. 0.05% aqueous chlorhexidine
- Suture silk with needle holder
- Catheter securing device, e.g. stat lock or brown tape
- Clear occlusive IV dressing (e.g. tegaderm)

UVC/UAC insertion technique

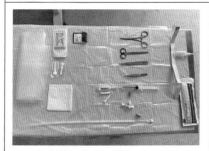	**1.** Prepare equipment. If possible, identify an assistant. Prime the umbilical line lumen(s) with 0.9% saline. Attach a three-way tap or bung to each lumen to avoid introducing air into the vascular system.
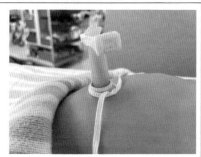	**2.** Place the fabric tape around the base of the umbilical cord using a locking knot (double knot) and adjust so that the tape is resting against the cord but is not tight. The tape should be around the skin at the base of the cord and NOT the jelly matter of the cord itself. The only purpose of the tape is haemostasis in the event of bleeding from the umbilical arteries.
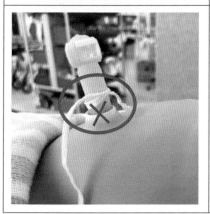	Tightening the tie around the Wharton's jelly of the cord may 'cheese-wire' through the jelly rather than control the bleeding. The umbilical tie is NOT for securing the line.

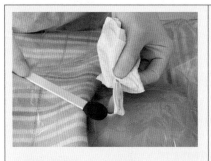

3. Place a sterile dressing over the baby with a central hole for the cord.

Clean the skin, cord and cord clamp using a chlorhexidine/alcohol mix. Some infants suffer chemical irritant burns from chlorhexidine solutions. In the case of premature infants, consider diluting solution with sterile water (0.05% aqueous chlorhexidine) or only using sterile water to clean.

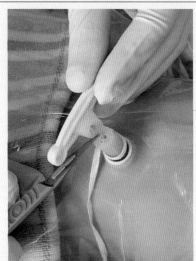

4. Apply gentle traction to the cord clamp and tilt it caudally.

Using the scalpel make a single clean incision below the umbilical clamp, until the vessel appears. It is not necessary to fully transect the cord and it can be useful to use the clamp to control the cord.

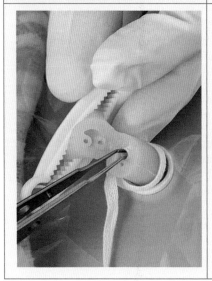

5. Identify vessels:

There are usually two arteries and one vein.

The arteries may stand proud of the jelly due to contraction of their muscular wall.

The vein is usually larger diameter with a thinner, floppier wall and may be collapsed.

The closer to the skin, the more the vein will come into a 12 o'clock position.

Gently rolling the cord between thumb and forefinger may help in opening up the vein.

Using the curved forceps, gently dilate the vessel. This DOES NOT require pressure. Simply insert the tips of the forceps into the vessel lumen and leave them there for a minute.

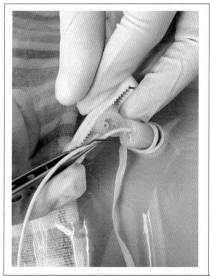

6. Insert the line using either your fingers or the curved forceps. Draw back on one lumen to confirm flash-back of blood. Insert to the pre-calculated depth.
The order of insertion (artery or vein first) is immaterial.
In this photo, the catheter has been inserted into the umbilical vein.

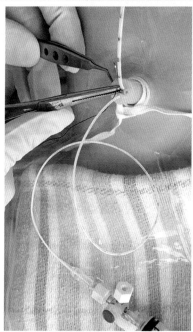

7. Secure the line. This may be done by suturing the line to the Wharton's jelly of the cord. Take a bite through the cord and tie off with a locking knot. Wrap the suture 2–3 times around the line and then secure to the anchored suture or with a second bite and locked knot.
This may be repeated for the second line.
A purse string suture of the exposed end of the umbilical cord may be used but should be wrapped around the lines to secure them within the stitch.

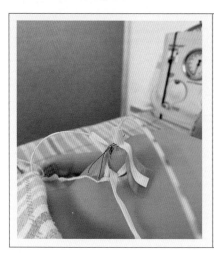

8. If suture is not available, then placing a tegaderm dressing over the whole stump may be the most practical method. Using the 'sandwich technique' or 'goal posts' – ultimately the aim is that the line does not dislodge and there is no definitive way to do this.

Ensure that the line is secured by PUSHING the line into the baby to see if there is any movement.

Stat-lock dressings may be used to additionally secure to the skin. This provides greater stability in a transport setting.

Rapid UVC insertion for use during resuscitation:

Notable differences from formal, sterile procedure described above:

- Clean rather than aseptic technique.
- Cut approximately halfway through from the superior aspect of the cord, **very close to the skin**. At the point of entry to the abdominal cavity the umbilical vein, which has been corkscrewing and coiling through the cord, straightens and sits at the 12 o'clock position. Exposing only this point ensures the greatest likelihood of a successful first attempt.
- By not cutting through the arteries the risk of blood loss in a resus setting is reduced.
- Not removing the umbilical clamp provides a useful handle for manipulating the cord in an emergency setting.

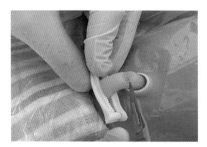

- The line should be inserted to approximately 5 cm of depth plus the stump and flash-back of blood confirmed. This does not require X-ray confirmation of position. It will be a 'low' UVC and sit distal to the portal vein in the umbilical vein.
- It is not necessary to stitch an emergency UVC in place. Using tegaderm or stat-locks is acceptable.

References

Starship. Umbilical artery and vein catheterization in the neonate. 2019. Online. Available: https://starship.org.nz/guidelines/umbilical-artery-and-vein-catheterisation-in-the-neonate/. 15 October 2021.

Sydney Local health District, Royal Prince Alfred Hospital. Women and babies: umbilical venous catheter insertion. 2015. Online. Available: https://www.slhd.nsw.gov.au/RPA/neonatal%5Ccontent/pdf/guidelines/RPAH_UVC_GL2015_025.pdf. 15 October 2021.

1.3 Simple thoracostomy

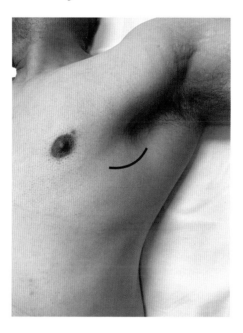

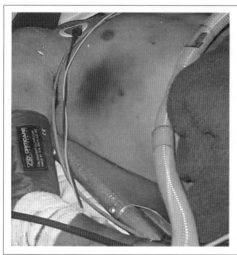

1. With the patient supine, abduct the arm to between 30 and 90 degrees. Use sterile gloves and prepare the area with antibacterial solution.

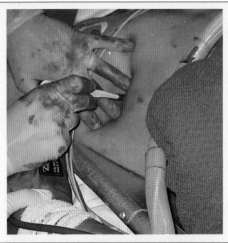

2. Make a 5 cm incision along the line of the ribs in the fourth or fifth intercostal space just anterior to the mid–axillary line (marked in picture above). Use a scalpel for the skin only.
   Note in this image, the thoracostomy site should be one or two rib spaces higher.

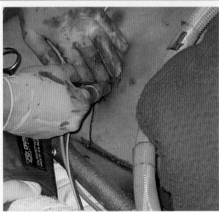

3. Use blunt dissection with forceps (e.g. Spencer Wells) to pass through the intercostal muscles.
   Try to be at 'eye level' with the incision to facilitate safe and accurate blunt dissection.

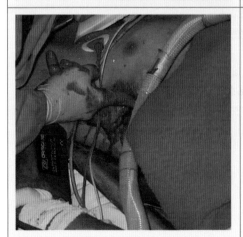

4. Make a hole sufficient to push one finger into the pleural cavity.
   Be careful at this point as there may be fractured ribs that are sharp.
   Palpate the lung to ensure it is up and expanded.
   Leave the soft tissues to fall back over the wound. These tissues will act as a flap valve.
   Re–clean the wound.
   Ensure safe sharps management.

Periodically, a sterile gloved finger should be re–inserted into the wound to ensure that intrathoracic pressure is not building up (tension pneumothorax).

1.4 Clam shell thoracotomy (see also Case 16)

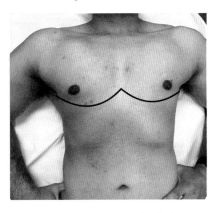

The photo above shows the landmarks for clamshell thoracotomy.

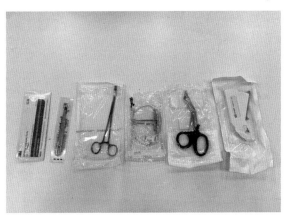

Minimum tools: antiseptic swab, broad blade scalpel, sterile forceps, Gigli saw, sterile shears, skin stapler

Procedure

- Undertake bilateral thoracostomies as described in Appendix 1.3.
- Make a broad skin incision along the line of the fifth rib joining up both thoracostomy wounds. This first incision should aim to get through all skin layers to fat/chest wall.
- Extend the original thoracostomy incisions in the intercostal space posteriorly to the posterior axillary line. This will allow the chest to be opened fully, maximising the exposure and identification of anatomy.
- Using a pair of strong scissors or shears (ideally sterilised), extend the original thoracostomy wounds on both sides up to the sternum. It may be possible to cut through the sternum with the shears. If not, the sternum must now be divided with a Gigli saw. Pass the Spencer Wells forceps behind the sternum, grab the Gigli wire and pull it behind the sternum. Attach the wire to Gigli handles and saw, keeping the operator's hands a metre or so apart to ensure the Gigli blade is not over angulated. It should take little more than two or three pulls to complete sternal division.
- Lift the chest open wide. Use suction if necessary to help clear the field and identify anatomy.

- Identify the heart. If cardiac tamponade is present, the pericardium will look purple and tense. Using two clips, raise a tent of pericardium on the anterior surface of the heart and cut a small vertical hole. Extend the hole vertically with scissors but try not to tear it. Ensure the opening in the pericardial sac is completely extended superiorly and inferiorly, avoiding the phrenic nerve.
- Remove blood clots with your hands. Identify any cardiac wounds and treat with staples or sutures, being careful to avoid the coronary vasculature. Following cardiac repair, blood (or IV fluid if blood unavailable) should be administered and the aorta transiently occluded manually below the heart.
- Internal cardiac massage should be commenced using a two–handed technique, while avoiding lifting the heart and causing kinking of the great vessels.
- The heart may fibrillate or beat spontaneously during this process. Fibrillation unresponsive to a finger flick to the myocardium should be defibrillated either with internal paddles (initial energy 10 joules) or with the clam shell closed using conventional external pads.
- Following return of spontaneous circulation (ROSC), the internal mammary arteries in the chest wall may start to bleed and should be clamped with forceps. Note also that following ROSC the patient may well start to show signs of life and will require adequate sedation and analgesia.
- Intermittent manual aortic compression may need to be performed en route, and the PHRM team should be aware of this when loading the patient into the transport vehicle.

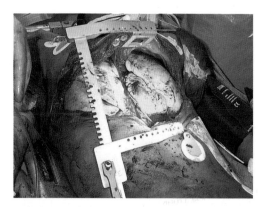

Key points to success

- Rapid access (ideally less than 1 minute to open pericardial sac).
- Extending the thoracotomy wound to the posterior axillary line to promote clam shell opening.
- Extending the opening of the pericardium as far cranially as possible.
- Two–handed quality internal cardiac massage; avoiding kinking of the heart anteriorly.
- Intermittent aortic occlusion against the spinal column.

1.5 Burns
1.5.1 Assessment chart

Adult Burns Patient
Assessment & Management

MEDICAL OFFICER:

PATIENT LABEL

UR NUMBER: _____

SURNAME: _____

GIVEN NAMES: _____

DOB: _____ Sex: _____

DATE OF BURN: _____ ESTIMATED TIME OF BURN: _____

MECHANISM [CIRCLE]: FLAME   SCALD   CONTACT   CHEMICAL   ELECTRICAL   EXPLOSION

Area of Burn
[Lund & Browder Chart]

Partial Thickness

Full Thickness

Note: Simple erythema is not included in %TBSA calculation

Weight: _____ kg

Region	% Burn
Head	
Neck	
Ant Trunk	
Post Trunk	
Right Arm	
Left Arm	
Buttock	
Genitalia	
Right Leg	
Left Leg	
Total	

ANTERIOR

POSTERIOR

IF CIRCUMFERENTIAL LIMB OR TRUNK BURNS – CHECK PERFUSION MAY NEED ESCHAROTOMY

Parkland formula for burns >15% TBSA elderly / co-morbid >20% TBSA adults

401

FIRST AID

☐ Cooling: 20 minutes of cool running water [effective up to 3 hours post injury]

☐ Burns cooling gel is NOT advised in >20% TBSA burns due to risk of hypothermia [EMSB 2021]

☐ Protect against hypothermia [maintain CORE BODY TEMP >36]

☐ Actively warm with blankets, Bair hugger, warmed IV fluids, ambient room temperature

AIRWAY [circle]

FACIAL BURNS   ENCLOSED   AREA VOICE   CHANGE   COUGH SOOT IN MOUTH / NOSE
If ANY of the above, NASENDOSCOPY findings: _____

PAIN MANAGEMENT

☐ Ensure adequate first aid has been given

☐ Fentanyl is the drug of choice for acute pain following burns in the ED

☐ Use IV pain protocol and reassess pain regularly

☐ For minor burns, oral analgesia [e.g. paracetamol / ibuprofen / oral opioids] may be adequate

FLUID MANAGEMENT

Modified Parkland Formula is calculated from the <u>time</u> of burn

3 mL × weight _____ [kg] × %TBSA = _____ mL/24 hours

Give half in first 8 hours = _____ mL = _____ mL/h [rate]

Remaining fluid over next 16 hours = _____ mL = _____ mL/h [rate]

☐ **Use Hartmann's solution**

☐ **Target urine output = 0.5 mL/kg/h**

☐ **All significant burns requiring fluid resuscitation must have <u>IDC with temperature probe</u>**

DRESSINGS

☐ Initially apply cling film to burned areas – DO NOT WRAP CIRCUMFERENTIALLY

☐ Do not de-roof blisters or apply formal dressings until review by the Burns team

DRESSINGS

All facial burns require staining with fluorescein in the ED to assess for corneal abrasions

LEFT EYE: RIGHT EYE:

TETANUS IMMUNISATION

Up to date?   YES / NO   Given?   YES / NO

!

BURNS UNIT CONTACT NUMBERS:

1.5.2 Escharotomy (chest and limb)

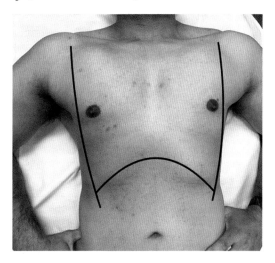

To enable effective ventilation in full–thickness circumferential burns to the chest, an escharotomy should be performed. The two initial incisions are from the shoulders down towards the mid–axillary line as far as the costal margin. An additional incision connecting the inferior end of the initial two incisions should then be made as demonstrated.

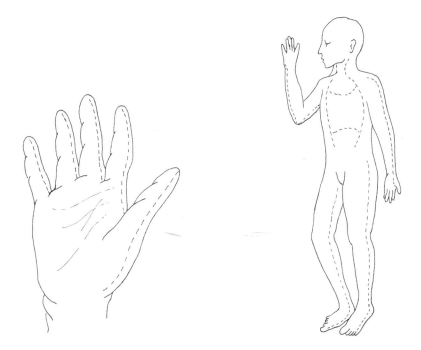

Escharotomy incisions for the limbs should be extended to the level of the thenar and hypothenar eminences for the upper extremity and to the level of the great toe medially and the little toe laterally for the lower extremity.

APPENDIX 2: EQUIPMENT

Suggested equipment for the pre–hospital and retrieval environment

Many services will differ regarding choice of equipment, depending on environment, case mix and transport modality. Space and weight are always at a premium and equipment should be carefully chosen with this in mind. The following list is not exhaustive but offers suggestions that can form the backbone of an appropriate PHRM equipment list.

2.1 General service kit

Generic equipment
Multipurpose monitor With capnography and capacity to defibrillate Spare batteries
Transport ventilator Ventilator tubing (pre–assembled as required) Heat and moisture exchanger (HME)/viral filter High–pressure oxygen hose
Suction unit Soft–suction catheters (variety of sizes) Hard–suction catheters (Yankeur, adult and paediatric)
Back–up portable monitor At least capable of recording saturations and capnography
Oxygen cylinder, lightweight Multi–purpose head (high–pressure attachment and flow meter)
Other Foldable femoral traction splint Stethoscope Shears Tracheal tube cuff manometer Manual hand–held sphygmomanometer Limb splints – variety of sizes (for splinting fractures) Carry sheet or vacuum mattress for moving/packaging patient Scoop stretcher Warming blanket/insulation for thermoregulation Extrication board Infusion pumps Spare batteries Portable ultrasound device Radio Mobile telephone Blood glucometer and testing strips Rapid reading thermometer Nebuliser masks (adult and paediatric)

Airway and breathing pouch

Adult bag valve mask with reservoir bag and oxygen tubing
Paediatric bag valve mask with reservoir bag and oxygen tubing
Supraglottic airway device (sizes 1–5)
Face masks (sizes 1–5)
PEEP valve
Non–re–breathe mask (adult and paediatric)
Extra oxygen tubing (2 m)
Yankauer sucker and Y suction catheter (sizes 6–14)
Oropharyngeal airway (sizes 00, 0, 1, 2, 3, 4)
Nasopharyngeal airway (sizes 4, 5, 7, 6)
Oro/nasogastric tube (variety of sizes) and drainage bag
KY jelly

Adult intubation pouch

Cuffed tracheal tubes (sizes 8, 7, 6)
Video laryngoscope blades (sizes 4, 3 and hyperangulated) and screen
Macintosh blade (sizes 4, 3, 2) and handles
Bougie
Intubating stylet (large)
20 mL syringe
Tube tie
KY jelly
Adult catheter mount
Adult HME/viral filter
Waveform capnography adaptor
Nasal cannula with oxygen hose
Yellow clinical waste bag
Adult Magill forceps
Yankeur sucker
Pre and post RSI checklist

Paediatric intubation pouch

Tracheal tubes (sizes 6, 5.5, 5, 4.5, 4, 3.5, 3, 2.5)
(tubes can be standard, cuffed or armoured)
Bougie (paediatric)
Intubating stylet (small and medium)
Macintosh blades (sizes 2, 3) and Miller blades (sizes 1, 0) and handles including
   options for videolaryngoscope screen
10 mL syringe

Paediatric intubation pouch—cont'd

KY jelly
Tube ties
Paediatric catheter mount
Paediatric HME/viral filter
Paediatric and infant waveform capnography adaptor
Elastoplast roll (2.5 cm)
Yellow clinical waste bag
Paediatric Magill forceps
Paediatric Yankeur sucker
Paediatric nasal prongs
Tongue depressors
Nasogastric tube (size 8 Fr) with ENFIT 10 mL purple syringe

Rescue and surgical airways

14–gauge cannula
10 mL syringe
Antibacterial swab
Needle cricothyrotomy kit including for jet insufflation
Scalpel (size 20 blade)
Cuffed tracheal tube (size 6.0)
Tracheal dilator
Gauze swabs
20 mL syringe
Cloth tie
Silk suture 2/0

C–spine

Adjustable cervical spine hard collar also for use in maxillofacial haemorrhage control

Chest drain pouch

Thoracostomy tube (x 3, varying sizes)
Drainage bags with inbuilt Heimlich valves x 2
Scalpel (22 blade)
Spencer Wells forceps (8 inch)
Hand–held silk 1/0 suture
Antibacterial swabs
Sterile gown, mask, theatre cap and drape
Gauze swabs

Circulation pouch

Intravenous cannulae (all sizes, 2 of each)
Blood–giving set
Intravenous fluid (500 mL)
Hypertonic saline
Elastoplast tape (2.5 cm width roll)
Cannula dressings
Tourniquet (for phlebotomy)
Long intravenous catheters
(large–bore, over–needle catheters for rapid central access)
Triple lumen central venous line (7.5 French gauge 20 cm)
Three–way taps with extension
Paediatric arm boards
Paediatric IV extension tubing
Intraosseous access devices
(mechanised or hand–held needles, adult and paediatric)
Arterial catheters 20 gauge (short)
Arterial catheters 20 gauge (long – femoral)
Steristrips
Pressure bag
Transducer set
Hand–held silk 1/0 suture
Sterile gloves, theatre cap and gown
BioPatch™ and Stat Lock™
Antibacterial swab

Haemorrhage control pack

Epistats (for severe maxillofacial haemorrhage)
Dental bite blocks (small, medium, large)
Large dressings
Gauze swabs
Haemorrhage control bandage
Foley Urinary catheter 18 Fr
1/0 Silk suture
Tourniquets (x2 arterial, for haemorrhage control)
(Consider) Haemostatic agents (e.g. Quikclot)

Thoracotomy pouch

Gigli saw and handles
Gauze swabs
Scalpel (20 blade)
Spencer Wells forceps (8 inch)
Mosquito clips (small)
Scissors (small)
Sterile gloves
2/0 suture and hand–held silk 1/0 suture
Skin stapler
Large dressing

Miscellaneous

Sharps box
Antibacterial swabs
Elastoplast rolls (varying sizes)
Strong tape
Cling film roll (for burns)
Safety razor
Yellow clinical waste bag
Shears (easily accessible)
Permanent marker pen
Syringes (all sizes from 1 mL to 50 mL)
Needles (variety)
Drawing–up needles
Drug labels (for syringes)
Minimal volume extension tubing (for infusions)

Optional additional kits (task specific)

Blood pouch (adequately temperature controlled)
2 to 4 units of O negative blood
Prothrombin Complex Concentrate
Fibrinogen concentrate
Portable blood/fluid warmer and giving set
(space to expand and carry other blood products as per service abilities)

Major incident/disaster pouch

Major incident record sheet
Log sheet or electronic dictation device
Triage cards/deceased labels
High–visibility tabards (e.g. Medical Incident Commander)
Major incident aide memoirs (triage sieve and sort)
Paediatric major incident guide
HAZMAT Identification and decontamination cards
Chemical light sticks
Permanent marker pens

Difficult airway pack

Fibre–optic intubating videoscope – large and slim with screen (e.g. AmbuScope)
Aintree intubating Catheter 19 Fr
100 mm Bermann Airway
Melker cricothyroidotomy kit
Catheter mount with suction port access
Endoscopy mask with securing strap and retaining ring
Lignocaine 2% and adrenaline 1:200,000 (20 mL)
EZ–100 airway atomiser
Lignocaine 4% (50 mL)
Co–phenylcaine forte spray
Glycopyrrolate 2 mL ampoules x 2 (200 microgams/mL)

Pacing kit

Pacing box with cables and spare battery
Introducer sheath 6 Fr
Percutaneous entry needle 18G
Flow–directed pacing catheter 5 Fr
Isoprenaline 200 micrograms/mL (5 mL total)
Transvenous cardiac–pacing aide memoire

Bariatric lifting pack

Hovermat and Hoverjack
240 Volt blower with hose
Lifting straps
Bariatric NIBP cuff
Power extension leads
Patient slide
Ground sheet

GI bleed pack

Sengstaken–Blakemore Tube (or equivalent)
Drainage bag
Cuff manometer
Pantoprazole 40 mg injection
Combine dressing 9 cm x 20 cm
Octreotide 100 mcg injection (5 x 1 mL ampoules) (refrigerated)

Neonatal/obstetric pack

Dressing pack
Woollen hat
Cord clamps
Neonatal bag–valve–mask and 50 mm / 60 mm masks
Tracheal tube uncuffed 2.5
Feeding tube 5 Fr
Laryngoscope handle (slimline) and Miller blade 0
Neonatal Magills forceps
Umbilical catheter (dual lumen) 4 Fr and catheter tapes
IV bungs
Neonatal aide memoires (e.g. neonatal life support)
Obstetric aide memoire
Syntocinon 10IU x 5 ampoules (refrigerated)
Ergometrine 500 mcg x 1 ampoule (refrigerated)
Misoprostol tablets 200 mcg x 10
Nifedipine tablets 20 mg x 4
Magnesium sulphate 50% 10 mL (10 mg) x 5
Vitamin K 1 mL ampoule (2 mg per 0.2 mL)

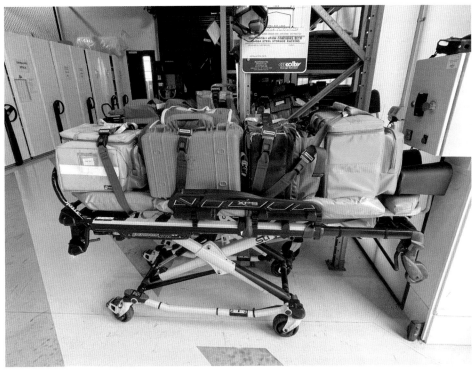

A full PHRM kit packaged and ready for deployment on any transport platform.

Drugs

Drugs have considerable regional variation in name, licensing and familiarity.

The following table attempts to divide drugs into arbitrary groups depending on type of service. While this caters for the variation in pre–hospital versus retrieval work, in many circumstances drugs from each category may be required.

Where relevant, drugs have also been included as part of the optional equipment packs listed above.

Urban/short range	Remote/long range	Special substances

ketamine, thiopentone
Propofol
Fentanyl
Succinylcholine,
  rocuronium
Benzodiazepines (e.g.
  midazolam)
Normal saline (0.9%)
Adrenaline
  (epinephrine)
Amiodarone
	Adenosine
	Other antiplatelet agents
	  (e.g. clopidogrel)
	Morphine
	Hypertonic saline (3%)
	Nitroglycerine IV
	Steroids (e.g
	  dexamethasone)
	  IV/IM/PO
	Ipratropium bromide NEB
	Glucagon, vasopressin
		Noradrenaline
		  (norepinephrine)
		Other vasoactive agents
		  (e.g. metaraminol,
		  hydralazine)
		Dobutamine
		Thiamine IV
		Insulin (Actrapid)
		Potassium chloride IV
		Acetazolamide IV
		antibiotics/antivirals*

Urban/short range	Remote/long range	Special substances
Calcium chloride, magnesium sulfate, sodium bicarbonate Local anaesthetics (e.g. lidocaine / ropivacaine) Salbutamol/albuterol or terbutaline IV and NEB Aspirin Nitroglycerine SL Low molecular weight heparin (e.g. enoxaparin) Loop diuretics (e.g. furosemide) Glucose IV Naloxone Oxytocin ondansetron Atropine Tranexamic Acid	β–blockers (e.g. metoprolol, labetalol) IV Nifedipine PO Haloperidol, droperidol Leviteracetam Ergot alkaloids (e.g. ergo-metrine) Fibrinolytics* Paracetamol	antimalarials* antivenin* antidotes*

*choice depends on regional recommendations
IV: intravenous, NEB: nebulizer, SL: sublingual, PO: oral, IM: intramuscular preparation
Some drugs require refrigeration.
Source: Modified from Sadewasser J, Potter A, Ellis D. Defining a standard medication kit for prehospital and retrieval physicians: a comprehensive review. Emerg. Med. J. 2010; 27(1): 62–71.

Priority drugs pouch

Controlled drugs can be carried in a separate pouch. Depending on case mix, it may be appropriate to have pre–drawn drug syringes to reduce the risk of drawing–up errors Such drugs are listed in the box below.

Priority drugs
Anaesthetic induction agent (e.g. ketamine, Propofol) Succinylcholine Non–depolarising neuromuscular blocking agent (e.g. Rocuronium) Morphine or Fentanyl Midazolam Ketamine (for analgesia and sedation)

Syringes containing drawn–up drugs should be signed, capped, labelled, timed and dated according to local drug guidelines.

2.2 Paediatric and neonatal kit

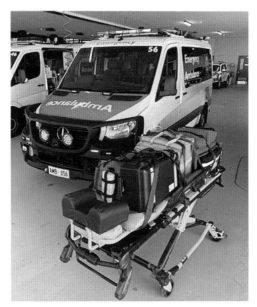

Paediatric kit: Black pelican drug case, red monitor bag, green ventilator bag, red main pack

Main pack
Paediatric stethoscope
Point of care blood test device (e.g. ISTAT) and cartridges
Tender foot lancet white (0.85 mm) and blue (1.0 mm)
Micro pipets, Pipet purple caps, Pipet Fleas
Case cards
Aide memoires
Airway bag
IGELs – 3, 2.5, 2, 1.5, 1
Oropharyngeal tubes – 5, 6, 7, 8 & 9 mm
Nasopharyngeal tube – 4, 6, 7 mm
14 g cannula (safety)
Laerdel fitted mask – 1, 3 & 4
Laerdel round mask – 60 mm & 72 mm
Anaesthetic T–piece (Mapleson C with Jackson Reece Modification)
Manometer set–up (for anaesthetic T–piece)
1 Manometer, 1 graduated connector, 2 x T–piece, 1 plastic adapter
Adult & paediatric HME
Paediatric self–inflating bag with PEEP valve
Nasal prongs – infant and paediatric
Non–rebreather face mask – paediatric

Intubation pack

Paediatric side
Yankeur sucker large
Intubation stylets – medium & large
Laryngoscope blades Mac 3, Mac 2, Miller 1
Sealed surgical airway kit
14 g cannula
10 mL syringe
10 mL 0.9% saline
Scalpel
Tracheal dilator
Insuflation adaptor
Brown tape 2.5 cm
Laryngoscope handle
Colourimetric ETCO$_2$ device (e.g. Easy Cap)
Cuff manometer
Cotton tape
Black silk
Lubricant
10 mL syringe
Paediatric Magills forceps
Rochester clamp with O$_2$ tubing (to clamp TT)
Croup tubes 3.0
Cuffed TT – 3.5, 4.0, 4.5, 5.0, 6.0, 7.0
Neonatal side
Uncuffed TT – 2.0, 2.5, 3.0, 3.5, 4.0
Brown tape 1 cm
Skin prep (e.g. Cavilon)
Adhesive removal wipes
Laryngoscope blades Miller 0 & 00
Laryngoscope handle slim–line neonatal
Colourimetric ETCO$_2$ device (e.g. Pedicap)
Yankeur sucker small *(Sterile)*
Intubation stylets small *(Sterile)*
Scissors *(Sterile)*
Surfactant administration kit
Neonatal Magills forceps
Lubricant
Neonatal HME
Paediatric bougie
Frova intubating catheter 14 Fr

Intubation pack—cont'd

Intubation checklist

Dump bag

Videolaryngoscope pack

Video laryngoscope (e.g. Glidescope)

Stylet – small & large

Blades Miller S0 & S1 and Mac S3

Blade LoPro S1, S2, S3

Additional paediatric monitor (e.g. Solaris NT1G Monitor), batteries and cables

Nasal CPAP (e.g.Medin Miniflow)
30 cm blue vent extension tubing and adapter

nCPAP Generator (Snorkle)

Hats – Small, Medium, Large & XXL

Cannulae – Small, Medium, Large & XL

Mini foam

Tape measure

Aide memoir

Mask CPAP
CPAP mask – Small

Latex head strap

Head strap prongs – Small & Large

Investigation bag
Hypoglycaemia investigation kit
Hypoglycaemia aide memoir

Newborn screening card

Urine bag

Grey top microbiology container

Yellowtop microbiology container

Small urine pots

Specimen bag

Small urine container

Bloods kit
Blood culture bottle (anaerobic & aerobic)

Tender foot lancet white (0.85 mm) and blue (1.0 mm)

Specimen bag

Nasogastric / suction bag
Nasogastric pot

Nasogastric drainage bag

Hydrocolloid dressing, e.g. Duoderm

Videolaryngoscope pack—cont'd

Hypafix dressing (10 cm tape, a 20 cm strip)
10 mL syringe & 10 mL purple syringe
Lubricant
pH sticks/roll (0–6)
Replogle tube Fr 10
Nasogastric tubes Fr 5, 8, 10, 12, 14
Suction catheters Fr 5, 6, 8, 10, 12, 14

Extreme low birth weight pack

Neonatal wrap bag (1–2.5 kg) (e.g. NeoHELP)
Silicone tape (2 cm x 3 m) (e.g. Mepitac)
IV Arm Board – Preemie (e.g. Argyle)
Nappy – 500–750 g infants
Face mask – round 35 & 42 mm
Miller 000 LED blade (purple) *Sealed Sterile*
Miller 00 LED blade (black) *Sealed Sterile*
Larygoscope handle LED (e.g. Parker Intubrite)

Central line/umbi–line/procedure pack

Multipurpose dressing pack
Lignocaine 1%

UVC/UAC insertion pack

Dressing towel
Plastic drape
Stat lock
Umbilical vessel dilator
Scapel blade size 11
Umbilical tape
Suture silk with needle – 4.0
Umbilical clamps
Three–way taps
Bungs
Tape measure
Pneumostat drains
Urine catheters – Fr 8

UVC/UAC insertion pack—cont'd

CVC 5.5 Fr triple lumen
Opsite dressing (10 cm x 12 cm)
Hypafix dressing – sterile (10 cm x 25 cm)
Large skin–prep wipes
Suture silk 2.0
Rochester clamp
Spencer wells

Umbi catheter pack

Umbilical cath – double lumen Fr 3.5 and 5.0
Umbilical cath – single lumen Fr 3.5 and 5.0

Chest drain pack

Intercostal catheters size 10, 12, 20
Pneumopericardial drain Set 6.0F 15 cm (e.g. Cook)
0.02% Chlorhex solution
Sam splint

Drugs and IV access pack

IV access
Tourniquet
Transpore tape and 1 cm brown tape
Interlink bung
IV cannula 16, 18, 20, 22, 24 (short and long)
Sterile clear plastic drape
Gauze swabs
Tegaderm dressing – Large & Small
Steri strips
Chlorhex & alcohol swabs
IV extension T–Piece
Neonatal armboards
Pre–prepared IV infusion kits (x4)
Extension tubing, three–way tap & blue BD thread lock, 50 ml syringe
0.9% Saline 10 mL
Water for injection 10 mL
Drug & infusion labels, e.g. Blue IV infusion & Red IA infusion

Drugs and IV access pack—cont'd

Blood–giving set
0.9% Saline 500 mL
10% Glucose 250 mL
EZ–IO needle + stabiliser kit – Adult
EZ–IO needle + stabiliser kit – Paediatric
EZ–IO drill
Large antiseptic swabs
Spare arrow guide wire
Mucosal atomisation device (Mad) / 1 mL syringe/drawing–up needle
Atrovent metered dose inhaler (MDI)
Salbutamol MDI
Spacer
Salbutamol obstetric IV 5 mg / 5 mL
Phenytoin 250 mg / 5 mL
Adrenaline (1:1000) 1 mg/mL
Salbutamol Nebs 5 mg
Glucose 50%
Phenobarbitone 200 mg/mL
Propofol 1% 20 mL
Infusion pumps
Transilluminator
50 ml syringe
Arterial line, transducer and cables
Hypertonic saline 7.5% (sealed in bag)
Syringe roll
   Needles 18 Fr blunt
   Needleless interlink bung access
   Needle 21 Fr, 25 Fr
   70% alcohol 1% Chlorhexidine swabs
   0.9% saline 10 mL
   5 mL Syringe (RED) – for muscle relaxants
   10 mL syringe
   1 mL syringe – Non–Luer lock
   3 mL syringe
   Red bungs
   IV access bungs

Drug zone
Amiodarone 150 mg/ 3 mL
Atropine 600 mcg / mL
Noradrenaline 4 mg / 4 mL

Drugs and IV access pack—cont'd

Calcium gluconate 2.2 mmol/ 2 mL
Caffeine citrate 40 mg / 2 mL
Hydrocortisone 100 mg
Naloxone 400 mcg / mL
Ondansetron 4 mg / 2 mL
Vitamin K 10 mg / mL
Frusemide 20 mg / 2 mL
Sucrose 24% 1 mL
Dopamine 200 mg / 5 mL
Dobutamine 250 mg / 20 mL
Adenosine 6 mg / 2 mL
Gentamicin 80 mg / 2 mL
Ampicillin 500 mg
Cefotaxime 1 g
Ceftriaxone 1 g
Vancomycin 500 mg
Potassium chloride 10 mmol / 10 mL
Adrenaline 1:10,000 1 mg /10 mL
with 10 mL syringe, red needle, bung access
Glucagon 1 mg
Heparinised saline 50 iu / 5 mL
Magnesium sulfate 2.47 mg / 5 mL (10 mmol / 5 mL)
Aminophylline 250 mg / 10 mL
Aciclovir 250 mg / 10 mL
Levetiracetam 500 mg / 5 mL
Drug book

Fridge drugs

Surfactant 80 mg / mL
Prostaglandin 500 mcg / mL
Suxamethonium 100 mg / 2 mL
Rocuronium 50 mg / 5 mL

Blood carriage bag (temperature controlled)

Blood
Blood/fluid warmer
Giving set

Monitor bag

Pedimate harness and 4 stretcher attachment buckles
Multi–purpose monitor
   ECG 4–lead cable
   Pulse oximeter lead and finger probe
   NIBP tubing and adult cuff
   NIBP cuffs 7, 9, 10
   Defib cable with test port attached
   Paediatric defib pads
   Adult defib pads
Compact suction unit
   Suction canister
   Suction tubing
   Large Yankaeur sucker
   Neonatal Yankaeur sucker
Child's toy
Invasive temperature lead
Monotherm disposable temperature probe
Fully charged spare monitor battery
Massimo SpO_2 sensor
ECG dots – adult
Thermometer
Pen torch
Microstream $ETCO_2$ FilterLine – Adult – orange
Microstream $ETCO_2$ FilterLine – Neonatal – yellow
Shears
Small sharps container

Ventilator pack

Ventilator, cables & accessories
Paed/adult ventilator circuit & block (**greater than 2 yo / 4.0 ETT**)
   HME filter – adult, child and neonate
   Superset catheter mount
   $ETCO_2$ microstream orange (adult/paed/neonate)
Neo/infant ventilator circuit & block (= **or less than 2 yo / 4.0 ETT**)
Ventilator aide memoir

Other specialised bags

These should be available, checked and ready to go if required. Examples of specialty packs include:

- Home birth pack
- Twin transfer pack
- Bilitron pack – for providing phototherapy during transport
- Cooling pack – cooling for neonatal encephalopathy
- Neonatal transport cot (an example of a neonatal transport cot can be seen in Case 61).

APPENDIX 3: PERSONAL PROTECTIVE EQUIPMENT (PPE)

3.1 Standard/aviation PPE

PPE is a cornerstone of pre–hospital and retrieval medicine. Many services will differ with choice of PPE depending on environment, case mix and transport modality. Equipment should be from a reputable source and should be approved nationally or internationally.

A suggested generic PPE list can be compiled according to anatomical site as outlined below.

Personal protective equipment
Head
Helmet – aviation and protective
Head torch
Ear defenders
Safety goggles
Body
High–visibility flame–retardant protective jacket and trousers
Protective vest ('stab resistant')
Limbs
Examination gloves (fluid resistant)
Debris gloves
Knee pads
Steel–cap boots
General
Radiation dosimeters/alert devices
Disposable dust/antimicrobial masks
Aviation
Constant wear life vest (e.g. Switlik) consisting of:
• Self–inflating life jacket
• Compact distress signal flares
• Emergency distress strobe light
• Fluorescent marine marker dye
• Emergency position–indicating radio beacon (EPIRB).

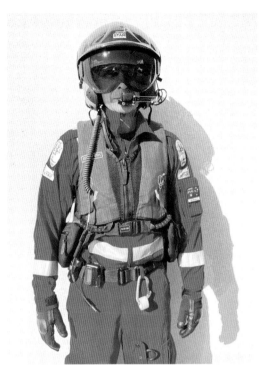

PHRM team member demonstrating aviation PPE

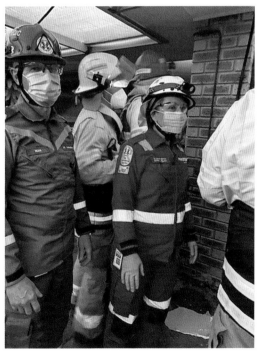

PHRM team member demonstrating 'on scene' PPE

3.2 On–scene PPE for 'clean' medical interventions

This includes a hat, face mask, sterile gown and gloves. Protective eyeware can be worn if required for the procedure.

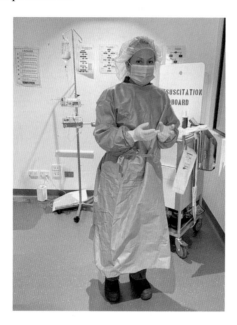

3.3 Medical intervention PPE for viral airborne diseases

The choice of PPE for appropriate circumstances should be dictated by a risk–assessment matrix. An example of PPE for a high–risk patient is an N95/99 mask, goggles, Tyvek suit, and gloves.

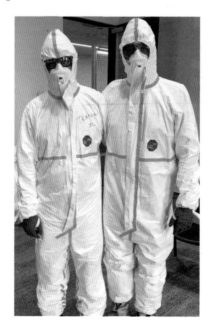

3.4 PPE for long–distance tasking over water (immersion suit)

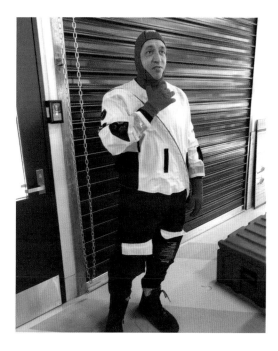

3.5 Other personal equipment

Some PHRM teams issue personal small kit bags to allow the clinician to carry some equipment that may be frequently used or that is unique to that clinician. As well as a specific bag, this kit can also be carried in pockets or on belt clips. It is essential this kit is kept to a minimum.

By definition, personal kit lists are highly variable, but certain items are popular in many cases as listed below.

Personal kit items
Intravenous cannulae (varying sizes)
Long intravenous catheters
(Large bore, over–needle catheters for rapid central access)
10 mL syringe
Sterile/examination gloves
Pen
Torch/head torch
Strong scissors/shears
Spencer Wells forceps (sterile)
Scalpel
Antibacterial swab

Personal kit items—cont'd
Nasopharyngeal and oropharyngeal airways
Documentation (for patient records)
Drug dose booklets (e.g. paediatric) or other compact medical texts
Handover template
Mobile telephones and radios

APPENDIX 4: TRANSFER AND RETRIEVAL CHECKLIST

4.1 Pre–hospital and inter/intra–hospital transfer and retrieval checklist

Following a familiar, generic structure can help to reduce the risk of omission or error. The 'ISBAR' process below is an example of such a structure. On PHRM tasks, an ISBAR handover is likely to be required on more than one occasion (e.g. on arrival at the patient's bedside, as a sitrep to the tasking agency, at final handover at destination). Further detail is likely to be required and additional information can be provided in a checklist format.

Identification	Self, role and patient
Situation	What is the issue/reason for transfer?
Background	Context, clinical background and relevant issues. May include time of injury, mechanism, injuries found, clinical signs
Assessment	Current issues and condition, including during transfer
Recommendation	Treatments required

Detailed patient issues (on arrival at patient's bedside)	
Identification	Name/Age/Sex/Date of birth
Respiration	Airway secure Ventilation adequate (e.g. $ETCO_2$ etc.) on transfer ventilator
Circulation	Haemodynamically stable Venous access adequate, patent and secure Arterial access patent and secure
Neurological	GCS recorded (with E, V, M breakdown)
	Pupils, size and reaction recorded
	Neuroprotection, if indicated
Monitoring (minimum)	ECG, blood pressure, SaO_2, $ETCO_2$, temperature
Other	Drains (wound, chest, urinary) patent and secure
	All non–essential infusions stopped
	Fractures stabilised and splinted
	Adequate precautions against transfer environment (blankets, ear protection)
	Resuscitation status established and confirmed

Information to confirm at referring hospital/location
Referral to receiving hospital made
Exact destination ascertained (e.g. radiology department, ward, bed number, theatre)
Notes, letters, radiographs and other tests prepared
Full handover taken
Relatives informed (patient as well, if feasible)
Contact numbers (mobile, pagers) of referring/receiving team recorded

Information required by the receiving hospital/location
Aware that patient arriving and exact destination
Estimated time of arrival (ETA) given
Contact numbers of coordinating agency
Aware of patient condition (lines/infusions/ventilatory status/monitoring)

Information for coordination agency
Liaison with land ambulance/pilots
Route planned
Return journey considerations

4.2 Final pre–departure checklist
(To be done when patient loaded onto ambulance/aircraft)

Patient identity confirmed
Patient stable and secured on suitable trolley
Sitrep to coordinating agency
Resus equipment present, accessible and secured
Sufficient oxygen for trip duration
Monitors and ventilators visible, alarms activated
Infusion pumps functional and sufficient for duration of trip
Equipment now powered by mains or extra batteries visualised

Vehicle/aircraft oxygen supply utilised and sufficient
Medical documentation / radiology / laboratory tests to hand
Documentation for use during transfer (paper or electronic)
Transfer consent / family / next of kin / partner briefing
Final check that all team equipment present (including radios, etc.)
Clinical coordination centre or Ambulance Service aware of departure
Destination aware of departure and revised ETA (via coordination agency)
Retrieval team seated and secured

Arrival at destination **(To be done at patient's bedside at receiving hospital)**
Immediate needs?
Patient stable?
Formal handover to receiving hospital (e.g. ISBAR)*
Final observations and time noted
Notes from transfer (including observations, drugs, fluids) written and photocopied
Notification of coordination agency

*The formal handover process will often be dependent on the type of PHRM case. For example, a trauma handover of a primary tasking in the emergency department should be succinct, concise and brief (less than 60 seconds). However, for an ICU to ICU PHRM case, a more detailed handover will be required.

To reduce the risk of error or omission, reminders and checklists can be incorporated into the patient clinical documentation.

Examples of Pre–departure checklists and handover tools can be seen in the sample case card in Appendix 6.

Additional reading

Association of Anaesthetists of Great Britain and Ireland. Interhospital transfer. 2009. Online. Available: https://anaesthetists.org/Home/Resources–publications/Guidelines/Interhospital–transfer–AAGBI–safety–guideline. 20 October 2021.

Australasian College for Emergency Medicine, Australian and New Zealand College of Anaesthetists and College of Intensive Care Medicine of Australia and New Zealand. Guidelines for transport of critically ill patients. 2015. Online. Available: https://acem.org.

au/getmedia/0daba691–5e60–4a88–b6a8–24f2af3e5ebf/Guidelines_for_the_Transport_of_
Critically_Ill_Patients. 20 October 2021.

Intensive Care Society. Guidance on: The transfer of the critically ill adult, 2019. Online.
Available: ficm.ac.uk/sites/default/files/transfer_critically_ill_adult_2019.pdf. 18 October
2021.

Nathanson M H, Andrzejowski J, Dinsmore J et al. Guidelines: safe transfer of the brain–
injured patient: trauma and stroke. Association of Anaesthetists of Great Britain and
Ireland, 2019.

Courtesy of WA office of chief psychiatrist: https://www.chiefpsychiatrist.wa.gov.au/wp-content/uploads/2017/03/20161128-updated-MH-Transport-Risk-Assessment-Form-V1.3-with-barcode.pdf

Government of **Western Australia**
Department of **Health**

St John

Mental Health Transport Risk Assessment Form

This form is intended to be used by services in order to identify the following:

Section 1: Assessed by   Section 2: Personal Particulars   Section 3: Risk Assessment Matrix   Section 4: Result of Assessment

THIS FORM IS USED TO ASSESS RISK ASSOCIATED WITH MENTAL HEALTH TRANSPORTATION ONLY AND SHOULD NOT REPLACE INDIVIDUAL AGENCY OPERATIONAL OR CLINICAL PROTOCOLS.

The purpose of information sharing is to ensure each agency has sufficient information to enable them to provide effective and appropriate services. Collection and disclosure should be limited to personal information that is necessary and relevant to these purposes and occur in accordance with Section 576 and 577 of the **Mental Health Act 2014.**

Referrer's Name:_____   **Contact Number:**_____

Please inform receiving site when the patient departs pick up location. This will ensure necessary resources can be in place to support the patient admission.

SECTION 1 – Assessed by

Medical or Authorised Practitioner: _____

Centre / Clinic / Hospital: _____

Treated On: _____/_____/_____

SECTION 2 – Personal Particulars

Surname: _____   **Given Names:** _____

Date of Birth: _____/_____/_____   **Language Spoken:**_____

Address: _____

Add the patient's current residential address in this field. If the patient is located at another place, record the address and location in the notes field supplied in Section 4.

Is the patient currently receiving treatment for a mental illness?   Yes ◯   No ◯

SECTION 3 – Risk Assessment Matrix

Complete Attachment A

• Indicate risk for each criterion by placing a tick in the applicable box.

• Each matrix is a tool to record information and provide guidance on a suitable transport option. If the majority of boxes ticked align to one risk category, the clinician's informed judgement should be used to determine if this is the most appropriate risk rating and transport option.

• Reasons for not selecting the risk rating that aligns to the majority of boxes ticked should be recorded in the Risk Rating Rationale section on the following page.

SECTION 4 – Result of Assessment

Form 4A - Transport Order: **Completed**

Transport Type: Inter-Hospital ◯   Community to Hospital ◯

Transport by: Mental Health Transport Officer ◯   Police Officer ◯
                        (Metropolitan area only)

NEXT STEPS

1. Identify bed availability (contact local inpatient service Bed Manager or delegate)
2. Book transport with appropriate provider (or refer to WA Police where appropriate)
3. Provide appropriate documentation to transport providers and others involved

Mental Health Transport Risk Assessment

SMHMR990

RISK ASSESSMENT NOTES

This section has been provided to record notes relevant to the risk assessment. Details such as next of kin/trusted friend, location of crisis, patient's behaviour and/or demeanour, current or history of mental illness/treatment, severity of situation and agency response can be recorded here.

MEDICAL OR AUTHORISED PRACTITIONERS REQUESTING THE TRANSPORT ARE REQUIRED TO RECORD A COMPREHENSIVE RISK ASSESSMENT (INCLUDING APPROPRIATE DETAIL). ALL STAFF INVOLVED IN TRANSPORTATION ARE REQUIRED TO UTILISE UNIVERSAL PRECAUTIONS TO MITIGATE THE RISK OF INFECTIOUS DISEASES.

Risk Rating Rationale:

Delusional systems that may impact on safe escort (e.g. fear of authority figures):

Access to weapons, concealed or otherwise:

Sensory impairment (e.g. sight, hearing, intoxication):

Medical considerations that may impact on safe escort (e.g. heart condition, epilepsy):

Has the patient's Family/Carer been notified regarding the transfer? Yes ◯ No ◯
Family/Carer Contact Name: _____ **Number:** _____
Does the patient have children that need care? Yes ◯ No ◯ (please specify arrangements made)

Notes:

Name: _____ Signature: _____ Designation: _____
Date: _____/_____/_____ Time: _____

XY600426

Mental Health Transport Risk Assessment

SMHMR990

Attachment A - Mental Health Patient Transport Matrix

Risk Category Inter Hospital and Community (Contacts)	Clinical	Mental State	Violence / Aggression to others	Self-Harm	Resistance	Absconding	Past Behaviour
Low • National Patient Transport (Metro Inter Hospital only) • St John Ambulance	Physically uncompromised; Ambulating without assistance ☐	Low risk of aggression, self-harm; Judgement intact ☐	Patient reports no intent to harm others ☐	Patient reports no intent to harm self ☐	Patient compliant to transfer ☐	Patient reports nil intent to abscond ☐	Past compliance to private transfer; Nil or distant past episodes of violence / aggression / resistance / absconding related to transfer ☐
Medium • National Patient Transport (Metro Inter Hospital only) • St John Ambulance	Physically uncompromised; Ambulating without assistance ☐	Low risk aggression and self-harm; No cognitive impairment Cooperative ☐	No identified intent to harm others; No current access to weapons ☐	No identified intent to self-harm / suicide ☐	Patient reluctant to engage but demonstrates willingness to transfer with transport personnel present ☐	Patient reports willingness to remain with transport personnel during transfer ☐	Past compliance to transfer with nurse escort/transport personnel present ☐
High • St John Ambulance	Physically uncompromised; Ambulating without assistance ☐	Poor cooperation but not physically resistive; Mild cognitive impairment ☐	Past aggression but not currently escalating; No clear plan to harm others ☐	Past attempts to self-harm / suicide but not currently escalating; No clear plan to self-harm / suicide ☐	Reluctant to engage in transfer but no clear plan to resist ☐	No clear plan identified to abscond ☐	Past compliance to transfer with security/ Special Constable/ transport personnel present ☐
Significant (Extreme) (WA Police)	Sedated but able to be roused; Not under the influence of alcohol or drugs; Medically cleared ☐	Not cooperating; High risk of aggression or self-harm; Significant cognitive impairment (not from alcohol or drugs). ☐	Currently displaying violence/ aggression to others requiring physical restraint; History of concealing weapons; Patient reports intent to harm others ☐	Currently attempting self-harming / suicidal behaviour; Patient reports intent to self-harm / suicide; Patient indicates clear plan to self-harm / suicide. ☐	Patient reports intent to resist transfer; Patient identifies clear plan to resist transfer ☐	Patient reports intent to abscond; Patient identifies clear plan to abscond ☐	Patient has required police escort previously (due to violence/ aggression / resistance / absconding related to transfer) ☐

433

APPENDIX 6: SAMPLE DOCUMENTATION AND CASE CARDS

6.1 General service case card

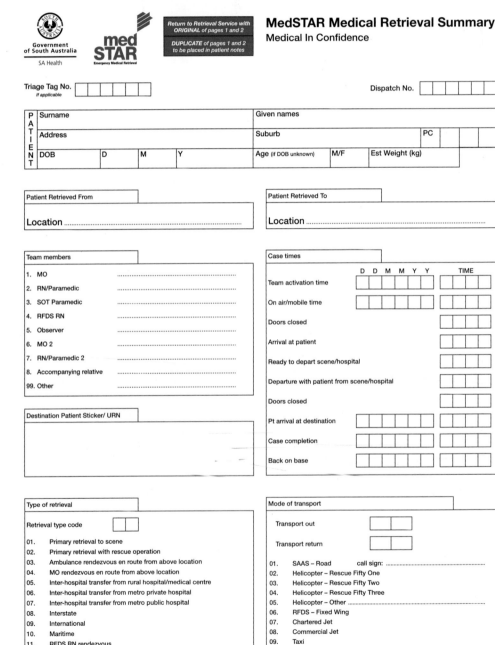

Government of South Australia
SA Health

med STAR
Emergency Medical Retrieval

Return to Retrieval Service with **ORIGINAL** of pages 1 and 2

DUPLICATE of pages 1 and 2 to be placed in patient notes

MedSTAR Medical Retrieval Summary
Medical In Confidence

Triage Tag No.
If applicable

Dispatch No.

P A T I E N T	Surname				Given names				
	Address				Suburb			PC	
	DOB	D	M	Y	Age (if DOB unknown)	M/F	Est Weight (kg)		

Patient Retrieved From

Location ....

Patient Retrieved To

Location ....

Team members

1. MO ....
2. RN/Paramedic ....
3. SOT Paramedic ....
4. RFDS RN ....
5. Observer ....
6. MO 2 ....
7. RN/Paramedic 2 ....
8. Accompanying relative ....
99. Other ....

Destination Patient Sticker/ URN

Case times

	D	D	M	M	Y	Y		TIME
Team activation time								
On air/mobile time								
Doors closed								
Arrival at patient								
Ready to depart scene/hospital								
Departure with patient from scene/hospital								
Doors closed								
Pt arrival at destination								
Case completion								
Back on base								

Type of retrieval

Retrieval type code

01. Primary retrieval to scene
02. Primary retrieval with rescue operation
03. Ambulance rendezvous en route from above location
04. MO rendezvous en route from above location
05. Inter-hospital transfer from rural hospital/medical centre
06. Inter-hospital transfer from metro private hospital
07. Inter-hospital transfer from metro public hospital
08. Interstate
09. International
10. Maritime
11. RFDS RN rendezvous

99. Other ....

Mode of transport

Transport out

Transport return

01. SAAS – Road   call sign: ....
02. Helicopter – Rescue Fifty One
03. Helicopter – Rescue Fifty Two
04. Helicopter – Rescue Fifty Three
05. Helicopter – Other ....
06. RFDS – Fixed Wing
07. Chartered Jet
08. Commercial Jet
09. Taxi
10. MedSTAR Fleet ....

99. Other ....

Return to Retrieval Service with ORIGINAL of pages 1 and 2 | DUPLICATE of pages 1 and 2 to be placed in patient notes

MedSTAR Medical Retrieval Summary cont
Medical In Confidence

Treatment interventions

Pre = commenced prior to team arrival   Post = commenced or continued by team

Pre	Post	Respiratory		Pre	Post	Circulation		Pre	Post	Medication		Pre	Post	Other
☐	☐	Oxygen		☐	☐	Peripheral IV		☐	☐	Opioid analgesia		☐	☐	Urinary catheter
☐	☐	NIV		☐	☐	Intraosseous		☐	☐	Sedation/GA		☐	☐	Temperature
☐	☐	PEEP		☐	☐	Fluid bolus		☐	☐	Relaxant		☐	☐	Cervical collar
☐	☐	Intubation		☐	☐	Blood transfusion		☐	☐	Anticonvulsant		☐	☐	Limb splints
☐	☐	Surgical airway		☐	☐	Cardiac pacing		☐	☐	Bronchodilator		☐	☐	Pelvic splint
☐	☐	IPPV		☐	☐	Cardioversion		☐	☐	Antiarrhythmic		☐	☐	Vacuum Mattress
☐	☐	Nitric		☐	☐	Defibrillation		☐	☐	Inotrope		☐	☐	Naso/orgo gastric tube
☐	☐	Pleural drain		☐	☐	CPR		☐	☐	Vasodilator		☐	☐	Thoracotomy
		☐ L ☐ R		☐	☐	Aortic balloon pump		☐	☐	Thrombolytic		☐	☐	Ultrasound FAST
☐	☐	Needle thoracocentesis		☐	☐	CVC		☐	☐	Heparin		☐	☐	Ultrasound Other:
		☐ L ☐ R		☐	☐	Arterial Line		☐	☐	Antibiotics				
☐	☐	Finger thoracostomy		☐	☐	PA catheter		☐	☐	Antivenom				
		☐ L ☐ R		☐	☐	Rapid infuser		☐	☐	Prothrombinex		☐	☐	Enrolled Clinical Trial:
☐	☐	S_aO_2		☐	☐	CVP		☐	☐	Tranexamic Acid				
☐	☐	E_tCO_2		☐	☐	ECG		☐	☐	Other medications				
				☐	☐	NIBP								

Diagnostic Category

Primary Diagnostic Category ☐☐   Secondary Diagnostic Category ☐☐   Additional Diagnostic Categories ☐☐ ☐☐

Cardiovascular
01 Cardiac arrest
02 Myocardial Infarction
03 MI post thrombolysis
04 Unstable angina
05 Arrhythmia
06 Cardiogenic shock
07 Pulmonary oedema/CCF
08 Vascular (e.g. AAA)
09 Other cardiovascular
Respiratory
10 Asthma
11 COAD

Respiratory (cont)
12 Pneumonia ± shock
13 Other respiratory
Neurological
14 Epilepsy
15 CVA - not SAH
16 SAH
17 Infection ± shock
18 Other neurological
Surgical/Anaesthetic Complication
19 Emergency
20 Elective

Gastrointestinal
21 Bleed - varices
22 Bleed - other
23 Pancreatitis
24 GI perforation
25 Other gastrointestinal
Metabolic/Endocrine
26 Diabetes
27 Other endo/metabolic
Renal
28 Infection ± shock
29 Other renal

Miscellaneous
30 Obstetric
31 Substance abuse/poisoning
32 Sepsis - site unknown
33 Allergy/drug side effect
34 Psychiatric
35 Envenomation
36 Decompression illness
37 Trauma - motor vehicle
38 Trauma - other
99 Other:

Retrieval outcome

Retrieval outcome code ☐☐

01	Admitted to CCU direct	05	Admitted to HDU/SDU direct	09	Died at scene - post team arrived	13	Retrieval cancelled
02	Admitted to ED - non resus	06	Admitted to ICU direct	10	Died during transport	99	Other:
03	Admitted to ED - resus	07	Admitted to OT	11	Died prior to team arrival		
04	Admitted to general ward	08	Admitted to Cardiac angio	12	Remained at scene/hosp (scene assist)		

Clinical issues / Incidents / Problems (inc equipment failure)

SLS Actioned ☐ Yes   ☐ No

Logistic issues / Incidents / Problems (inc transport & packs)

SLS Actioned ☐ Yes   ☐ No

435

Government
of South Australia
SA Health

med
STAR
Emergency Medical Retrieval

Medical Retrieval Record

Medical in Confidence

Surname		Time	Date
Given names		M/F	Date of Birth
Referring MO	Location	Retrieval MO	Retrieval RN/Para

ORIGINAL of pages 1 and 2 return to retrieval service

DUPLICATE of pages 1 and 2 to be placed in patient notes

Allergies:

Past Medical History

Current Medication List

Last ate:

Infectious status

Patient Assessment

Investigation / Results

CT / Xray / FAST

ABG / Bloods / BSL / ECG

Diagnosis / Differential

Management Plan

RSI Induction Time

TT size

TT Length at teeth

Grade of intubation

Number of passes

Patient weight

Medical Officer Surname ....

Medical Officer Signature ....

Detention sighted ☐ Yes ☐ No   Consent ☐ Yes ☐ No   Advanced care ☐ Yes ☐ No

MVC Information
⊗ Patient position

Direction
of impact

Time ....
Approx Speed ....
Intrusion ☐ Yes ☐ No
Seatbelt/Restraint ☐ Yes ☐ No
Protective gear ☐ Yes ☐ No
Type ....

Page 1

Government of South Australia
SA Health

med STAR
Emergency Medical Retrieval

Retrieval Observations Chart	Surname
	Given names
	Date of Birth / M/F

Medical in Confidence — DUPLICATE of pages 1 and 2 to be placed in patient notes   ORIGINAL of pages 1 and 2 return to retrieval service

	Time (24 hr)	On arrival										On handover
Systolic BP ▼	200											
	190											
	180											
	170											
	160											
	150											
Diastolic BP ▲	140											
	130											
	120											
	110											
MAP ●	100											
	90											
	80											
	70											
	60											
Heart Rate ✕	50											
	40											
	30											
General Obs	Rhythm											
	S_pO_2											
	Cap refill (seconds)											
	Temperature											
	Blood Glucose											
	Pain score											
Respiratory	Resp rate											
	F_iO_2											
	E_tCO_2											
	Tidal volume											
	PS											
	PEEP											
	PIP/Plat pressure											
	ETT cuff pressure											
Neurological	Eyes /4											
	Verbal /5											
	Motor /6											
	GCS /15											
	Pupils (mm) R / L	/	/	/	/	/	/	/	/	/	/	/
Neurovascular	Pupils / Sensation RA / LA											
	Pulse / Sensation RL / LL											
Access												
Arterial line												
Drug infusion	Conc^N / volume											
Fluid infusion / type												
L Litres												
mL Millilitres												
Fluid out	Urine/Gastric/Wound (mL)											

Medications given	Name	Dose	Discard	Route	Time	MO	RN / Paramedic
g Grams							
mg Milligrams							
mcg Micrograms							

....
Nurse / Paramedic Signature   Date ....

....
MO Signature   Date ....

● 2mm (pinpoint)
● 4mm
● 7mm (dilated)

Eye Opening:
4 - Spontaneous
3 - To speech
2 - To pain
1 - Nil

Verbal Response:
5 - Orientated
4 - Confused
3 - Inappropriate words
2 - Incomprehensible
1 - Nil

Best Motor Response:
6 - Obeys commands
5 - Purposeful movement
4 - Withdraws to pain
3 - Flexion to pain
2 - Extension to pain
1 - Nil

437

Government
of South Australia
SA Health

med
STAR
Emergency Medical Retrieval

Retrieval Follow up

(Return to Retrieval Service with Pages A, B and C, and originals of 1 and 2)

LMO feedback (usually completed the next working day)

To: LMO / Other ....

By ....

Dated ....

Final diagnosis / injuries

....
....
....
....
....
....
....
....
....
....
....
....
....
....
....
....
....

Government of South Australia
SA Health

med STAR
Emergency Medical Retrieval

Checklist / Handover

Standard Checklist	Pre - departure patient location	Pre - departure final destination
Equip ⟍ Location		
EOC / MRC sitrep	☐	☐
Radio	☐	☐
Resus kit (inc BVM)	☐	☐
Procedure kit	☐	☐
Monitor	☐	☐
Ventilator	☐	☐
Ultrasound	☐	☐
Blood	☐	☐
Special kits	☐	☐
Notes / XR / CT / Labs	☐	☐
Family / NOK / Partner briefing	☐	☐

Must have access to	O_2 ☐	Suction ☐	BVM ☐	Drugs / IV kit ☐	Intubation kit ☐	Fluids ☐

HANDOVER - Draft your ISBAR handover here:

Immediate needs Y / N –
Identify (self, role, and patient)

Situation (what is going on with patient)

Background (what is the clinical background / context)

Assessment (what is the current problem)

Response – Recommend – Read back (recommended treatments, check back for shared understanding)

6.2 Multi–casualty template

Mass Casualty Patient Record Sheet

Date: _____

Patient Name	Patient No. or Triage Tag No.	Age	M/F	Triage Cat	Injuries	Dest	Transport Call Sign	Depart Scene	Notes

Government of South Australia
SA Health

med STAR
Emergency Medical Retrieval

APPENDIX 7: PAEDIATRIC AND NEONATAL KEY INFORMATION

7.1 Paediatric common drug doses and infusions

Common emergency resuscitation drugs	
Drug	**Dose**
Adenosine (SVT)	1st dose 0.1 mg/kg IV 2nd dose 0.2 mg/kg IV 3rd dose 0.3 mg/kg IV
Adrenaline (arrest)	10 mcg/kg (0.1 mL/kg of 1:10,000) IV 100 mcg/kg (0.1 mL/kg of 1:1000 in 5 mL saline) ETT
Adrenaline (anaphylaxis)	10 mcg/kg (0.01 mL/kg of 1:1000) IM
Amiodarone	5 mg/kg IV
Atropine	20 mcg/kg IV/IM, ETT
Bicarbonate	1 mmol/kg IV
Calcium Chloride 10% (arrest)	0.15 mmol/kg IV (0.2 mL/kg)
Calcium Gluconate 10% (hyperkalemia)	0.1 mmol/kg IV (0.5 mL/kg)
Fentanyl (intubation)	1–2 mcg/kg IV
Glucose	2 mL/kg of 10% dextrose IV
Insulin (hyperkalemia)	0.1 units/kg IV (with 10% dextrose 5 mL/kg, dextrose administered 1st followed by insulin)
Ketamine (intubation)	1–2 mg/kg IV
Lignocaine (arrythmia)	1 mg/kg IV
Magnesium Sulfate (asthma)	0.2 mmol/kg IV over 20 mins
Magnesium Sulfate (torsades)	0.05 mmol/kg
Mannitol 20%	0.5–1 g/kg IV

Continued

441

Common emergency resuscitation drugs—cont'd

Drug	Dose
Metaraminol (Aramine)	0.01 mg/kg IV
Midazolam (seizure)	0.15 mg/kg IV/IM 0.3 mg/kg buccal
Naloxone (Narcotic overdose)	5–10 mcg/kg IV/IM, ETT
Propofol	1–4 mg/kg IV
Rocuronium (intubation)	0.6–1.2 mg/kg IV (1.2 mg/kg RSI dose)
3% sodium chloride (hypertonic saline)	Traumatic brain injury: 3–5 mL/kg over 10 mins Hyponatremia + seizure refer to drug dose guideline
Surfactant	200 mg/kg (via tracheal tube, round up to nearest vial)
Suxamethonium (intubation)	2 mg/kg IV
Thiopentone (intubation)	2–5 mg/kg IV (use alternative drug if signs of shock)
Vecuronium	0.1 mg/kg IV

Common emergency resuscitation drug infusions

Drug	Dilution	Infusion drug	Start rate
Adrenaline 1:1000 Noradrenaline	0.3 mg/kg / 50 mL 5% dextrose	1 mL/h = 0.1 mcg/kg/min	0.05 mcg/kg/min 0.05 mcg/kg/min
Aminophylline	Loading dose 10 mg/kg over 30 mins		
Aminophylline	1 gram / 1000 mL 0.9% NaCl		<9yo 0.9 mg/kg/hr >9yo 0.7 mg/kg/hr
Calcium chloride 10%	Neat	0.1 ml/kg/hr = 240 mg/kg/day	120 mg/kg/day
Dopamine Dobutamine	15 mg/kg/ 50 mL 5% dextrose	1 mL/hr = 5 mcg/kg/min	5–10 mcg/kg/min

Common emergency resuscitation drug infusions—cont'd

Drug	Dilution	Infusion drug	Start rate
Fentanyl	50 mcg/kg / 50 mL	1 ml/hr = 1 mcg/kg/hr	1 mcg/kg/hr
Isoprenaline	0.3 mg/kg/ 50 mL 5% dextrose	1 mL/hr = 0.1 mcg/kg/min	0.05 mcg/kg/min
Ketamine	15 mg/kg / 50 mL 0.9% Sodium Chloride	1 mL/hr = 5 mcg/kg/min	5 mcg/kg/min
Midazolam	3 mg/kg / 50 mL 5% dextrose	1 mL/hr = 1 mcg/kg/min	1 mcg/kg/min
Morphine	1 mg/kg / 50 mL 5% dextrose	1 mL/hr = 20 mcg/kg/hr	20 mcg/kg/hr
Nitroprusside	3 mg/kg / 50 mL 5% dextrose	1 mL/hr = 1 mcg/kg/min	0.5 mcg/kg/min
Potassium Chloride	20 mmol potassium chloride / 40 mL water	0.2 mL/kg/hr = 0.1 mmol/kg/hr	0.1 mmol/kg/hr
Prostaglandin E1 (Alprostadil)	150 mcg/kg / 50 mL 0.9% NaCl	1 ml/hr = 50 nanograms/kg/min	50 ng/kg/min
Salbutamol	Neat 1 mg/mL	Weight x 0.06 mL/hr = 1 mcg/kg/min	5 mcg/kg/min
Vecuronium	5 mg/kg / 50 mL 5% dextrose	1 mL = 100 mcg/kg/hr	100 mcg/kg/hr

DC shock: SVT or pulsatile VT: 1 J/kg then 2 J/kg for all doses synchronous
VF or pulseless VT: 4 J/kg all doses, asynchronous

Hyperkalemia with ECG changes
Remove exogenous potassium
Start Salbutamol nebuliser
Calcium Gluconate 0.1 mmol/kg IV
Dextrose 10% 5 mL/kg IV, consider Actrapid 0.1units/kg IV (use with caution in infants)
Bicarbonate 1 mmol/kg
Resonium 1 g/kg Q6hr PO/PR

Drug doses courtesy of Dr Andrea Christoff

7.2 Paediatric and neonatal key physiologic values (APLS)

Normal ranges:

Age	Guide weight (kg) Boys	Guide weight (kg) Girls	Resp rate 5th–95th centile	Heart rate 5th–95th centile	BP Systolic 5th centile	BP Systolic 50th centile	BP Systolic 95th centile
Birth	3.5	3.5	25–50	120–170	65–75	80–90	105
1 month	4.5	4.5					
3 months	6.5	6	25–45	115–160			
6 months	8	7		110–160			
12 months	9.5	9			70–75	85–95	
18 months	11	10		100–155			
2 years	12	12	20–30	100–150	70–80	85–100	110
3 years	14	14		90–140			
4 years	16	16		80–135			
5 years	18	18			80–90	90–110	111–120
6 years	21	20		80–130			
7 years	23	22					
8 years	25	25	15–25	70–120			
9 years	28	28					
10 years	31	32					
11 years	35	35					
12 years	43	43	12–24	65–115	90–105	100–120	125–140
14 years	50	50		60–110			
Adult	70	70					

Samuels M, Wieteska S. (Eds) Advanced Paediatric Life Support: a practical approach to emergencies. 6th edn. Advanced Life Support Group, BMJ Books, Wiley Blackwell, 2016

7.3 Common emergency paediatric calculations

Weight: (age + 4) x 2
TT size: age/4 + 4 (uncuffed)
TT size: age/4 + 3.5 (cuffed)
TT length: age/2 + 12 (oral), age/2 + 15 (nasal)
Fluid bolus: 10–20 mL/kg and re-assess
Defibrillation: 4 J/kg (asynchronous)
Emergency drug doses:
   Glucose bolus: 2 mL/kg 10% dextrose
   Adrenaline: 10 mcg/kg
   Amiodarone: 5 mg/kg
   Tranexamic acid: 15 mg/kg (max 1 g)
Maintenance fluids:
   4 mL/kg per hour (1st 10 kg)
   2 mL/kg per hour (2nd 10 kg)
   1 mL/kg per hour (each subsequent kg)
   Default isotonic crystalloid: Normal saline + 5% dextrose

7.4 Apgar score

Score	0 points	1 point	2 points
Appearance • Skin colour	Cyanotic/Pale all over	Peripheral cyanosis only	Pink
Pulse (Heart rate)	0	<100	100–140
Grimace • Reflex irritabililty	No response to stimulation	Grimace (facial movement)/weak cry when stimulated	Cry when stimulated
Activity • Tone	Floppy	Some flexion	Well flexed and resisting extension
Respiration	Apnoeic	Slow, irregular breathing	Strong cry

Major incident aide memoire

METHANE REPORT

M Major incident STANDBY/DECLARED

E Exact location – grid reference/GPS

T Type of incident

H Hazards – present and potential
Is this a CBRN incident?

A Access to scene and egress route
including helicopter landing site

N Number and severity of casualties

E Emergency services – present/required

CSCATTT

C **COMMAND AND CONTROL**

S **SAFETY – of self, scene and survivors**
- Wear PPE plus tabard/vest to identify yourself
- Take responsibility for safety of self and all medical staff
- Delegate to a Safety Officer once available
- Is this a CBRN incident? More PPE + Decontamination

C **COMMUNICATIONS**
- Provide METHANE report
- Find Ambulance Commander and start log
- Keep in regular contact using vertical chain of command
- Liaise regularly with all emergency commanders
- Alert potential receiving hospitals
- Brief doctors/nurses arriving on scene
- Later, brief media with Police Commander

A **ASSESSMENT OF SCENE**
- Asses accurate casualty numbers
- Consider need for additional personnel/equipment
- Delegate specific roles to medical staff if available
- Set-up scene plan

T **TRIAGE**
- Oversee triage but delegate to triage officer(s)
- Consider use of P4/expectant category

T **TREATMENT**
- Casualty clearing station (CCS) set-up
- Where available, appoint a doctor to run the CCS
- Concentrate doctors/nurses in CCS

T **TRANSPORT**
- With Ambulance Commander, organise transport and decide destination for each patient
- Provide medical escorts where necessary

ADULT TRIAGE SIEVE^

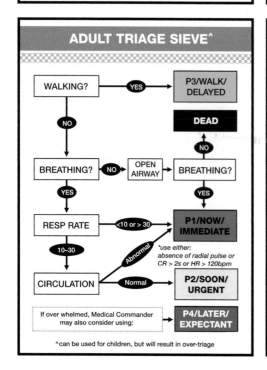

^can be used for children, but will result in over-triage

PHONETIC ALPHABET

A	alpha	N	november
B	bravo	O	oscar
C	charlie	P	papa
D	delta	Q	quebec
E	echo	R	romeo
F	foxtrot	S	sierra
G	golf	T	tango
H	hotel	U	uniform
I	india	V	victor
J	juliet	W	whiskey
K	kilo	X	X-ray
L	lima	Y	yankee
M	mike	Z	zulu

SITE PLAN

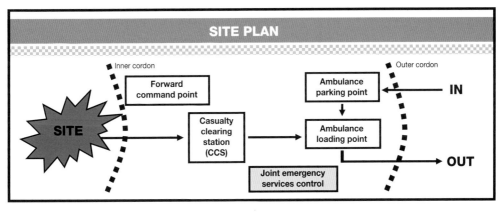

CBRN HAZARDS

Is there anything unusual about this incident – are there any CBRN hazards?
If so, approach from UPWIND & UPHILL. KEEP YOUR DISTANCE.
WAIT FOR SPECIALIST ADVICE. Consider need for PPE + DECONTAMINATION.

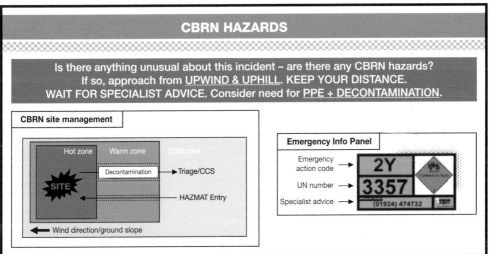

TRIAGE SORT (in CCS)

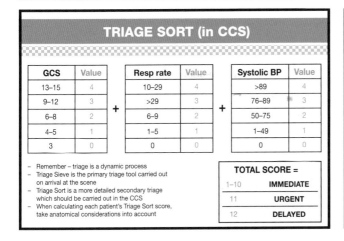

GCS	Value
13–15	4
9–12	3
6–8	2
4–5	1
3	0

Resp rate	Value
10–29	4
>29	3
6–9	2
1–5	1
0	0

Systolic BP	Value
>89	4
76–89	3
50–75	2
1–49	1
0	0

- Remember – triage is a dynamic process
- Triage Sieve is the primary triage tool carried out on arrival at the scene
- Triage Sort is a more detailed secondary triage which should be carried out in the CCS
- When calculating each patient's Triage Sort score, take anatomical considerations into account

TOTAL SCORE =	
1–10	IMMEDIATE
11	URGENT
12	DELAYED

USEFUL NUMBERS

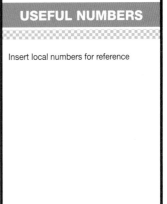

Insert local numbers for reference

Advanced Life Support Group. Major Incident Medical Management and Support (MIMMS). 2nd edn. BMJ Books, 2002.

447

KEY TO CASES

List of questions and key issues covered
Section A: Pre-hospital medicine

1. Scene safety I
   - the approach to scene

2. Scene safety II: a series of six scenarios related to scene safety
   - vehicle fire
   - vehicle rollover
   - scaffold collapse
   - car versus building
   - fuel tanker
   - hazard plate
   - approaching the helicopter

3. Entrapment I
   - the pre-hospital plan
   - interaction with emergency services
   - defining entrapment

4. Entrapment II
   - emergent extrication

5. Pre-hospital anaesthesia I
   - patient selection for emergency anaesthesia
   - builder's yard extrication (via crane)

6. Pre-hospital anaesthesia II
   - performing rapid-sequence intubation

7. Pre-hospital equipment
   - extrication board
   - scoop stretcher
   - pelvic splint
   - intraosseous access
   - vacuum mattress
   - femoral traction splint

8. Preparing for transport I
   - packaging the pre-hospital patient
   - use of scoop stretchers

9. Preparing for transport II
   - decisions at the scene and communication with hospital
   - the potentially complex airway
   - hospital pre-alert calls

10. Polytrauma I
    - traumatic brain injury (paediatric)
    - neurological deterioration

See also definitions of PHRM, clinical coordination, primary tasking, etc., in the Introduction.

Healthcare facilities

Clinic
Nurse or family doctor-led facility, often geographically isolated and minimally equipped.

Major trauma hospital
Large urban tertiary/quaternary referral facility with specialist trauma capability (e.g. neurosurgery, paediatric, etc.) and on-site helipad.

Regional hospital
Regional facility, maybe within metropolitan boundaries. Able to provide initial resuscitation and stabilisation of critically ill or injured patients. May have obstetric and surgical capabilities as well as on-call anaesthesia. Assume no specialist trauma capability.

Tertiary/Quaternary referral hospital
Large urban hospital with most medical and surgical specialties on-site.

Definitions

A-, B-, C-post
Front, middle and rear structural pillars that support the roof in most passenger vehicles.

Ambulance response vehicle
Road vehicle not capable of patient carriage conveying an Ambulance Service team member with generic paramedical skill set.

Challenge and response
A two-person technique for carrying out critical checks. One person reads the item from a checklist (challenge), the other checks the item then confirms its presence and functionality (response).

Fire & Rescue Service
Personnel, vehicles and equipment cache able to address scene safety (where relevant), fire hazards and assist in the extrication of trapped or poorly accessible patients. Assume basic medical skill set only.

Fixed-wing aircraft
Aeroplane dedicated and equipped for patient transport. The aeroplane may be turbo-prop or jet powered and may have capacity for carrying more than one patient.

Flash team
A flash team is one in which most members of the team have not worked together before or may do so very infrequently. Usually there is a core group (two or three people) within the team who are accustomed to working together, but the remainder of the team (can be several or even dozens of people) will be new to that team structure.

Gigli saw
Hand-held wire saw used for cutting bone.

Hippus
Spasmodic, rhythmic irregular dilating and contracting of the pupils (papillary athetosis).

ISBAR
A handover tool for ensuring the effective transmission of information from one person/team to another. Stands for: Identify, Situation, Background, Assessment, Response/recommendation.

Karabiner
Metal loop with hinged gate used to secure one item to another. The gate allows rapid and safe connection or disconnection of the items.

Land ambulance
Road vehicle capable of patient carriage and an Ambulance Service team of two with generic paramedical skill set.

Moulage
A mock practical scenario involving the whole PHRM team. Moulage should be as realistic as possible and utilise real kit, monitors, stretchers, etc.

Paramedic
Ambulance Service professional able to independently perform clinical assessment and advanced life support (e.g. supraglottic airway insertion, vascular access and drug administration).

Personal protective equipment (PPE)
Regionally accepted equipment provided to ensure personal safety in the pre-hospital and retrieval environment. Relevant PPE is required for potential aviation, medical and environmental risks (see Appendix 3).

PHRM team
Pre-hospital and retrieval medicine team. A physician-led team responding to pre-hospital and retrieval tasks via the clinical coordination agency. Usually, a team of two people with the second clinician as either a paramedic or a nurse trained to work in the PHRM team.

Police service
Personnel, vehicles and equipment able to ensure scene safety (where relevant). Assume basic medical skill set only.

Rapid-sequence induction and intubation (RSI)
A three-stage process of patient selection, drug-assisted intubation of the trachea and subsequent management of the ventilated patient.

Rendezvous point
Prearranged location away from the primary incident at which emergency services meet prior to scene attendance.

Rotary-wing aircraft
Helicopter dedicated and equipped for patient transport. The helicopter may have the capacity to carry up to two stretcher cases.

Sit rep
A 'situation report'. A brief report usually by telephone or radio to update the coordination agency on the situation during the task. May contain medical or logistical information or both.

Spencer Wells forceps
Type of artery forceps.

Measurements in aviation practice

- Altitude or height is measured in feet.
- Horizontal distance in meteorology is measured in metres (e.g. visibility).
- Distance in navigation is measured in nautical miles (1 nm = 1.15 statute miles).
- Speed is measured in nautical miles per hour (knots).

Abbreviations

ABG	arterial blood gas
ACS	acute coronary syndrome
AGE	arterial gas embolus
AIC	ambulance incident commander
AIMS	advanced incident management system
AME	air medical evacuation
ARDS	acute respiratory distress syndrome
BiPAP	bi-level positive airways pressure
BP	blood pressure (mmHg)
BPM	breaths per minute
BSA	burns surface area
BSL (or BM)	blood sugar level
BVM	bag valve mask
CAGE	cerebral arterial gas embolus
CBRN	chemical, biological, radiological, nuclear
CHD	congenital heart disease
CK	creatine kinase
COPD	chronic obstructive pulmonary disease
CPAP	continuous positive airways pressure
CPR	cardiopulmonary resuscitation
CRM	crew resource management
CRRT	continuous renal replacement therapy
CRT	capillary refill time
CT	computed tomography scan
CVA	cerebral vascular accident ('stroke')
CVP	central venous pressure
DCS	decompression sickness
DIC	disseminated intravascular coagulation
ECMO	extracorporeal membrane oxygenation
ECPR	extracorporeal cardiopulmonary resuscitation

ETA	estimated time of arrival
ETCO$_2$	end tidal carbon dioxide
FAST	focused abdominal ultrasound in trauma
FiO$_2$	fraction of inspired oxygen
FRC	functional residual capacity
GCS	Glasgow Coma Score (consisting of Eyes, Verbal response and Motor response [EVM]; score range 3–15)
GP	general practitioner
HEMS	helicopter emergency medical service
HFNC	high flow nasal cannulae
HLZ	helicopter landing zone
HME	heat and moisture exchanger
KPI	key performance indicator
IA	intra-arterial
IABP	intra-aortic balloon pump
ICS	internal communication system
ICU	intensive care unit
IM	intramuscular
IN	intranasal
IO	intraosseous
IPPV	intermittent positive pressure ventilation
IV	intravenous
LMA	laryngeal mask airway
MAP	mean arterial pressure
METAR	meteorological aviation report
MI	myocardial infarction
MIC	medical incident commander
mmHg	millimetres of mercury
MV	minute volume
MVA	motor vehicle accident
MVR	mitral valve replacement
NAC	N-acetyl cysteine (drug)
NGT	nasogastric tube
NIV	non-invasive ventilation
NMBA	neuromuscular blocking agent
NOTAM	notice to airmen
NRBM	non-rebreather mask

NVG	night vision goggles
O_2	oxygen
OIC	officer in charge
OGT	orogastric tube
P	pulse rate (beats per minute)
$PaCO_2$	partial pressure of carbon dioxide in the arterial blood
PCR	polymerase chain reaction (for microbiological tests)
PEEP	positive end expiratory pressure
PIP	peak inspiratory pressure
POC	point of care
POCUS	point of care ultrasound
PPE	personal protective equipment
Pplat	plateau pressure
PS	pressure support
PV	per vaginum
RCA	root cause analysis
REBOA	retrograde endovascular balloon occlusion of the aorta
RFDS	Royal Flying Doctor Service
RIC	rapid infusion catheter
ROSC	return of spontaneous circulation
RR	respiratory rate (breaths per minute)
RSI	rapid-sequence induction and intubation
RVP	rendezvous point
SaO_2	oxygen saturation
SBP	systolic blood pressure (mmHg)
SCUBA	self-contained underwater breathing apparatus
SGA	supraglottic airway device
SI	seriously injured (military terminology)
SIMV	synchronised intermittent mandatory ventilation
SIRS	systemic inflammatory response syndrome
SOP	standard operating procedure
TAF	terminal aerodrome forecast
TCA	tricyclic antidepressant (drug)
TRM	team resource management
TT	tracheal tube
TV	tidal volume
TXA	tranexamic acid

UAC	umbilical arterial catheter
UVC	umbilical venous catheter
VBG	venous blood gas
VC	volume control
VSI	very seriously injured (military terminology)

Index